T0222688

War Against Smallpox

Michael Bennett provides the first history of the global spread of vaccination during the Napoleonic Wars, offering a new assessment of the cowpox discovery and Edward Jenner's achievement in making cowpox inoculation a viable and universally available practice. He explores the networks that took the vaccine around the world and the reception and establishment of vaccination among peoples in all corners of the globe. His focus is on the human story of the horrors of smallpox, the hopes invested in vaccination by medical men and parents, the children put arm-to-arm across the world and the early challenges, successes and disappointments. He presents vaccination as a quiet revolution, genuinely emancipatory, but also the sharp end of growing state power. By the end of the war in 1815, millions of children had been vaccinated. The early success of the war against smallpox paved the way to further advances towards eradication.

MICHAEL BENNETT is Emeritus Professor of History at the University of Tasmania. He is the author of four books on late medieval England and is a Fellow of the Australian Academy of Humanities and a Life Member of Clare Hall, Cambridge.

War Against Smallpox

Edward Jenner and the Global Spread of Vaccination

Michael Bennett

University of Tasmania

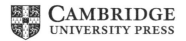

CAMBRIDGE
UNIVERSITY PRESS

University Printing House, Cambridge CB2 8BS, United Kingdom

One Liberty Plaza, 20th Floor, New York, NY 10006, USA

477 Williamstown Road, Port Melbourne, VIC 3207, Australia

314–321, 3rd Floor, Plot 3, Splendor Forum, Jasola District Centre, New Delhi – 110025, India

79 Anson Road, #06–04/06, Singapore 079906

Cambridge University Press is part of the University of Cambridge.

It furthers the University's mission by disseminating knowledge in the pursuit of education, learning, and research at the highest international levels of excellence.

www.cambridge.org
Information on this title: www.cambridge.org/9780521765671
DOI: 10.1017/9781139019569

First published 2020

A catalogue record for this publication is available from the British Library.

Library of Congress Cataloging-in-Publication Data
Names: Bennett, Michael, 1949- author.
Title: War against smallpox : Edward Jenner and the global spread of vaccination / Michael Bennett, University of Tasmania.
Description: Cambridge, United Kingdom ; New York, NY : Cambridge University Press, 2020. | Includes bibliographical references and index.
Identifiers: LCCN 2019060150 (print) | LCCN 2019060151 (ebook) | ISBN 9780521765671 (hardback) | ISBN 9780521147880 (paperback) | ISBN 9781139019569 (epub)
Subjects: LCSH: Smallpox–Vaccination–History–18th century. | Smallpox–Vaccination–History–19th century. | Jenner, Edward, 1749-1828.
Classification: LCC RA644.S6 B46 2020 (print) | LCC RA644.S6 (ebook) | DDC 614.5/21–dc23
LC record available at https://lccn.loc.gov/2019060150
LC ebook record available at https://lccn.loc.gov/2019060151

ISBN 978-0-521-76567-1 Hardback
ISBN 978-0-521-14788-0 Paperback

For Fatimah, Masni and Amy

Contents

Figures

Preface and Acknowledgements

The germ of this book goes back almost two decades to two encounters, one in a second-hand bookshop and the other in an open access library, cultural spaces now almost of another era. In the shop, I bought a copy of *Lady Nugent's Journal* and was soon reading of her anxiety in 1802 about having to give her baby smallpox. Browsing in the library, I came across Michael M. Smith's remarkable study of the Royal and Philanthropic Vaccine Expedition to New Spain in 1803–5. Although I knew about Jenner's cowpox and the final eradication of smallpox in 1980, I had no awareness of the first years of cowpox inoculation and the early spread of the practice around the world. I began to discover the surprising richness of the sources relating to vaccination in its first years that revealed aspects of human life rarely documented. Above all, I was enthralled by the discovery of a fascinating episode of humanitarian endeavour and global connectedness that had been somewhat overlooked.

For my research on the early history of vaccination, I was supported by Australia Research Council grants for a pilot-study (2004) and a major project (2008–10). The grants were used to fund research assistance and translation. I was fortunate to have as collaborators: Glynn Barrett, who sought out and translated Russian sources; Rebekah McWhirter, who completed a PhD thesis on vaccination in Australia; Diana Barnes who worked on Mary Wortley Montagu and assisted in the compilation of a database of Jenner's correspondence; Jacqueline Gratton, who completed an MA thesis on inoculation in Spain, undertook most of the research on vaccination in Spain, read through early drafts of this book, and was responsible for many improvements; and Jennifer Penschow, who completed a PhD on inoculation in northern Germany, read through the penultimate draft of the book, and saved me from many errors. For work in note-taking and translating foreign language sources, I thank Jacqueline Fox (German), Nell Tyson (Dutch), Ella Ashley (Polish), Håkan Arvidsson (Swedish) and Al Taskunas (Lithuanian). I was especially pleased that my sister Margaret Le Blanc was able to do some early proofreading.

It has been my good fortune to work in the School of History and Classics (now the History and Classics Discipline in the School of Humanities) at the University of Tasmania, and thank my former and current colleagues for creating a stimulating and supportive environment, namely Kate Brittlebank, Peter Chapman, Gavin Daly, Peter Davis, Tom Dunning, Elizabeth Freeman, Hamish Maxwell-Stewart, Anthony Page, Stefan Petrow, Mike Powell, Cassandra Pybus, Henry Reynolds, Michael Roe, Asim Roy, Pam Sharpe, Rod Thomson and Elisabeth Wilson.

As a historian who has spent most of his career working on late medieval and early modern history, I have enjoyed engaging with new communities of scholars. I benefitted from the vaccine network brought together by John Buder, the hospitality of Sanjoy Bhattarcharya in London and York, the generosity of Peter Sköld who sent a copy of his monograph, and the expert advice of Gerda Bonderup, Chang Chia-Feng and José Rigau-Pérez. I have received valuable references from Edward Duyker, Jennifer Spinks, James Walvin and Richard Yeo.

I have had the pleasure of working in wonderful libraries and archives, with the Wellcome Library and the British Library in London having pride of place. I was made welcome in the libraries of the Royal College of Physicians, the Royal College of Surgeons and the Royal Society of Medicine, in London; the New York Academy of Medicine; the Countway Library in Boston; the Medical Center Library, Duke University; the Bibliothèque de l'Académie nationale de médecine, Paris; and elsewhere. I am grateful for photocopies of rare material supplied by the Arxiu Comarcal de la Cerdanya, Puigcerdà, Catalunya; the Lietuvos nacionaline Martyno Mažvydo biblioteka, Vilnius, Lithuania; and the Württembergische Landesbibliothek, Stuttgart.

While I have been working on this book for some fifteen years, I have had many other commitments. I made most progress during three periods of study leave but, during this time too, I was dividing my time between a series of other smaller but often more pressing projects. For a time, my project of vaccination was borne aloft, but then almost swamped by the vast amount of information made available through digitalisation. I found myself making notes from far more material than I could possibly use.

I presented an early outline of my book as lectures to the University of the Third Age, Hobart, and am grateful to Leone Scrivener for her invitation to give the lectures and her continuing interest. I have had the opportunity of presenting papers on aspects of the project at several conferences and symposia, including three of the biennial conferences of the Australia and New Zealand Society for the History of Medicine.

I am grateful to Michael Watson at Cambridge University Press for his enthusiasm for the project and his patience as it proved a longer enterprise than originally anticipated. I am very appreciative of the valuable suggestions made by the press's anonymous reader. I thank Lucy Rhymer and James Baker for their support and courtesy, Liz Steel for her careful and constructive attention to the text, and Ruth Boyes and Vinithan Sethumadhavan for overseeing the production process.

Above all, I would like to thank my wife Fatimah, my daughters Masni and Amy and my family and friends for their love and support while writing this book.

Abbreviations and Acronyms

AN	Archives Nationales, Paris
BB, S&A	*Bibliothèque britannique, sciences et arts*
BHM	*Bulletin of the History of Medicine*
BL	British Library, London
BMJ	*British Medical Journal*
GM	*Gentleman's Magazine*
HRA	*Historical Records of Australia*
HRNSW	*Historical Records of New South Wales*
JHM	*Journal of the History of Medicine and Allied Sciences*
MH	*Medical History*
MPJ	*Medical and Physical Journal*
NVE	National Vaccine Establishment
PTRS	*Philosophical Transactions of the Royal Society*
RCP	Royal College of Physicians, London
RCS	Royal College of Surgeons, London
RJS	Royal Jennerian Society
TNA	The National Archives, London
WHO	World Health Organisation
WLL	Wellcome Library, London

1 A Tale of Two Diseases

Smallpox and Cowpox

In Jamaica in 1801, Lady Maria Nugent was seeking to start a family. Born in New Jersey in 1771, she was the daughter of Cortlandt Skinner, who raised a regiment to serve on the British side in the American War of Independence and sent his family as refugees to Britain. In late 1797, she married Sir George Nugent, fourteen years her senior, who after rising through the ranks in America served as commander of the British forces in the northern sector during the Irish Rebellion of 1798 and was appointed Governor of Jamaica in spring 1801. Though Britain was at war with France, and the Caribbean was a theatre of conflict, Maria went with her husband to assume the role of governor's wife. Amidst her pert observations of Jamaica, however, there began to appear in her journal, month by month, more sombre reflections and, at year's end, a confession of her 'misery that the dear name of mother will never greet my ear'. In early 1802, however, she became pregnant and, after an anxious confinement, gave birth to a healthy boy in October. A week later, she recorded her thanks to God for 'the great blessing' and 'the joy that now fills my heart'. She embarked on a note-book 'to keep an account of my dear baby's health, and know, from hour to hour, how he goes on, that I may be ready in case of any illness'. On 17 November, after reporting that her baby was 'prospering', she gloomily notes, 'but, alas, we must soon think of giving him the small-pox'.[1]

Maria's statement is chilling and shocking. After her concern that she might never be a mother and anxieties about having her first child far from family and friends, the idea that she would give her baby smallpox appears perplexing and disturbing. It soon becomes apparent, of course, that she is referring to having him inoculated with smallpox. Over eighty years earlier, Lady Mary Wortley Montagu, the wife of another British official in foreign parts, had observed how Greek women in Istanbul inserted smallpox matter under the skin on a child's arm in the hope that the child would develop a mild case of smallpox which would then provide security against future infection. Trials of smallpox

---

[1] *Lady Nugent's journal: Jamaica one hundred years ago*, ed. Frank Cundall, 2nd ed. (London, 1934), pp. 65, 169, 171.

inoculation (variolation) in England in the 1720s showed that inoculated smallpox was generally less severe than smallpox acquired casually. In the second half of the eighteenth century, it became a familiar practice in the English-speaking world. Since it was used extensively during the smallpox epidemic that raged during the war in America, it is likely enough that Maria herself had been inoculated. Still, the procedure involved some risk. A mild case of smallpox could not be counted on, and a small percentage of children died of inoculated smallpox, making it an awful decision for parents. As it was not usual to inoculate a neonate, the presence of smallpox in Jamaica was probably a determining factor. Sir George may have been especially resolute, but Maria's words suggests that it was a joint decision. The Nugents could call on medical men who were experienced in the procedure as it was extensively deployed on the plantations. Their physician found a child in Spanish Town with a mild case of smallpox and brought him or her to the house to provide fresh lymph for the operation. There followed an anxious fortnight. After being advised that her son's infection was approaching the critical time, Maria abandoned a ball to hurry to his side. Shortly afterwards, she was happy to report that her child was back in good health.[2]

Maria's anguish about smallpox inoculation is hardly surprising, but referring to the procedure as giving a child smallpox, though apposite, is very unusual. The likely explanation is that variolation was no longer the only option for smallpox prophylaxis. In 1798, the first year of their marriage, Edward Jenner published his thesis that inoculating cowpox was a much safer and just as effective means of protection against smallpox.[3] Trials of cowpox (vaccine) in London in 1799 generated publicity and cowpox inoculation (vaccination) was introduced in the British army and navy in 1800. Seeking to start a family, the Nugents would have invested some hope in the new procedure, read reports of its success in Europe, and heard about attempts to establish the practice locally with imported vaccine. In 1803, Maria was pregnant again, giving birth to a daughter in October. The likely availability of vaccine evidently eased her mind. She reported that the doctor brought 'a nice little mulatto child, from whose arm my dear baby was vaccinated'. The outcome was disappointing, raising the concern that 'perhaps, after all, we must give her the smallpox'. Fortunately, a new supply of vaccine arrived in November. 'We agreed', Maria wrote in high spirits, 'to have the puncture made in her dear little leg; for if the present fashion for excessive short sleeves lasts till she grows up, it will not be becoming to expose a scar on the arm,

---

[2] *Nugent's Journal*, pp. 173–4, 177, 179.

[3] Edward Jenner, *An inquiry into the causes and effects of the* variolæ vaccinæ, *or cow pox, a disease discovered in the western counties of England, and known by the name of the cow pox* (London, 1798).

which I now see disfiguring many pretty young ladies'.[4] The anguish of giving a child smallpox already seemed to belong to another age.

War on Smallpox and the World Arm-to-Arm

This book is the first full-length history of the spread of vaccination around the world in the early nineteenth century. The first generation of practitioners often saw themselves as making history by introducing, establishing and promoting the practice in their communities. In seeking a supply of vaccine, in sharing observations and insights about the new prophylaxis with colleagues, they were consciously or unconsciously participating in networks that, though locally based, were ultimately transnational. The promoters of vaccination certainly looked to developments elsewhere in the world for instruction and inspiration.[5] Writing a history of vaccination at the end of the Napoleonic Wars, James Moore included a sketch of its global career, and popular histories of smallpox and smallpox prevention, usually ranging from the earliest times until the declaration of the eradication of smallpox in 1980, have tended to include a similar outline of its early spread around the world.[6] Over the past fifty years, there has been an impressive body of scholarship on the history of vaccination, largely national and regional studies.[7] More recently, there has been a growing recognition of the interest of the global dimension, especially the common and the distinctive challenges and responses to the problems of delivering vaccine and embedding the practice in different climes and cultures around the world.[8] This book draws on an immense range of primary sources, published and unpublished, and builds on the available scholarship in a dozen languages, to present a richer and more comprehensive picture of the beginnings of vaccination, one that reveals the value of seeing the connectedness of developments around the world. The approach is more that of a general historian than a historian of medicine. An inspiration was the quality and richness of the documentation generated by the cowpox discovery and the

---

[4] *Nugent's Journal*, pp. 231–2, 236, 240.

[5] James Moore, *The history and practice of vaccination* (London, 1817), pp. 226–73.

[6] E.g. Donald R. Hopkins, *The greatest killer: smallpox in history, with a new introduction* (Chicago, 2002), first published as *Peasants and princes: smallpox in history* (Chicago, 1983); Ian Glynn and Jennifer Glynn, *The rise and fall of smallpox* (London, 2004); Gareth Williams, *Angel of death. The story of smallpox* (Basingstoke, 2010).

[7] Early leaders in the field were Yves-Marie Bercé, *Le chaudron et la lancette. Croyances populaires et médecine preventive (1798–1830)* (Paris, 1984) and Pierre Darmon, *La longue traque de la variole. Les pionniers de la médecine preventive* (Paris, 1986). More generally see the Select Bibliography.

[8] John Z. Bowers, 'The odyssey of smallpox vaccination', *BHM*, 55 (1981), 17–33; Ann Jannetta, *The vaccinators. Smallpox, medical knowledge, and the 'opening' of Japan* (Stanford, CA, 2007); Andrea Rusnock, 'Catching cowpox: the early spread of smallpox vaccination, 1798–1810', *BHM*, 83 (2009), 17–36.

advent of early vaccination, and the insights and perspectives it offered on aspects of life that are otherwise rarely documented. Vaccination, like variolation before it, has to be seen not only as a medical and sanitary intervention but as a technology, a social and cultural practice and an emotion-laden rite of passage. This study seeks to explore how the new prophylaxis was not only shaped by the broader historical forces but was also constitutive of them. As some literary scholars have shown, for example, the enthusiasm for cowpox and the cult of Jenner reflect and inform the sensibilities of the age of Romanticism.[9] The scale of the mobilisation in relation to vaccination in its first decade needs to be especially stressed. Millions of people around the world played their part in the vaccination revolution and experienced its emancipatory power.

The early global spread of vaccination involved more than the flow of information and a simple technology. It required the distribution of cowpox (vaccine) in a good state of preservation, its successful propagation on arrival, and measures to maintain the supply of vaccine. Even in England, cowpox was found only occasionally on dairy-farms, and from the outset the supply of cowpox lymph depended on the vaccination process itself, that is lymph drawn from the vaccine vesicle that had risen on the arm of a child vaccinated around nine days previously. Often enough, the previously vaccinated children would be put, almost literally, arm-to-arm with the next batch of children. It may be that many mothers found the use of vaccine that had passed through other children, without obvious harm, somewhat reassuring. To extend the practice and set it on the firm foundations, of course, required the collection and preservation of vaccine for future use. Cowpox lymph in its liquid state did not survive long, even when stored in a sealed glass bottle. The standard method for maintaining a supply of vaccine was to soak cotton threads in the cowpox lymph, allow the cowpox-imbued threads to dry, wrap them in paper, and perhaps even store them in bottles. In the early years of vaccination, packets of dried vaccine threads were dispatched from London and other centres of early practice in almost diasporic profusion. Dried vaccine wrapped in paper, however, had a short life span, especially in conditions of heat and humidity. There were remarkable successes, especially in sending dried vaccine to Vienna in 1799, but it proved surprisingly difficult to deliver vaccine in any form to France. There was a rapid address, in which practitioners around the world contributed, to the technical problems of storing and transporting vaccine. State-of-the-art solutions, like sealing lymph between sealed plates or in vacuum sealed capillaries, were expensive, not easily transported, and delivered only marginally better results than sending large numbers of threads

---

[9] Tim Fulford, Debbie Lee and Peter J. Kitson, *Literature, science and exploration in the Romantic era: bodies of knowledge* (Cambridge, 2004), ch. 9.

in packets. As Andrea Rusnock has shown, the spread of vaccination was more than a matter of the world, in her happy phrase, simply 'catching cowpox'.[10]

One method for delivering vaccine over long distances and in challenging environments was to move children under vaccination. It built on the routine practice of using a previously inoculated child as the source of vaccine for other children. As early as 1800, children were being taken to be vaccinated in towns where the practice was established and brought home to go arm-to-arm with other children. It was found that on a sea-voyage it was possible to maintain a supply of fresh lymph for delivery at the destination by the successive vaccination of young people who had not had smallpox. Within a few years, vaccination chains were being used to introduce and extend the practice in many parts of the world, most notably in the Spanish empire. Although it drew on the techniques used for storing and variolous matter, vaccination faced the new challenge of needing to have to hand a supply of a virus that was hard to find in England and not available at all in most other parts of the world. The maintenance and extension of the practice therefore depended on a higher level of organisation. The availability of vaccination as an option to the individual depended on other people adopting the practice. The spread of vaccination around the world required massive mobilisation, rarely coercive but often involving a degree of pressure and hustle. Millions of people were to be enlisted or dragooned into the war against smallpox. Unlike variolation, which kept smallpox alive, vaccination offered the prospect of a world free from smallpox.

As historians of medicine, health policy analysts, and philosophical patients have often observed, the language of wars and battles against diseases can have unfortunate connotations. It is noteworthy, though, that the use of military metaphors in medicine gained traction in the eighteenth century with the perception of smallpox as an invasive agent, and the idea that inoculation assisted bodily resistance. Although he confided his thoughts to a manuscript unpublished until modern times, Cotton Mather was probably not alone in imagining 'unseen armies of numberless things, ready to seize and prey on us', figuring smallpox as an enemy that the body needs to be 'very strong' to resist, and inoculated smallpox as attacking only the 'outer works' of the citadel.[11] The coincidence of the beginnings of vaccination with the Revolutionary and Napoleonic wars may have further encouraged the use of military metaphors in the new form of prophylaxis. Jenner, no enthusiast for the war, used them very often. In a letter to two ladies inoculating cowpox in Wales, he congratulated them on opening 'the vaccine campaign so successfully' and

---

[10] Rusnock, 'Catching cowpox', 17–36.
[11] Cotton Mather, *The Angel of Bethesda*, ed. Gordon W. Jones (Barre, MA, 1972), pp. 47, 94, 112.

continued, 'May this species of warfare never terminate till you have driven from your country the most formidable foe that ever invaded it'.[12] The prospect of banishing smallpox led naturally to the language of war and conquest. In Napoleonic France, Minister of the Interior Chaptal wrote in martial tones about disputing 'every inch of ground with the enemy whom we wish to exterminate'.[13] In embattled Britain, some of the most bellicose language was used not about smallpox itself, but about the men who sought to undermine confidence in vaccination and spread smallpox by inoculation. Jenner's cowpox discovery proved to be the occasion of the first great confrontation in Britain and elsewhere between expert opinion and popular denialism. Still, in promoting the new prophylaxis in an age of global warfare, Jenner could be presented as a humanitarian hero, who saved lives rather than sacrificed them.

This history, then, is a story of humanitarian endeavour. From the outset, cowpox was presented as a boon to mankind, both a providential blessing and fruit of the Enlightenment. It was obvious that just as smallpox was a near universal affliction so there was no reason to doubt that cowpox would be a universal panacea. The moves to make vaccine available more broadly, in terms of geographical range, and more deeply, in terms of social reach, were by no means wholly philanthropic. There were material interests at play in protecting colonial enclaves and plantation economies as well as in projecting images of western superiority and imperial paternalism. Closer to home, the need to propagate a supply of vaccine, the economic benefits of suppressing smallpox and the reputational return on aristocratic and professional philanthropy were important motives for sponsoring vaccination. A harder edge was only revealed when popular prejudice and apathy made it hard to maintain the supply of vaccine on which the practice depended. In general, the enthusiasm with which cowpox was promoted, and the delight in what was seen to be a common good are all too apparent. The idea of vaccination as a humanitarian cause is most evident in the manner that, in a time of war, no advantage was taken to restrict access to information about the practice, and considerable efforts were made to make it available across enemy lines and among peoples of different races and religions. Even in the age of war and imperial rivalry, cowpox found in English dairies and propagated on English children was sent both to Austria, Britain's ally, and France, its mortal foe. From Vienna, vaccine lymph was communicated through intermediaries to Moscow and Bombay, and provided the stock for vaccination in the Russian empire and British India, passing through the

---

[12] W. W. Francis and L. G. Stevenson, 'Three unpublished letters of Edward Jenner', *JHM*, 10 (1955), 359–68, at 361–3.

[13] *Circulaires, instructions et autres actes émanés du Ministère de l'interieur, ou relatifs à ce département de 1797 à 1830 inclusivement*, 2nd ed. (Paris, 1821), 1, p. 309.

bodies of Europeans and non-Europeans, Christians, Moslems, Hindus and animists. From Paris, vaccine was made available in Spain, and three years later a Spanish expedition was launched to carry vaccine, by the successive vaccination of children, across the Atlantic, through South America and across the Pacific. Vaccination discloses connection and trust even in an age of imperial conflict and exploitation. Between 1800 and 1805, millions of the people around the world came together, almost literally, arm-to-arm. For the first time, smallpox's empire was brought within bounds and the means became available, given sufficient resource and application, to eradicate it. In a letter to Jenner in 1806, President Thomas Jefferson assured him that he had 'erased from the calendar of human afflictions one of its greatest'.[14]

The study considers the first phase in the history of vaccination, which saw the introduction and the establishment of the practice, the wide acceptance of the potential of the new prophylaxis and millions of people vaccinated. By the last decade of Jenner's life, however, the initial momentum had been lost. The early expansion of the practice had been carried forward with a great deal of enthusiasm and after the first few years it proved hard in many places to make vaccination a routine practice. Some governments provide support and some even sought to make it compulsory. Pockets of anti-vaccination sentiment were often inflamed rather than soothed by medical hectoring or government pressure, especially when the populace had little trust in the elite. By the 1820s, medical men were starting to acknowledge that vaccination did not provide life-time protection and that periodic revaccination might be necessary, making it more difficult to promote. The main problem, then as perhaps now, was not active denial of the value of vaccination but complacency and apathy. The success of vaccination in the first decade of its adoption had played a part in suppressing the disease and, in turn, in making it less feared and less pressing. Lady Nugent may not have been untypical as a parent in moving from fear of smallpox, anxious acceptance of the calculated risk of giving smallpox by inoculation, to expectation of the availability of vaccination and the less serious concern about the vaccination mark. It would be all too easy and all too common for parents to move to the next step and not to assign vaccination any priority at all. Thomas Jefferson's vision of smallpox eradication would be realised only slowly. There were advances, punctuated and then accelerated by smallpox epidemics, through the nineteenth and early twentieth centuries in the western world. It would take a well-funded international campaign to suppress smallpox in its last redoubts in the 1970s, making it possible for the WHO to formally announce the global eradication of smallpox in 1980. 'Future nations will know by history only that the

---

[14] John Baron, *The life of Edward Jenner*, 2 vols. (London, 1827 and 1838), 2, p. 95.

loathsome smallpox has existed', Jefferson pronounced in 1806.[15] It is to that history that it is now necessary to return.

The Rise of Smallpox

Smallpox (*orthopoxvirus variola*) is known to be an ancient disease. It flourished in the civilisations in the Fertile Crescent and the Indus Valley three thousand years ago. The first historical record of a disease clearly identifiable with smallpox occurs in China in the second century CE. It was neither distinctly described nor named in the Greek or Roman world, but the plague that swept westward from Persia into the Roman empire in 166–172 CE was probably smallpox.[16] In China, clinical descriptions of the disease date back to the fifth century CE. Five centuries later, the Persian physician known as Rhazes offered a description of the disease that remained influential in Europe into the seventeenth century. Over this period smallpox gained in profile throughout the Old World. The growth of population and the locking together of systems of trade and empire from the twelfth century made it possible for smallpox to become endemic in core regions, especially in China, India and the Middle East, and to circulate with increasing frequency through large areas of Asia and Europe. It was carried along the caravan routes across the Sahara and on Arab dhows down the east coast of Africa, eventually gaining hold in the African kingdoms on the savannah grasslands either side of the Equator. In Europe, it was believed that smallpox came from the Arab world at the time of the Crusades. During the later middle ages, it appeared more regularly in the more densely settled regions and became increasingly associated with children. Though a nasty disease, distinguished by fever, pain and, above all, its 'pox', it was probably milder than it later became. In the sixteenth century, the arrival of syphilis in Europe brought a new scourge often described as the 'great pox'. The English term 'smallpox', and its equivalents in other languages, was then applied to the more persistent and troubling of the lesser poxes. By this time, however, the *variola* virus was not only spreading more rapidly, but also acquiring a new virulence.

Smallpox arrived in the New World not long after Columbus, proving a potent ally of the Spanish conquistadors in the conquest of the Aztec empire. Scholars have generally assumed high rates of infection and mortality in 'virgin-soil populations' in Mesoamerica and South America.[17] The size of the original population of Mexico, the scale of the demographic collapse and the role of smallpox in the devastation, however, are matters of some debate.

---

[15] Baron, *Life*, 2, p. 95.   [16] Vivian Nutton, *Ancient medicine* (Abingdon, 2004), p. 24.
[17] E.g. Alfred W. Crosby, *Ecological imperialism. The biological expansion of Europe, 900–1900* (Cambridge, 1993), pp. 200–1.

Early Spanish sources may have given undue emphasis to smallpox because of the visibility of the disease, and because the high susceptibility of the indigenous people could be presented as a providential mandate for European rule.[18] It has been rightly observed that smallpox was 'not a cloud of infection that descends from on high' and did not move 'with seven-league boots'.[19] Still, even if less cataclysmic than has often been assumed, the epidemic in Mexico in the 1520s almost certainly involved higher mortality rates than in Europe.[20] Furthermore, it spread widely, though largely dependent on colonial commerce and penetration. In the mid-1520s it ravaged Peru, de-stabilising the Inca empire and making it more vulnerable to Spanish adventurism.[21] There is little evidence of its spread northwards beyond central Mexico before the eighteenth century.[22] Epidemic smallpox reappeared several times in Mesoamerica and South America in the sixteenth century. 'They died by scores and hundreds', a colonist reported of an epidemic in Peru in 1585, 'Villages were depopulated. Corpses were scattered over the fields or piled up in the houses or huts'.[23] Over the course of the seventeenth century, it appeared more regularly and spread more widely, though with the colonial activity still providing the crucial links in the chain of infection. In the early decades of the eighteenth century, its lethal impact is well documented in the Jesuit missions in Paraguay, where there was a severe epidemic in 1738–40.[24] The importation of African slaves increased the opportunities for disease transmission. Brazil was especially exposed to infection brought on slave ships from west Africa.[25]

By 1600, *variola* virus was entrenched in the heartlands of Asia and Europe. It was long endemic in the cities and flood plains of China, where it became largely a childhood illness. The peoples beyond the Great Wall, who were still highly susceptible to smallpox, lived in fear of the contagion, describing China as 'a house on fire'.[26] In their campaigns in Ming China in the early

---

[18] Francis J. Brooks, 'Revising the conquest of Mexico: smallpox, sources and populations', *Journal of Interdisciplinary History*, 24 (1993), 1–29.

[19] Brooks, 'Revising the conquest', 12; Paul Kelton, *Cherokee medicine, colonial germs: An indigenous nation's fight against smallpox, 1518–1824* (Norman, OK, 2015), pp. 21–2.

[20] Robert McCaa, 'Spanish and Nahuatl views on smallpox and demographic collapse in Mexico', *Journal of Interdisciplinary History*, 25 (1995), 397–431; Mark Harrison, *Disease in the modern world: 1500 to the present day* (Cambridge, 2004), pp. 74–5.

[21] Hopkins, *Greatest killer*, pp. 208–12.   [22] Kelton, *Cherokee medicine*, p. 25.

[23] Hopkins, *Greatest killer*, p. 213.

[24] Robert H. Jackson, *Missions and the frontiers of Spanish America: a comparative study of the impact of environmental, economic, political, and socio-cultural variations on the missions in the Rio de Plata region and on the northern frontier of New Spain* (Scottsdale, AZ, 2005), pp. 337–8.

[25] Dauril Alden and Joseph C. Miller, 'Out of Africa: the slave trade and the transmission of smallpox to Brazil, 1560–1831', *Journal of Interdisciplinary History*, 18 (1987), 195–224.

[26] Hopkins, *Greatest killer*, p. 119.

seventeenth century, the Manchus saw the disease as a more formidable obstacle than fortifications and armies.[27] Crossing to Japan as early as the sixth century, smallpox became endemic in major population centres from the fourteenth century. The Dutch observed its heavy toll of children in Nagasaki in the 1640s. Even in the mountainous provinces of Honshu, where it reappeared every three or four years, it was becoming a disease of childhood.[28] In the seventeenth century, there were serious smallpox epidemics in the Philippines and the Indonesian archipelago.[29] On the western edge of the Eurasian landmass, smallpox was also appearing more often and with greater severity. It was becoming endemic in London, roaming the English countryside, and making forays into remote parts of the British Isles. After the Great Plague of London in 1665, smallpox displaced bubonic plague as the most feared scourge. Around this time, the author of *Medela Medicinæ* claimed that smallpox had been quite mild until about forty years earlier.[30] From the mid-seventeenth century, other European countries experienced epidemics of increasing virulence. An outbreak in 1736 is regarded as the first very severe epidemic in Sweden.[31] The eighteenth century in Europe began and was to end in the shadow of smallpox.

Smallpox was also becoming fully global. In 1733, a student returning from Denmark unwittingly carried the virus across the north Atlantic to Greenland. The consequences were cataclysmic. In one settlement missionaries found no survivors other than a small girl and her infant brothers. After burying his neighbours, their father 'had laid himself and his youngest child in a grave of stones, bidding the girl to cover him with skins' and to share the remaining food with her brothers until help arrived.[32] The expansion of the Russian empire east of the Urals facilitated the spread of smallpox from central Asia to the nomadic peoples of Siberia and across the Bering Strait to Alaska. In the late 1770s, smallpox was carried westwards from the British colonies and northwards from Mexico into the interior of North America, along the Mississippi-Missouri river system and across the Prairies. In the early 1780s the Hudson's Bay Company began to receive reports of the dreadful mortality spreading northward. In visiting Nootka Sound in 1792, George Vancouver

---

[27] Jiafeng Zhang, 'Disease and its impact on politics, diplomacy, and military: the case of smallpox and the Manchus (1613–1795)', *JHM*, 57 (2002), 177–97.

[28] Jannetta, *Vaccinators*, p. 19.

[29] Hopkins, *Greatest killer*, pp. 112–13; Peter Boomgaard, 'Smallpox, vaccination, and the *Pax Neerlandica*, Indonesia, 1530–1930', *Bijdragen tot de Taal- en Volkenkunde*, 159 (2003), 590–617, esp. 591–5.

[30] R. A. Anselment, *The realms of Apollo. Literature and healing in seventeenth-century England* (Newark, NJ, 1995), p. 174.

[31] Peter Sköld, *The two faces of smallpox. A disease and its prevention in eighteenth- and nineteenth-century Sweden* (Umeå, 1996), p. 61.

[32] Hopkins, *Greatest killer*, p. 52.

observed evidence of recent depopulation.[33] In the eighteenth century, small-pox was likewise extending its range in the southern hemisphere. Its spread through South America, especially through Brazil, was assisted by the import-ation of African slaves.[34] By the 1760s it was causing havoc as far south as Santiago in Chile. During this time, too, smallpox completed its conquest of Africa. The slave-trade brought it from the interior to Angola in the late seventeenth century.[35] European trade with Asia was responsible for the first outbreak at the Cape of Good Hope in 1713. Spanish and Dutch commerce and colonisation quickened and broadened the circulation of smallpox in the Philippines and the Indonesian archipelago. In the early 1780s, fishermen from Sulawesi may have brought *variola* to the northern coast of Australia. In 1789, a smallpox epidemic decimated the Aboriginal people living around the British colony at Sydney Cove.[36]

The Experience of Smallpox: Fear and Fatalism

The *variola* virus generally entered the body through the mouth or nose. For around twelve days the virus multiplied, nesting in the lymph nodes and then spilling out into the bloodstream. It was only then that the carrier of smallpox felt unwell and became infectious. After a few days of high fever, sickness and lassitude, a rash appeared, usually on the face and the body's extremities. The rash developed into pustules which emitted a sickening smell as they suppurated (see Figure 1.1).[37] They frequently formed in the mouth and throat, making eating and drinking painful, sometimes impossible, occasion-ing a choking death. In more serious cases the pustules were so numerous as to run together, that is they became 'confluent'. After a week, they started to dry and form scabs. For two weeks from the first fever to the loss of the last scab, the patient was highly infective, spreading millions of infective particles from the pustules on his skin and sores in his throat into the immediate environment. In the 1780s, Dr Haygarth wrote in terms of particles of 'variolous poison' forming a miasma around the patient. He presented evi-dence that the chance of a susceptible person in close contact with a smallpox case becoming infected was rather less than was often imagined, not much

---

[33] Elizabeth A. Fenn, *Pox Americana. The great smallpox epidemic of 1775–82* (New York, 2001), pp. 227–31.

[34] Hopkins, *Greatest killer*, p. 179.

[35] P. Verger, *Trade relations between the Bight of Benin and Bahia from the seventeenth to the nineteenth century* (Ibadan, 1976), p. 577.

[36] Michael Bennett, 'Smallpox and cowpox under the Southern Cross: the smallpox epidemic of 1789 and the advent of vaccination in colonial Australia', *BHM*, 83 (2009), 37–62, at 43–50.

[37] J. R. Smith, *The speckled monster. Smallpox in England, 1670–1970, with particular reference to Essex* (Chelmsford, 1987), p. 15.

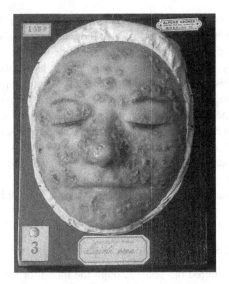

Figure 1.1 Variola (Smallpox). Plaster cast
(Universitäts-Hautklinick Münster)

more than fifty-fifty. The *variola* virus, however, could also survive in fomites – for example, clothing and blankets – and sometimes – though Haygarth believed only rarely – spark an outbreak at some distance in time and space from a live case.[38]

Few people in eighteenth-century Europe and Asia escaped smallpox. The fatality rate was variable, generally ranging between one in ten and one in five. If smallpox became 'confluent', the prognosis was bleak. Survivors would often be badly scarred and a few left blind or with their health otherwise seriously impaired. In addition to its impact on mortality, smallpox had a deleterious impact on life-chances, including marriage prospects.[39] It was dreadful to witness a loved one, especially a child, with the disease. Dr Eberhard Munch af Rosenschöld, a pioneer of vaccination in Sweden, observed that the suffering in a severe case had to be witnessed to be fully appreciated. 'The face is terribly swollen and disfigured', he observed, 'the eyes are deprived of the light; the nose the air; the infected rattling throat thirsts after water and cannot swallow it'; the lungs exhale a rotten stench; the orifices of the body discharge noxious matter; the whole body is an abscess that cannot

[38] John Haygarth, *An inquiry how to prevent the small-pox and proceedings of a society for promoting general inoculation at stated periods* (Chester, 1784), pp. 18–31, 67–86.
[39] Peter Sköld, 'The beauty and the beast – smallpox and marriage in eighteenth and nineteenth-century Sweden', *Historical Social Research*, 28 (2003), 141–61.

be touched. A brown scab forms over the body and face, he continued, and it is no longer possible to discern humanity in the monstrous form. The patient's loved ones can do no more than pray for the suffering to end, and sometimes the patient survives, sadly deprived of all that Nature provides for the enjoyment of life.[40]

The nature of smallpox was poorly understood. According to the classical paradigm associated with Galen (130–210), it arose from an imbalance of humours. In the tenth century, Rhazes explained it as the product of the blood's inherent tendency to ferment and expel waste matter through the pores of the skin.[41] According to this theory, smallpox was innate and ineluctable, with the severity of the disease varying according to the individual's state of health and circumstances. Major outbreaks of smallpox were explained not by contagion but by an 'epidemic constitution' in the environment. The Renaissance saw a re-engagement with the classical tradition but also some criticism of Galen. The arrival of plague and syphilis in Europe provided new challenges, practical and theoretical, and prompted new thinking about epidemic disease. Girolamo Fracastoro (1478–1553) attempted to bring analytical rigour to understandings of contagion. Associating specific diseases with specific seeds, he proposed three modes of infection, namely from person to person, through fomites and through the air, which served as a medium for 'disease-specific *seminaria*'.[42] Still, many physicians prior to the late eighteenth century regarded smallpox as innate. Even the iconoclastic Dr Thomas Sydenham (1624–89) allowed contact with a prior case of smallpox only a precipitating role in the disease. This thinking survived the early introduction of inoculation: the procedure was initially explained as a means of provoking the body to purge itself of the poison of smallpox. Awareness that there were peoples in the world who had no or only recent experience of smallpox, however, made it hard to sustain the notion that the disease was innate. Growing experience with inoculation likewise sharpened the focus on infection and the idea of a specific disease agent. Cotton Mather, who championed inoculation in Boston in the 1720s, imaginatively presented the seeds of the 'variolous miasma' as an invading army. Given the limited power of microscopes, of course, there could be no more than the haziest intimations of microbial pathogens until the late nineteenth century. It was not until the 1930s that the *variola* virus and *vaccinia* virus were seen under a microscope and not until several more decades more that progress began to be made towards an understanding of the immune system.[43]

---

[40] Sköld, *Two faces*, p. 77.   [41] Hopkins, *Greatest killer*, p. 9.

[42] Vivian Nutton, 'The seeds of disease: an explanation of contagion and infection from the Greeks to the Renaissance', *MH*, 27 (1983), 1–34, esp. 28–30.

[43] Glynn and Glynn, *Rise and fall*, ch. 13.

There was no cure for smallpox. All that could be done was to ease the patient's path through the disease. On Galenic principles, Rhazes recommended purging through the application of 'heat'. Common to both Asian and European medical cultures, this therapy remained remarkably resilient, persisting into modern times. Physicians were not called in for smallpox cases and some confessed their lack of experience in managing it. 'It is no slight reflection the world makes', Dr Gideon Harvey wrote in 1696, 'that motherly women, nurses and midwives, by their petty inspection of diseases of their family and of those whom they neighbourly go to visit' gain more knowledge of smallpox than 'a whole herd of doctors'.[44] Dr Sydenham was unusual in taking time to observe smallpox patients and experiment with new therapies.[45] His advocacy of a cool regimen proved controversial and only gradually won acceptance. The fierceness of the debate was stoked by the professional stress of dealing with smallpox in elite families. In Britain, the house of Stuart was largely destroyed by smallpox, with two of Charles I's children felled by the disease and his granddaughter, Mary II, falling victim to a rare and horrific case of haemorrhagic smallpox in 1694. Smallpox took a heavy toll on all of Europe's ruling families. Among the Bourbons, Louis XIV lost his eldest son to smallpox in 1711 and several of his great-grandchildren, including Luis I of Spain and Louis XV of France, died of the disease. Especially significant was the death of the Habsburg Emperor Joseph I from smallpox in 1711. This changed the course of the War of the Spanish Succession and set the stage for the extinction of the house of Habsburg in the male line.[46]

If medical theory played down contagion, common sense did not. Among nomadic peoples, the response to smallpox was often flight, sometimes leaving infected family members to look after themselves. The phenomenon was observed in a range of contexts, including among the Khoikhoi in Cape Colony in 1713 and, by the botanist Carl Linnaeus, among the Saami of northern Sweden.[47] In the more settled parts of Europe and Asia, responses were more varied. For people living in more populous districts, engaged in agriculture or manufacturing, flight was not an option. The best hope was to keep smallpox out. Rural communities might escape smallpox for long periods, but then suffer an epidemic with high levels of mortality in all age groups. In cities and large towns, where smallpox was endemic, poorer families had little real prospect of shielding their children from contagion

---

[44] Gideon Harvey, *A treatise of the small-pox and measles: describing their nature, causes, and signs, diagnostick and prognostick, in a different way to what hath hitherto been known* (London, 1696), pp. 1–2.

[45] Hopkins, *Greatest killer*, p. 33.   [46] Hopkins, *Greatest killer*, pp. 43–4.

[47] George McCall Theal, *History of South Africa 1691–1795* (London, 1888), p. 59; Sköld, *Two faces*, p. 190.

and, in an environment of high infant mortality, banked on early exposure delivering lifelong immunity. According to Dr Haygarth, country-dwellers were more anxious about smallpox than townsmen, many of whom had some immunity.[48] Most people in the early modern world accepted smallpox with a degree of fatalism but believed that it was best to get it over as a child. As an English observer wrote, smallpox 'is found to be safer [in childhood] than in riper years'.[49] Perversely, the more successful parents were in shielding a child, the greater the risk of a severe case in later life, a point that helps to explain the many high-profile deaths. For poorer folk, the death of an older child, on the verge of contributing to the family income, added economic loss to the emotional pain. Peasants in Livonia had a saying that 'It is better for a child to die when it ought to die rather than first eating a lot of bread and then dying'.[50]

Few people in eighteenth-century Europe could wholly avoid smallpox. The Genevan physician Jean-Antoine Butini claimed in the 1750s that less than five per cent of adults died without having had smallpox.[51] The scourge hung like the sword of Damocles over all who escaped it as children. On recovering from smallpox in 1716, the thirteen-year-old Duke of Chartres, son of Philippe of Orleans, Regent of France, was overjoyed at having put it behind him.[52] It was a custom for French aristocratic women to go into seclusion with husbands who fell ill with smallpox. In 1716, the young Duchess d'Olonne accepted her fate stoically, informing her relatives: 'I shall surely take smallpox and die of it; but one must do one's duty'.[53] Physicians sometimes expressed concern that people were too reckless in visiting the sickrooms of loved ones and friends. Fear of contagion, on the other hand, was socially inhibiting. In 1724, a clergyman refused a desirable position in London because he had not had smallpox, only to die of shock when his son, who had accepted the post, took the disease fatally.[54] Belief that smallpox was innate led some people to believe that their own anxiety would provoke the disease.[55] After her mother's smallpox death, Isabella of Parma had premonitions that she would share her fate. She indeed died of smallpox in 1763, shortly after her marriage to the future Emperor Joseph II. Given the smallpox toll in the house of Austria in the

---

[48] John Haygarth, *A sketch of a plan to exterminate the casual smallpox*, 2 vols. (London, 1793), 1, p. 186.

[49] *GM*, 7 (1737), p. 561.

[50] Erich Donnert, *Johann Georg Eisen (1717–1779). Ein Vorkämpfer der Bauernbefreiung in Rußland* (Leipzig, 1978), pp. 120–1.

[51] Léon Gautier, *La médecine à Genève jusqu'à la fin du dix-huitième siècle* (Geneva, 2001), p. 387.

[52] *Journal du marquis de Dangeau*, vol. 16, ed. E. Soulié and L. Dussieux (Paris, 1839), p. 457.

[53] *Journal du marquis de Dangeau*, 16, p. 475.   [54] *Weekly Journal*, 17 April 1725.

[55] David E. Shuttleton, *Smallpox and the literary imagination 1660–1820* (Cambridge, 2007), pp. 28–31.

1760s, a level of anxiety about the disease would seem wholly appropriate. For Count Kaunitz, Austria's chief minister, however, the phobia was pathological. After witnessing the Empress Maria Theresa's suffering in 1767, he wrote that he was 'so keenly affected by the thought of this illness that since then I have not been able to hear its name without shuddering, to the point that I am at once seized with shortness of breath and a general trembling which give me considerable pain'. He issued a circular ordering his staff never to speak of the malady in his presence.[56]

Belief that smallpox was inevitable or nearly so encouraged parents to consider exposing their children to the disease at an opportune time. Allowing a child's contact with a sibling who was ill with smallpox was not unknown in seventeenth-century England. Dr Sydenham made a point of exposing children of relatives and friends to mild cases of the disease.[57] In 1695 Anne Finch, Countess of Nottingham, encouraged her daughter to visit and kiss her infected brother.[58] This sort of arrangement is also recorded in Holland, Germany and France in the 1760s.[59] In addition, there were some traditional practices, quasi-magical, that involved the transference of smallpox, usually through scabs, from one person to another in the hope of a milder case. In 1673 Thomas Bartholin, a Danish physician, wrote that he knew 'more than a few people who have bought smallpox for themselves'.[60] The growing profile of inoculation elicited reports of similar customs across Europe.[61] According to Dr Perrot Williams, it was an 'immemorial custom' in southwest Wales for parents to procure smallpox scabs, in return for a coin or token, to press into the hands of their children.[62] Unknown to most medical men, 'buying the smallpox' may have been a practice surviving from a time when the disease was less severe. In eighteenth-century Europe, it does not appear to have been practised on any scale.

---

[56] Derek Edward Dawson Beales, *Joseph II: in the shadow of Maria Theresa, 1741–1780* (Cambridge, 1987), p. 142.

[57] Richard Blackmore, *A treatise upon the small-pox* (London, 1723), pp. 110–11.

[58] *Correspondence of the family of Hatton, being chiefly letters to Christopher Hatton*, 2 vols., ed. E. Maunde Thompson (London, 1878), 2, pp. 211–12.

[59] Augustin Roux, *Mémoire sur l'inoculation de la petite verole* ... (Amsterdam, 1765), p. 9; Willibrord Rutten, 'In de schaduw van de pest: Reacties op pokkenepidemieën in de Republick in de zeventiende en achttiende eeuw', in W. de Blécourt, W. Frijhoff and M. Gijswijt-Hofstra (eds.), *Grenzen van genezing: Gezondheid, ziekte en genezen in Nederland zestiende tot begin twintigste eeuw* (Hilversum, 1993), pp. 172–202, at 190.

[60] Geneviève Miller, *The adoption of inoculation for smallpox in England and France* (Philadelphia, 1957), p. 43.

[61] E.g. Pierre Louis Gandoger de Foigny, *Traité-pratique de l'inoculation* (Nancy, 1768), p. 29; Sköld, *Two faces*, p. 230.

[62] *The correspondence of James Jurin (1684–1750)*, ed. Andrea Rusnock (Amsterdam, 1996), pp. 129–31.

Exotic Practices and Western Borrowings

In Asia, there were more sophisticated forms of smallpox prophylaxis whose origins are likewise lost in the mists of time. The peoples of central Asia may have pioneered the prophylactic practices that subsequently spread eastwards, southwards and westwards. By the eighteenth century, there were robust traditions of inoculation in China, northern India and parts of the Middle East. In China, the practice of insufflation is first described in medical texts in the sixteenth century.[63] Described in poetic language as 'planting the heavenly flowers', this mode of communicating smallpox involved blowing processed smallpox dust through a pipe into the nostril of the patient. The Manchu warlords who conquered China quickly adopted the practice. Prior to his death from smallpox in 1654, the first Emperor of the Xing dynasty barred from the succession anyone still susceptible to smallpox. His successor Xangsi (K'ang Hsi), a smallpox survivor, promoted insufflation in and around the imperial capital.[64] 'Although it is an act seemingly going against nature', a Chinese scholar wrote in 1727, 'it has great merits for the people in the world'.[65] It is hard to be sure how extensively and routinely it was used in China. According to a contemporary Chinese text, the procedure was not practised in Beijing in the late eighteenth century.[66] In India, smallpox inoculation first gained profile in the seventeenth century. In the hands of specialists and somewhat ritualised, it involved a puncture on the arm or forehead and the insertion of smallpox matter in a manner not unlike that observed in Istanbul.[67]

Around 1700, Europeans became active in collecting knowledge from all corners of the globe, especially the *materia medica* of Asia.[68] The increasing severity of smallpox encouraged interest in exotic forms of prophylaxis. Peter the Great of Russia reportedly sent medical men to China to learn about insufflation.[69] Two reports of the Chinese practice reached the Royal Society in England early in 1700.[70] There was curiosity in London, too, about inoculation in the Ottoman empire. Emanuele Timoni, a native of Chios and

---

[63] Hopkins, *Greatest killer*, pp. 109–10; Joseph Needham, *Science and civilisation in China*, vol. 6: part 6, ed. Nathan Sivin (Cambridge, 2000), pp. 134–40 and 169–74.

[64] Zhang, 'Disease', 181–2.   [65] Needham, *Science in China*, 6: 6, pp. 137–8.

[66] Chang, Chia-Feng, 'Aspects of smallpox in Chinese history', Unpublished PhD thesis, University of London, 1996, p. 142.

[67] Ralph W. Nicholas, *Fruits of worship: practical religion in Bengal* (New Delhi, 2003), pp. 175–6.

[68] Hal Cook, *Matters of exchange. Commerce, medicine, and science in the Dutch Golden Age* (New Haven, 2007).

[69] Needham, *Science in China*, 6: 6, p. 149. The evidence for the dating is a little suspect: Renate Burgess, 'Thomas Garvine – Ayrshire surgeon active in Russia and China', *MH*, 19 (1975), 91–4.

[70] Miller, *Adoption*, pp. 48–9.

graduate of Padua, was asked about the procedure on a visit to London in 1703. Encouraged by Dr Skraggenstierna, physician of Charles XII of Sweden, he wrote a brief account of *variolarum insitio* ('grafting smallpox') that was subsequently published in the *Ephemerides* of the Leopoldine Academy in 1715. He also sent a copy to Dr Woodward, secretary of the Royal Society in London, that was translated into English for publication in the *Transactions*.[71] According to Timoni, inoculation originated in Circassia and Georgia, was introduced in Istanbul about forty years earlier, and had been used to treat thousands of people without mishap in the previous eight years. He describes the procedure as involving a slight incision with a needle or lancet on the arm or leg, the insertion of smallpox matter taken from a healthy child, and bandaging the incision for several hours.[72] Dr Woodward sought further information from the British consul in Smyrna, who in turn encouraged Dr Jacob Pylarini, who had been taught by a Greek woman and assisted in an inoculation in 1701, to write his own report. Published in Venice in 1715 and translated for the *Transactions* in 1716, Pylarini describes the inoculator as scratching the skin and then applying lymph on the forehead, cheeks and chin. This mode, sketching out a cross, presumably reflects Christian usage. In a dissertation on inoculation in 1722, Antoine Le Duc, a native of Istanbul, adds the detail that the Greek woman who inoculated him, along with 3,000 others, requested the payment of wax candles as an offering to the Virgin Mary.[73]

By this time a few children from western Europe had been inoculated. Among the first Britons were two sons of Mr Hefferman, secretary of Sir Robert Sutton, the British ambassador to the Ottoman empire, who were inoculated before their return home in March 1716 and were made available for inspection by medical men in London.[74] Lady Mary Wortley Montagu, whose husband succeeded Sutton in the post, was presumably aware of the occurrence. One of the brightest women at the Hanoverian court, she had good reason to be interested in prophylaxis. After losing her brother to the disease in 1713, she declined to lease a house in London that had stood empty after a lady and her child died there from smallpox. 'I know tis two or three years ago', she wrote, 'but tis generally said, that infection may lodge in blankets etc. longer than that'.[75] She was seriously ill with smallpox in 1715 and was badly scarred. In a poem about her trauma, she described how she became 'A frightful spectre to myself unknown!'[76] Travelling with her husband and

---

[71] Miller, *Adoption*, pp. 55–9.

[72] Emanuel Timoni, 'An account, or history, of the procuring the small pox by incision, or inoculation; as it has for some time been practiced at Constantinople', *PTRS*, 29 (1714), 72–84.

[73] Miller, *Adoption*, pp. 59–63.   [74] Miller, *Adoption*, p. 51.

[75] Isobel Grundy, *Mary Wortley Montagu* (Oxford, 1999), p. 80.

[76] Grundy, *Montagu*, pp. 100–2; Smith, *Speckled monster*, p. 19.

son to Istanbul in 1717, she observed the practice of smallpox inoculation and declared her intent to bring it 'into fashion' in England.[77] In spring 1718, she took the bold step of having her only son inoculated by an old Greek woman, with Charles Maitland, her surgeon, in attendance.[78] Back in London, she awaited an opportunity to have her daughter inoculated. In April 1721, with smallpox spreading 'like a destroying angel', she asked Maitland to undertake the procedure.[79] She readily agreed that two physicians should be called to attend the child and 'be eye-witnesses of the practice, and contribute to the credit and reputation of it'.[80] Though the first inoculation in Britain was not reported in the newspapers, news of the success of the procedure spread rapidly among the chattering classes.

In a remarkable conjuncture, smallpox inoculation was introduced in another part of the English-speaking world at this very time. British slave-traders, who had reason to be attentive to pockmarks on slaves, presumably noted the scarification marks on some of them, and may have pondered their significance. In Boston, Massachusetts, Dr Cotton Mather, a Fellow of the Royal Society, learned about the African practice of smallpox prophylaxis from an African slave or servant named Onesimus. Asked whether he had ever had smallpox, Onesimus replied that he had 'undergone an operation that gave him something of the smallpox' and showed the marks on his arm. After making enquiries of merchants and other Africans in Boston, Mather learned more about smallpox prophylaxis in Africa and was confident that it provided security against subsequent infection. After reading Timoni's account in the *Transactions*, he reported his findings to Dr Woodward in London and declared his intent to make a trial of the practice when smallpox next broke out in Boston, adding that if we could 'hear that you have done it before us, how much would that embolden us!'[81] A serious smallpox epidemic in May 1721 provided the incentive for Zabdiel Boylston, Mather's surgical colleague, to make a trial of inoculation, beginning with his own children. The bold initiative outraged many people. Dr William Douglass argued that the practice was unsafe and was fuelling the infection. Over summer, Boylston inoculated fifty-eight people, seemingly with success, but then one of his patients died. The arrival of a report of the success of a formal trial of inoculation in London did little to settle minds.[82] The controversy continued to rage in Boston, and indeed fed popular anxieties about the practice in Britain. In 1722, Boylston's detailed account of his inoculation activity in Boston, in which he cogently

---

[77] Miller, *Adoption*, p. 69.   [78] Grundy, *Montagu*, p. 162.   [79] Grundy, *Montagu*, p. 209.
[80] Miller, *Adoption*, p. 72.
[81] *Selected letters of Cotton Mather*, ed. Kenneth Silverman (Baton Rouge, LA, 1971), pp. 213–14.
[82] Arthur W. Boylston, *Defying providence. Smallpox and the forgotten eighteenth-century medical revolution* (North Charleston, 2012), pp. 53–7.

argued for its utility, proved an important foundation for the practice on both sides of the Atlantic.

In Britain, the inoculation of Lady Wortley Montagu's daughter encouraged the Royal Society to seek opportunities for experimentation. Caroline, Princess of Wales, proved a persuasive advocate. At her request, George I granted a pardon to six condemned felons conditional on their submitting to inoculation in a trial supervised by the Royal Society.[83] In August 1721, Maitland successfully inoculated three male and three female convicts at Newgate.[84] In the meantime, Dr Richard Mead made a trial of insufflation, the distinctive mode of prophylaxis in China, finding that the inhalation of smallpox dust occasioned a more severe response than inoculating smallpox on the arm.[85] Eager to see more trials prior to the inoculation of her own children, Princess Caroline offered to pay for the inoculation of poor children in Westminster. In spring 1722, royal physicians inoculated five orphans and exhibited them to the public and, in a further experiment, a child was inoculated with lymph from one of the inoculated children.[86] After George I indicated his willingness to leave the decision to his son and daughter-in-law, the stage was set for the inoculation of his grandchildren. In April 1722, Princesses Amelia and Caroline passed safely through the procedure.[87] Despite the recent death of the Earl of Sunderland's son following inoculation, many elite families were encouraged by the royal family's example to adopt the practice.

Elite endorsement by no means allayed ethical and medical concerns. Although leading churchmen took the line that it was not a sin to accept a surgical procedure that could save their children's lives, the Reverend Edmund Massey, an influential preacher, condemned it as an impious affront to Providence.[88] Dr William Wagstaffe broke ranks with his medical colleagues in the Royal Society to express bewilderment that 'an experiment practised only by a few ignorant women, amongst an illiterate and unthinking people, should of a sudden ... so far obtain in one of the politest nations in the world, as to be received into the royal palace'.[89] Drawn into the controversy, Lady Montagu championed the practice in a letter written under the guise of a 'Turkey Merchant', but castigated 'the knavery and ignorance' of doctors for making a deep incision with a lancet rather than pricking the skin with a needle, and

---

[83] Grundy, *Montagu*, pp. 211–12.   [84] Miller, *Adoption*, pp. 84–5.

[85] Miller, *Adoption*, p. 86.

[86] Geneviève Miller, 'Smallpox inoculation in England and America: a reappraisal', *The William and Mary quarterly*, third series, 13 (1956), 476–92, at 478–81.

[87] Miller, *Adoption*, pp. 96–7.

[88] Miller, *Adoption*, pp. 130–1; John Wilmot, *The life of John Hough, successively bishop of Oxford, Lichfield and Coventry, and Worcester* (London, 1812), p. 321.

[89] Grundy, *Montagu*, p. 216.

imposing on the patient an expensive regimen of preparation and aftercare.[90] The critical issue was the risk involved in a procedure that was tantamount to fighting fire with fire. The promoters of inoculation argued that, if one's house were on fire, a sensible person would take the risk of jumping from the window. Francis Howgrave, an apothecary and critic of inoculation, conceded the point, but asked, 'Did ever any man leap out of a window at Charing Cross for fear of a fire at Temple Bar?' In any case, he continued, 'smallpox is the fire you are to avoid, and [inoculation] is leaping out of the frying pan into the fire'.[91] Steadily, this aspect of the debate moved from rhetoric and trading anecdotes to attempts at statistical analysis. In 1722, Thomas Nettleton of Halifax acknowledged that one of the sixty-one patients he had inoculated had died, but observed that the mortality rate among people who caught the disease naturally was one in five. For him, it was a matter of applying merchant's logic: 'state the account of profit and loss to find on which side the balance lies ... and form a judgement accordingly'.[92] James Jurin, secretary of the Royal Society, began to collect data on smallpox and smallpox inoculation from across England and calculated that one in seven or eight cases of natural smallpox proved fatal but only one in ninety-one people inoculated died.[93] It was countered that the people who were inoculated were more generally people in otherwise good health, and that some might have avoided smallpox entirely. There was also the danger that smallpox inoculation posed for the broader community. Many Bostonians and many Londoners believed that the practice increased the number of smallpox cases, added to the contagion and increased the overall mortality.

Britain's experiment with inoculation was followed with interest in continental Europe. Dr Johann Eller, who claimed to have acquired the technique from a Greek friend and inoculated a child in Paris in 1719, made a demonstration of the practice, at the request of the Prince of Anhalt-Bernberg, in Bernberg in 1721.[94] The dynastic connection between Britain and Hanover increased the profile of inoculation in northwest Germany. Dr Johann Georg Steigherthal, George I's physician, was involved in the trial at Newgate, and Dr Matthias Boretius, a German visitor to London in 1721, witnessed the trial and published an account of it.[95] In early 1723,

---

[90] Diana Barnes, 'The public life of a woman of wit and quality: Lady Mary Wortley Montagu and the vogue for smallpox inoculation', *Feminist Studies*, 38 (2012), 330–62, at 351–2.

[91] Francis Howgrave, *Reasons against the inoculation of the small-pox* (London, 1724), pp. 43–4.

[92] Andrea Rusnock, '"The merchant's logick": numerical debates over smallpox in eighteenth-century England,' in E. Magnello and A. Hardy (eds.), *The road to medical statistics* (Amsterdam, 2002), pp. 37–54, at p. 38.

[93] Andrea Rusnock, *Vital accounts. Quantifying health and population in eighteenth-century England and France* (Cambridge, 2002), pp. 53–4.

[94] Miller, *Adoption*, pp. 67–8.   [95] Miller, *Adoption*, pp. 81, 84–5.

J. E. Wreden began inoculating in the electorate of Hanover, setting the scene for the inoculation there of the eldest son of the Prince of Wales in 1724.[96] The early inoculations in Germany, with less than optimal outcomes, failed to overcome the hesitancy and prejudice that was nourished by some adverse reports from Britain. Initially, France looked a promising field for the new prophylaxis. Philippe of Orleans, Regent of France, showed interest in sponsoring a trial. The royal physician prepared the ground and Dr Jean Delacoste, a Huguenot exile in England, returned to France eager to introduce the practice. In autumn 1723, a murderous smallpox epidemic in Paris helped the cause for a time. Reports of the controversy in Britain and America, however, stiffened the opposition of the old guard in the Faculty of Medicine, and the death of Philippe of Orleans in December deprived the practice of a potential patron.[97] For a time it looked as if the duchy of Lorraine might embrace prophylaxis. Duke Leopold and his wife, a sister of Philippe of Orleans, lost three children to smallpox in 1711, and then his eldest son in 1721. Although he was in correspondence with Lady Montagu and commissioned a French translation of Timoni in 1725, he seemingly made no move to introduce the practice.[98]

By the late 1720s inoculation was losing ground in Britain. Some aristocratic and professional families continued to have their children inoculated but there was little or no extension of the practice. In the 1730s, it was even neglected in the British royal family. The future George III, born in 1738, caught the disease accidentally when he was five years old.[99] Geneviève Miller has argued that the notion that inoculation lapsed between 1728 and 1740 was a 'historical myth' promoted by Dr James Kirkpatrick, who wished to associate the practice's revival in Britain with his success with the procedure in South Carolina in the late 1730s and his championship of it on his return.[100] He was by no means, though, the only or earliest witness to a decline of interest from the late 1720s. Dr John Andrew, who practised inoculation on a small scale in the provinces in the 1730s, observed that the practice 'was in decline in London'.[101] Asked about inoculation early in 1738, Bishop Hough of Worcester replied that 'the method loses ground, even in this country'.[102] In claiming that the practice remained in good repute, Miller refers to three

---

[96] Miller, *Adoption*, pp. 177–8.   [97] Miller, *Adoption*, pp. 180–92.

[98] Pierre-Joseph Buc'hoz, *Lettres périodiques curieuses, utiles et interessantes: Sur les avantages que la société économique peut retirer de la connoissance des animaux, pour servir de suite aux lettres sur les végétaux*, vol. 2 (Paris, 1769), p. 13.

[99] *The letters of Horace Walpole, Earl of Orford*, vol. 1, ed. Peter Cunningham (London, 1857), p. 277.

[100] Miller, 'Reappraisal', 476–92.

[101] John Andrew, *The practice of inoculation impartially considered* (Dublin, 1765), p. xii.

[102] Wilmot, *Bishop Hough*, pp. 321–2.

physicians who wrote positively about inoculation in the 1730s. Their books were published early in the decade, however, and none refer to inoculations after 1727. Dr Lobb, the best informed of the three, declared that he only recommended inoculation when infection was otherwise inevitable.[103] Though Miller was right to point out that smallpox was less of a threat in the 1730s, there were certainly significant outbreaks, including in Bury St Edmunds in 1733, the only English town in Miller's brief list of places where inoculation activity is documented. Far from supporting Miller's case, the response to smallpox in Bury would seem to undermine it: a well-reasoned proposal to use inoculation to suppress the outbreak was strongly opposed, and only three people were inoculated.[104]

A recognition of the decline in inoculation in Britain in the 1730s makes it easier to understand its failure to make early headway on the continent. While Voltaire championed inoculation in his *Letters from England*, first published in French in 1734, his fellow-countrymen were becoming more circumspect. In opposing the practice in 1740, Julian Ofray de La Mettrie, physician and *philosophe*, observed that the English had wisely abandoned it.[105] In presenting the decline of the practice as a 'myth', Miller does less than justice to the American contribution to its revival in the 1740s. Although they carried only occasional notices of individuals inoculated in London, British newspapers in the 1730s reported the inoculation of hundreds of people during smallpox outbreaks in Philadelphia and Charleston in North America, and in Barbados and St Kitts in the Caribbean.[106] The inoculation of large numbers of workers and slaves served to extend the social range of the practice and brought improvements in efficiency and outcomes.[107] The decision to inoculate children admitted to the new Foundling Hospital in London in 1744 and the establishment of the Smallpox and Inoculation Hospital in 1746, signal events in the revival of inoculation in Britain, need to be seen in the context of the use of inoculation on large population groups on the other side of the Atlantic.

---

[103] Thomas Fuller, *Exanthematologia* (London, 1730); Thomas Dover, *The ancient physician's legacy to his country* (London, 1732), pp. 87–90; Theophilus Lobb, *A treatise of the small pox* (London, 1731), pp. 184–5.

[104] Miller, *Adoption*, p. 137; Sloane MS. 4053, item 163, BL.

[105] Julien Offray de La Mettrie, *Traité de la petite vérole avec la manière de guérir cette maladie* (Paris, 1740), p. 9; Kathleen Wellman, *La Mettrie: Medicine, Philosophy, and Enlightenment* (Durham, NC, 1992), pp. 93–4.

[106] *Daily Gazetteer*, 6 December 1737; *Weekly Miscellany*, 14 July 1738; *Daily Post*, 18 July 1738; *London Evening Post*, 15–17 March 1740.

[107] Larry Stewart, 'The edge of utility: slaves and smallpox in the early eighteenth century', *MH*, 29 (1985), 54–70.

The Broader Disease Environment, Human and Animal

Smallpox was not the only threat to life and well-being in the eighteenth century and the level of the threat varied over time and place. In England, it was endemic in London and other large cities and towns, but there were still villages, not especially remote, that managed to escape it for a decade or so. The London bills of mortality show that the proportion of deaths attributed to smallpox was one in eight in 1725, but did not reach that level again for two decades. During an epidemic in 1752, however, it was responsible for one in six deaths.[108] In parishes across England, there were peaks in mortality that were specifically identified with smallpox in registers of births, marriages and deaths. For a village untroubled by smallpox for a decade or more, and a high proportion of the population consequently at risk, an outbreak could be devastating. Even in larger population-centres where smallpox was endemic, its destructive force ebbed and flowed with epidemics, some associated with high mortality, others relatively mild. The 'speckled monster' was evidently much less menacing in the 1730s than in earlier and subsequent decades. During this time, too, food prices were relatively low and average standards of living were on the rise. Broader cultural changes, including growing awareness of the role of contagion, the value of sanitary measures and personal cleanliness, may likewise have proved helpful in the fight against disease in Britain and elsewhere. It is important, then, to consider smallpox and smallpox prophylaxis in the context of the larger disease environment.

From 1348, bubonic plague was the source of most concern in western Europe. It prompted much of the new thinking about contagion and experimentation with measures to contain outbreaks, notably quarantine and sanitation.[109] The Great Plague in London of 1665 and the epidemic in Marseille in 1720, however, proved to be the last outbreaks in their respective countries. It remained a dreadful menace in eastern Europe, north Africa and the Middle East, with Russia experiencing a major epidemic as late as the 1770s. As the decades passed, however, the retreat of the plague was a source of quiet satisfaction in the western world, giving grounds for hope that other diseases might be controlled and banished. In the meantime, smallpox and other crowd diseases were becoming more salient. Typhus was a major source of morbidity and mortality in large towns and other places, like army camps, prisons and ships, where people were crowded together. It was not seen as a single entity, attributable to a single disease agent, but observed as a range of environmentally determined fevers. Even less understood was the

---

[108] Miller, *Adoption*, appendix C.
[109] Mark Harrison, *Contagion. How commerce has spread disease* (New Haven, CT, 2012), chs. 1 and 2.

identity and infectiousness of tuberculosis, described by reference to its symptoms as the wasting disease or consumption. There were soon other major killers on the loose, notably yellow fever and cholera, which took advantage of the increase in global commerce from the late eighteenth century. In this context, it was smallpox's misfortune to be so readily identifiable. Though superficially like measles and chickenpox, its symptoms and *sequelae* clearly marked it out in typical cases. Like the bubonic plague, it acquired a distinct cultural identity.[110] Some features of the disease, including its genetic stability, its lack of a non-human reservoir of infection, and its visibility at the infective stage, proved advantageous to humanity in its struggle to contain it. Above all, the fact that people took smallpox only once allowed survivors to nurse the sick and made it worth considering the advantages of acquiring the disease by artifice.

Europe's understanding of infection was informed, too, by observing non-human diseases. From Antiquity through to the Renaissance, the observation of plants and animals enriched and challenged medical understandings. Few people living on the land needed to be told to take rotten apples out of a barrel or that a sick animal might infect the herd or flock. The specificity of diseases was most evident when considered across species: there were pests that attacked some plants and animals but not others.[111] The observation of outbreaks of animal disease in Europe – which arose from the very conditions, namely the increase in population, commerce and communication, that spread infection among humans – offered insights on the nature of disease, patterns of infection, and modes of containment that could be applied more generally. In the early eighteenth century, Europe was under siege from a deadly cattle disease, known as the cattle plague or rinderpest. Spreading eastward from the Steppes, it decimated herds in northern Germany and Italy in 1711 and France and the Netherlands in 1713–14. The mortality was on an epic scale: the Netherlands lost some 300,000 head of cattle.[112] After a lull in the late 1720s and 1730s, the disease reappeared in the 1740s and 1750s. Aware of the economic costs, governments responded with rare energy and resource. Regulations to isolate infected animals and limit the movement of herds showed a practical understanding of the aetiology of the disease. Although it was generally described as a plague, many people saw a likeness to smallpox. In 1711 Bernardino Ramazzini, professor of medicine at Padua, stressed the similarities in appearance and aetiology.[113] Familiarity with smallpox

---

[110] Shuttleton, *Smallpox and literary imagination*, esp. introduction; Catriona Seth, *Les rois aussi en mouraient. Les Lumières en lutte contre la petite vérole* (Paris, 2008), pp. 28–34.

[111] Lise Wilkinson, *Animals and disease. An introduction to the history of comparative medicine* (Cambridge, 1992), p. 26.

[112] C. A. Spinage, *Cattle plague. A history* (New York, 2003), pp. 104–11.

[113] Wilkinson, *Animals and disease*, p. 41; Spinage, *Cattle plague*, p. 111.

doubtless encouraged the insight that cattle surviving an outbreak were safe from subsequent infection. Familiarity with smallpox inoculation prompted an English physician, Daniel Layard, to make a trial of inoculating cattle with cattle plague in the 1740s. Though it proved more feasible in England to suppress cattle plague by quarantine and culling, Layard's publication of his researches in 1754 attracted interest in the Netherlands. In experiments in 1755 and the late 1760s, Pieter Camper, professor of medicine at Groningen, unfortunately killed more animals by inoculation than he saved. In the mid-1770s, however, Gerd Reinders, a dairy-farmer, drew on best practice in smallpox inoculation to use only lymph from cows that had survived the disease and, after achieving promising outcomes, formed a society to extend rinderpest inoculation. The use of inoculum from mild cases likewise proved successful in Mecklenburg and led to the large-scale inoculation of cattle in the district, supported by insurance schemes to spread the risk.[114] By the end of the eighteenth century, though, the threat of rinderpest in western Europe receded and the practice fell into abeyance.

Costly in economic terms, animal diseases received serious attention and provided opportunities for speculation and experimentation. The recognition of similarities between human and animal diseases led to speculation, too, that transferring a disease from an animal might protect a human from a cognate human disease. Veterinary science, of course, was even less well developed than medical science. Animal distempers were less precisely named and described than human diseases, and observations were less well documented and integrated into systems of knowledge. If the challenge presented by cattle plague in the early eighteenth century intrigued some medical men, comparative pathology brought as much confusion as clarity. The cattle plague was variously described as a plague, a pox or a sort of typhus. In his papers to the Royal Society in the 1750s, Daniel Layard simply named it 'the distemper among horned cattle'. There were other contagious livestock diseases that were also a matter of high concern. Foot-and-mouth disease was highly communicable and appeared in severe epidemics. Though rare in Britain, clavelée or sheep-pox was a serious menace to flocks in the foothills of the Alps and Pyrenees. Its seeming affinity to smallpox made it an additional focus of interest. There were many other livestock ailments that were insufficiently common or serious to attract close attention, including several pustular conditions on the teats of cows, known generally in England as 'cowpox'.

Cowpox is not attested before the 1760s, and only then in retrospect. Though known to dairy-farmers in parts of England and western Europe, it appeared only sporadically and caused little apparent distress to cattle. It could

---

[114] C. Huygelen, 'The immunization of cattle against rinderpest in eighteenth-century Europe', MH, 41 (1997), 182–96.

be communicated to dairy workers, occasioning a local lesion and swelling, but rarely warranting professional attention. One apparent property of cowpox attracted attention. Some people believed that cowpox infection protected them against smallpox. Edward Jenner was among a small number of practitioners who started to look closely at the correlation between cowpox infection and insusceptibility to smallpox. From the 1770s, he collected evidence of cases and examined the progress of the disease on cattle and humans. A careful observer, he saw it was necessary to distinguish between the several forms of cowpox communicable to man. One that is now known as pseudo-cowpox is a parapoxvirus that has no prophylactic value, while another, still known as cowpox, is an orthopoxvirus that provides protection against smallpox but produces a very severe reaction.[115] There is no certainty as to the identity of the cowpox that Jenner used, with one longstanding argument being that it was modified smallpox.[116] As Derrick Baxby and others have shown, however, extant strains of *vaccinia*, all of which have been used for some time, show no recent affinity either with smallpox or modern cowpox.[117] Baxby's speculation that *vaccinia* was derived from horsepox, extinct in Europe, has recently received strong support from the genomic sequencing of a sample of the disease from Mongolia.[118] Interestingly, Jenner himself believed that the source of his 'cowpox' was a pustular disease on the legs of horses. Given the wide host range of *vaccinia* it is very conceivable that a similar virus was the infective agent of both Jenner's cowpox and horsepox. To add to the confusion, since the horse and the cow were merely the incidental hosts of the virus, it is probable that the natural reservoir of the ancestor of *vaccinia* was a rodent or other small mammal in occasional contact with them.[119]

The Uses of Inoculation

From the outset, inoculation was more than a surgical procedure. It was originally called 'grafting' in England, a direct translation of '*insitio*' or '*inoculatio*' in Latin. The term, used in horticulture, commended itself as a description of the process of cutting into a trunk and inserting matter. Early

---

[115] Frank Fenner, Riccardo Wittek and Keith R. Dumbell, *The orthopoxviruses* (San Diego, CA, 1989), pp. 187–8.

[116] Peter Razzell, *Edward Jenner's cowpox vaccine: the history of a medical myth* (Firle, 1977).

[117] Derrick Baxby, *Jenner's smallpox vaccine: the riddle of vaccinia virus and its origin* (London, 1981).

[118] José Esparza, Livia Shrick, Clarissa R. Damaso and Andreas Nitsche, 'Equination (inoculation of horsepox) and the potential role of horsepox virus in the origin of the smallpox vaccine', *Vaccine*, 35 (2017), 7222–30; Clarissa R. Damaso, 'Revisting Jenner's mysteries, the role of the Beaugency lymph in the evolutionary path of ancient smallpox vaccines, *The Lancet. Infectious Diseases*, 18 (2018), e55–63.

[119] Baxby, *Jenner's vaccine*, p. 168; Fenner, Wittek and Dumbell, *Orthopoxviruses*, ch. 6.

modern Europe witnessed significant advances in horticulture through grafting, and even fanciful speculation as to its use on animals as well as plants. In 1659, Joseph Sharrock, a churchman fascinated by horticulture, humorously dismissed calls 'to apply ourselves by these rarer ways of insition to the improvement of animal bodies'.[120] The conception of 'grafting' as improving on nature provided figurative support for the idea that inoculation of smallpox from a milder case reduced the natural severity of smallpox. In 1783 Gadso Coopmans, physician and classical scholar at the University of Franekar in the Netherlands, made the idea the centrepiece of a long Latin poem on smallpox entitled *Varis, sive Carmen de variolis*. Inspired by Fracastoro's *Syphilis*, it tells of a shepherd named Lycidas and his sweetheart Amaryllis. A malicious nymph named Varis sought to seduce Lycidas, and smarting from his rejection of her inflicted a disease that took away his good looks. His sweetheart likewise took the disease and died in agony. The disease then traversed the world, killing some and leaving others badly scarred. Eventually a pious old man turned to Apollo for aid. The oracle replied: 'A fruit loses its sourness when a graft has been implanted in another tree'.[121]

In the 1720s, inoculating smallpox was promoted as a protection against casual infection. Early supporters of practice sought to demonstrate its relative safety and utility, embed the new procedure in medical practice, and allay ethical and religious objections. The basic task was to demonstrate the value of the procedure. If it was revealed to be beneficial, medical men would make it available and people could adopt it in good conscience. The clinical trials showed it to be reasonably safe. In the first major use of medical statistics, data was presented to show that the case-fatality rates of inoculated smallpox were significantly lower than for casual smallpox. In terms of understanding how inoculation worked, the priority was to fit the practice into the existing humoural paradigm rather than unsettle it. The assumption was that smallpox was innate and that a range of factors, including infection, caused it to break out. Inoculated smallpox could be seen as acting in this fashion, provoking ebullition and serving to 'deplete' the body's store of variolous poison. Still, the growing familiarity with inoculation served to advance understandings of infection. Inoculation made it possible to establish the moment of infection and demonstrate the specificity of the disease. In the 1720s, Cotton Mather sought to explain the milder nature of inoculated smallpox by reference to the inoculation of the disease on an outer limb.[122] As Geneviève Miller observed,

---

[120] Ken Mudge, Jules Janick, Steven Scofield and Eliezer E. Goldschmidt, 'A history of grafting', *Horticultural Reviews*, 35 (2009), 437–93, at 466.

[121] D. Sacré, 'An imitator of Fracastorius's *Syphilis*: Gadso Coopmans (1746–1810) and his *Varis*', *Humanistica Lovaniensia. Journal of Neo-Latin Studies*, 45 (1996), 520–38.

[122] Mather, *Angel of Bethesda*, ed. Jones, p. 112.

inoculation had the capacity 'to provide the capital to the column of evidence supporting the doctrines of contagion and specificity'.[123]

The success of smallpox inoculation gave rise to attempts to inoculate other human diseases as well as animal diseases. It was a matter of some interest whether inoculation could be used to prevent the bubonic plague, but the disappearance of plague in western Europe left no opportunity to experiment. During a plague epidemic in the Russian empire in 1770–2, however, medical men in Moscow and Bucharest made a serious trial of inoculation as a form of plague prophylaxis. Though the inoculated patients survived, they can have derived little benefit from the procedure, given that it was possible for people to contract plague, a bacterial rather than a viral disease, more than once.[124] A more obvious candidate for inoculation was measles, a disease that some-times took a heavy toll of children. Since it produced no vesicles, though, it was hard to obtain matter for inoculation. Francis Home rose to the challenge by turning to 'the magazine of all epidemic diseases, the blood'. In experi-ments in Edinburgh in 1759 he reportedly succeeded in producing milder cases of measles by inoculating blood from infected patients.[125] In 1774 Dr Cook, his pupil, followed up on this practice, recommending the tears of patients as the inoculum, and John Hunter, Jenner's mentor, also experimented with measles.[126] No one thought the operation worthwhile. The infective agent was hard to obtain and the resulting illness was only slightly milder than natural infection. Inoculation was nonetheless increasingly recognised as a valuable tool in pathology. It offered insights into the interaction between infections: when smallpox and measles were inoculated together, for example, the two diseases came out separately, one ahead of the other. John Hunter sought to establish the relationship between gonorrhoea and syphilis by inoculating a patient's penis with gonorrhoea and monitoring for signs of syphilis. Unfortunately, he acci-dentally communicated both diseases, presumably through a contaminated lancet, and his ill-founded conclusion that syphilis was an advanced stage of gonorrhoea misled several generations of practitioners.[127]

Above all, inoculation remained an invaluable tool for investigating small-pox itself. According to Dr Haygarth, the 'truth' of the proposition that smallpox was caused by infection only 'is proved, beyond all possibility of doubt, by the daily practice of inoculation'.[128] There was still little

[123] Miller, *Adoption*, p. 259.
[124] John T. Alexander, *Bubonic plague in early modern Russia: public health and urban disaster* (Oxford, 2002), pp. 293–5.
[125] Francis Home, *Medical facts and experiments* (London, 1759), pp. 266–88.
[126] *Town and Country Magazine*, 6 (1774), 300–2.
[127] Wendy Moore, *The knife man. The extraordinary life and times of John Hunter, father of modern Surgery* (London, 2005), pp. 192–8.
[128] Haygarth, *Inquiry*, p. 13.

understanding of the process of infection. The infective agent was understood, in a loose way, as a poison. Haygarth imagined variolous particles being absorbed in the atmosphere. Inoculation allowed precision with respect to the timing of infection and the number of days before the disease broke out. With no conception of the immune system, it was assumed that the patient became insusceptible to subsequent smallpox by the purging of variolous matter. Still, many medical men used the metaphor of resistance and some took their cue from the great Dr Boerhaave, who felt that smallpox 'left some positive and material quality in the constitution' that prevented subsequent infection.[129] On a more practical level, close attention to groups of patients undergoing the disease provided opportunities to experiment with different regimens and introduce them in anticipation of the fever. Some inoculators gained facility in diagnosing natural cases of smallpox before the disease broke out, enabling them to prescribe medicines earlier and to better effect.[130] The handling and storage of smallpox matter provided insight on the length of time it remained infective, a crucial point practically and epidemiologically. Variolation often proved useful as a test of susceptibility to smallpox. People who were unsure whether they had had smallpox as a child might have themselves inoculated to set their minds at rest. It was used sometimes to establish a diagnosis in uncertain cases in which chickenpox was assumed but smallpox needed to be ruled out. In a ghoulish experiment conducted by Dr George Pearson to test whether a pregnant woman could infect a child with smallpox in utero, a dead foetus reported to have pockmarks was exhumed from a grave-yard, and the pocky matter used in the inoculation of a young girl.[131]

Crucially, smallpox inoculation laid the foundations for cowpox inoculation. During the eighteenth century, practitioners gained experience and made significant improvements in the technical aspects of inoculation, including making a lighter incision or puncture on the outer limb, inoculating fresh lymph taken from mild smallpox cases, and devising methods for storing variolous matter, all of which helped to set the scene for the success of vaccination. In addition to the key elements of the procedure, the broadly-based culture of inoculation in Britain provided a common frame of reference that allowed the new prophylaxis to be recognised, assessed, and communicated by medical men and a broader constituency of interest. Most basically, it was inoculation that revealed that some people who had been previously exposed to cowpox resisted smallpox infection, and provided, in early trials

[129] Arthur M. Silverstein and Alexander A. Bialasiewicz, 'A history of acquired immunity', *Cellular Immunology*, 51 (1980), 151–67, at 161.
[130] Michael Bennett, 'Curing and inoculating smallpox: the career of Simeon Worlock in Paris, Brittany and Saint-Domingue in the 1770s', *French History and Civilization*, 7 (2017), 27–38.
[131] George Pearson, *Observations on the effects of variolous infection on pregnant women* (Reprint from *Medical Commentaries*, 19, no date), pp. 9–10.

of cowpox, the means of testing the resistance to smallpox of people who had been vaccinated. Most of the critical developments in smallpox inoculation, of course, took place in the late eighteenth century. Chapter 2, then, begins with the revival of the practice in Britain in the 1740s and 1750s and then focuses on the significant development of the practice and its rapid expansion, in terms of social reach and geographical range in the last quarter of the eighteenth century. This expansion in Europe and the Americas provided a platform for the new prophylaxis and generated enthusiasm for the potential of a practice that offered both the individual and the community safety from smallpox. It both anticipated and, in turn, gave momentum to the rapid global expansion of vaccination in the early nineteenth century.

2   Fire with Fire

Smallpox Inoculation in the Eighteenth Century

In March 1756, when smallpox threatened Wotton-under-Edge in Gloucestershire, residents gave thought to inoculating their children and using
parish funds to offer the procedure to the poor, including newcomers in
the textile mill. At a vestry meeting, fifteen of seventeen vestrymen agreed
to hire a local surgeon to inoculate the poor at 5s. per head. Over a couple
of weeks, the surgeon prepared, inoculated and attended to 336 patients,
two of whom died. The record of this 'general inoculation' only survives
because one ratepayer took the overseers of the poor to court, unsuccessfully, for using parish funds for this purpose.[1] There is other evidence that
the small town took smallpox prophylaxis seriously. In the following year,
an eight-year-old orphan attending the town school was inoculated with his
schoolmates. It was the full deal, with bloodletting, purgative medicine and
a deep incision. 'After this barbarism of human-veterinary practice,' as the
episode was recalled half a century later, 'he was removed to one of the
then usual inoculation stables, and haltered up with others in a terrible state
of the disease, although none died.'[2] It was just as well: the little boy was
Edward Jenner.

The coming of spring in 1756 also raised concerns about smallpox in Paris.
The Duke of Orleans resolved to have his son and daughter inoculated. When
asked for permission, Louis XV would neither approve nor prohibit his cousin's
plan of action. Dr Théodore Tronchin came from Geneva to perform the
operation. More experienced than any Frenchman in the practice, he had
developed a gentler procedure than was standard in England. His arrival in
Paris caused a great stir. On 25 March, he inoculated the eight-year-old
Philippe. The announcement of the happy outcome occasioned great rejoicing.[3]
The audience at the Opera was entranced by the sight of the Duke and Duchess

---

[1] Q/SO/8, f. 145v, Quarter Sessions, Gloucestershire RO, Gloucester.

[2] Thomas Dudley Fosbroke, *Berkeley manuscripts ... to which are annexed a copious history of
the castle and parish of Berkeley ... and biographical anecdotes of Dr Jenner* (London, 1821),
p. 221.

[3] Miller, *Adoption*, pp. 212, 217.

taking their box with their children in their arms, and loudly cheered them.[4] For the young boy, later Duke of Orleans, it was a formative experience. Always hungry for public acclaim, he led the liberal nobles in support of the French Revolution, under the name Philippe Égalité. However, security from smallpox did not save him from the guillotine.

The inoculations in Gloucestershire and Paris in 1756–7 reflect significant developments in the history of the practice. The initiative at Wotton-under-Edge is testimony to increasing popular interest in inoculation in the English-speaking world. For its part, Tronchin's success in introducing inoculation in the house of Orleans made it fashionable in aristocratic and liberal circles in France, helping to establish its credibility and prompting emulation elsewhere in Europe. The two developments, at either end of the social spectrum, were mutually supportive. Prior to accepting the procedure, European princes and nobles often sponsored trials among children in charitable institutions under their patronage. Enlightened self-interest likewise led them to promote the practice among their servants and tenants. The widening demand for prophylaxis made it possible for more medical men to build expertise and introduce improvements, most notably a simplification of the procedure that made it more affordable and less traumatic for patients. The growing body of experience of inoculation challenged and transformed understandings of disease and inspired new thinking about public health. Furthermore, the expansion of smallpox inoculation in the late eighteenth century not only made possible Jenner's cowpox discovery but also created the conditions for its rapid appraisal and adoption in many parts of the world.

Inoculation in England: Survival and Revival

By arranging the inoculation of her children and by publicising its benefits, Lady Mary Wortley Montagu brought smallpox inoculation into fashion in Britain. The Royal Society's experiments and Dr Jurin's collection of data showing its relative safety provided some basis for confidence in the procedure. Costly and time-consuming, however, the procedure initially had little social reach. The reports of some deaths and concern that inoculation spread the infection created anxieties and stoked outrage among the population at large. The chance of a severe or fatal outcome was a source of stress to the practitioners themselves. Physicians were disinclined to promote 'what so many are disposed to find fault with', and recommended it only when smallpox was an immediate threat.[5] Since the procedure was largely in the hands of surgeons, it

---

[4] *L'Année Littéraire*, 3 (1756), 232–4.
[5] James Kirkpatrick, *The analysis of inoculation: comprizing the history, theory, and practice ...* (London, 1754), pp. 271–82; Miller, *Adoption*, p. 131; Lobb, *Treatise*, pp. 184–5.

is instructive that Samuel Sharp, a leading London surgeon, did not include inoculation in the first three editions of his bestselling surgical treatise (1739–40).[6] Lady Montagu herself came to regret 'her patriotic undertaking' and claimed she would never 'have attempted it if she had foreseen the vexation, persecution, and even the obloquy it brought upon her'.[7]

In the early 1740s, however, smallpox inoculation staged a revival. The decade began with smallpox outbreaks across the British Isles, and in 1740–1 there was popular demand for inoculation in the southern counties of England.[8] The surgeon at Wotton-under-Edge in 1756 claimed that he 'had practised the method for sixteen years', that is, from around 1740.[9] John Ryder, Bishop of Down, reported in 1743 that in the last 'two or three years' 1,000 people had been inoculated in his diocese in northern Ireland.[10] In 1743, Sharp finally included a section on smallpox inoculation in the fourth edition of his textbook.[11] Although the revival in the practice was underway before Dr James Kirkpatrick's return to Britain in 1742, Geneviève Miller was perhaps too hasty in discounting his role in re-establishing its fortunes.[12] After all, reports of inoculation in the American colonies in the late 1730s, including Kirkpatrick's report of its success in Charleston in 1738, would have disposed British readers to reconsider its advantages.[13] In Britain, Kirkpatrick could claim an expertise in inoculation that was hard to match locally and his *Essay on Inoculation*, published in 1743, was unprecedented in ambition and scale.[14] His boast that 'several' people told him that his work 'had been of some effectual tendency to revive the practice in England' is entirely credible.[15] In dismissing the possibility of his influence on the decision of the Foundling Hospital to introduce inoculation, Miller mistakenly states that the decision was made in January 1743, before Kirkpatrick's return, when it was actually made early in 1744.[16] Another signal event in the revival of inoculation, suggesting at least the timeliness of Kirkpatrick's book, was its re-adoption

---

[6] Samuel Sharp, *A treatise on the operations of surgery* ... 3rd ed. (London, 1740).

[7] Isobel Grundy, 'Medical advance and female fame: inoculation and its after-effects', *Lumen*, 13 (1994), 13–42, at 29.

[8] *London Evening Post*, 11–13 September 1740; 29–31 October 1741.

[9] R. Perry, *Wotton-under-Edge. Times past – times present* (Wotton-under-Edge, 1986), p. 68.

[10] *Eighteenth century Irish official papers in Great Britain: private collections*, vol. 2, ed. A. P. W. Malcolmson (Belfast, 1990), pp. 14–15.

[11] Samuel Sharp, *A treatise on the operations of surgery* ... 4th ed. (London, 1743), pp. 224–8.

[12] Miller, *Adoption*, pp. 134–46; Miller, 'Reappraisal', 487–92.

[13] *Weekly Miscellany*, 14 July 1738.

[14] James Kilpatrick [Kirkpatrick], *An essay on inoculation, occasioned by the small-pox being brought into South Carolina in the year 1738* (London, 1743), pp. 32–5; Smith, *Speckled monster*, pp. 37–9.

[15] Kirkpatrick, *Analysis* (1754), p. 111.

[16] Ruth K. McClure, *Coram's children. The London Foundling Hospital in the eighteenth century* (New Haven, 1981), p. 206.

by the royal family. The five-year-old Prince George, the future George III, caught smallpox in November 1743, prompting the hurried inoculation of his older sister and younger brother.[17]

By the mid-1740s, there was a solid platform for the advance of inoculation. Established in 1746, the Smallpox Hospital in London included inoculation in its remit from the outset, and in 1752 began to offer the procedure at no charge. Thenceforward it provided an important focus for the practice, providing instruction and advice to practitioners, and generally building knowledge of the practice. Dr Richard Mead, who had been active in the early appraisal of inoculation, finally gave the procedure his endorsement in his long-awaited treatise on smallpox and measles in 1747.[18] A major smallpox epidemic in 1751–3 set the scene for further expansion in inoculation activity. In a sermon to the patrons of the Foundling Hospital in 1752, Bishop Madox of Worcester presented a positive account of the practice and allayed religious concerns about it.[19] In 1755, the Smallpox Hospital reported that, while around one in seven who caught smallpox died, only one of its 593 inoculations had proved fatal.[20] There was growing demand for inoculation in the provinces as well. Expressing concern that the practice 'as it is now managed, must necessarily exclude . . . the greatest part of mankind, from the benefit of it', a letter to *The Gentleman's Magazine* called on medical men to 'perform it out of charity to the poor, on moderate terms to others, in proportion to their circumstances.'[21]

In his *Analysis of Inoculation* (1754), Dr Kirkpatrick offered a fuller account of the practice than had hitherto been available. Dedicating it to King George II, he praised his 'sagacity and resolution' in having his children inoculated and saving by his example many thousands of his subject's children.[22] His ability to draw on the extensive notes of the practice by John Ranby, the king's surgeon, was another indication of his standing.[23] Kirkpatrick presented an interesting analysis of inoculation as a business, contrasting the 'œconomy of inoculation' in London, where it was overseen by physicians and qualified

---

[17] *Daily Advertiser*, 15 November 1743; [Charles-Marie de] La Condamine, *A discourse on inoculation, read before the Royal Academy of Sciences at Paris*, transl. Matthieu Maty (London, 1755), p. 7n.

[18] He observed that, though established for some time in England, inoculation had 'drawn our physicians into parties': Richard Mead, *A discourse on the small pox and the measles*, transl. Thomas Stack (London, 1748), pp. 82–98, at p. 82.

[19] Isaac Maddox, Bishop of Worcester, *A sermon preached before [the] governors of the Hospital for the Small-pox, and for Inoculation . . . 1752* (London, 1752).

[20] The circular is tipped in at the end of the BL's copy of James Killpatrick [Kirkpatrick], *A full and clear reply to Doctor Thomas Dale: wherein the real impropriety of blistering with cantharides in the first fever of the small-pox is plainly demonstrated* (Charleston, NC, 1739).

[21] *GM*, 22 (1752), 511–13.   [22] Kirkpatrick, *Analysis* (1754), p. iv.

[23] Kirkpatrick, *Analysis* (1754), xxiii–xxiv and *passim*; Maddox, *Sermon*, p. 19.

surgeons, and in the country-towns and villages, where it was in more mercenary and careless hands. Acknowledging that the procedure's cost put it out
of the reach of many people, he expressed the hope that his colleagues would
make it available to the poor at reduced or no cost. He also acknowledged that,
in seeking to protect themselves by inoculating smallpox, individuals could
endanger their neighbours. It was widely recognised that in urban settings
smallpox inoculation required careful control. In autumn 1752, medical men in
Salisbury inoculated 133 residents and almost 300 people from the district but,
as the epidemic began to subside, all but one practitioner agreed to cease the
practice, as it threatened to reignite the infection.[24] For rural communities,
Kirkpatrick recommended 'general inoculations' in which patients could go
through the infective stage together, but accepted that they could be difficult to
organise.[25]

The Inoculation Controversy in Europe

Smallpox was as great a scourge and inoculation as interesting a topic
in continental Europe as it was in Britain. The experiments by the Royal
Society in London in the 1720s attracted significant attention and there were
early trials in Germany and elsewhere. In 1722, the Dutch physician Hermann
Boerhaave acknowledged inoculation's potential value in a new edition of his
Aphorisms.[26] Francophone readers learned about inoculation from the *Journal
des Savants* and in the *Mémoires de Trévoux*, a Jesuit journal with a broad
circulation in Catholic Europe.[27] In Spain, the Benedictine monk Benito Feijóo
was inspired by the Jesuit journal to include a cautiously positive report of the
practice in the fifth volume of his popular compendium, *Teatro crítico universal*, in 1733.[28] In his *Philosophical Letters* (1734), Voltaire stoked interest
among *salonistes* and *savants*. Presenting inoculation as a boon to mankind, he
praised Lady Montagu for her boldness and good sense, and deprecated the
French nation for not following the English example. In fashionable circles,
approval of inoculation became emblematic of enlightened opinion. Prejudices
and doubts about the practice, however, were nourished by stories of mishaps
in England and reports that it had fallen into disrepute.[29] European visitors
who had recourse to prophylaxis in London did not always have a positive
experience: General Diemar, resident for the Principality of Hesse-Cassel, lost

---

[24] *PTRS*, 47 (1751–2), 570–1; *Salisbury Journal*, 4 December 1752, 2 July 1753.
[25] Kirkpatrick, *Analysis* (1754), p. 288.   [26] Miller, *Adoption*, p. 174.
[27] Miller, *Adoption*, pp. 181–4, 189–91.
[28] Jacqueline Gratton, '"Un mal pequeño para un gran bien": Smallpox prevention and the
dissemination of new ideas in Spain 1725–1775', MA thesis, University of Tasmania, 2012,
pp. 88–9.
[29] La Mettrie, *Traité*, p. 9.

a daughter to inoculated smallpox in 1734.[30] As in Britain, the return of epidemic smallpox in the early 1740s revived interest in inoculation. Dr Tronchin, who lived in London in the mid-1720s, studied under Boerhaave at Leiden, and built his career in Holland, inoculated his son and other children in Amsterdam in 1748 and, in the following spring, supervised Daniel Guiot's trial of the practice in Geneva. After an enquiry into inoculation, the Republic of Geneva authorised its use on children of the state in 1751.[31] The Genevans wasted no time in publicising their success with prophylaxis.[32] In Lausanne, the humane physician Samuel Auguste Tissot followed their lead. Published in 1754, Tissot's *L'Inoculation justifiée* was hailed by Voltaire as 'a service rendered to humankind'.[33]

A smallpox epidemic in Paris in 1753 prompted Charles-Marie de La Condamine, mathematician and naturalist, to champion the cause. During his travels in 1731, he observed inoculation in Istanbul and, on his geodetic expedition to South America in 1743, learned of its successful use, fifteen or so years earlier, on a Carmelite mission at the mouth of the Amazon.[34] On 14 April 1754, he delivered a powerful oration on inoculation to the French Academy of Sciences, presenting its advantages and inviting the audience to consider them. In a rhetorical *tour de force*, he described smallpox as a monster who had fed upon human blood for twelve centuries. Of a thousand persons, who had survived infancy, he observed, it often took 200 victims. Likening the deaths to the tribute in young lives that the Athenians paid the Minotaur, he declared that the happy deliverance of Athens by Theseus 'seems to be realised in our own time in England' through inoculation. If the practice were adopted in France, he continued, the monster would only take those 'who imprudently expose themselves to its attack.'[35] The oration was a hot topic in Paris and the kingdom at large. Rapidly put into print, his *Mémoire sur l'histoire de l'inoculation* went through three editions in the first year. In the provinces, La Condamine met members of the medical school in Montpellier, made a presentation at the court of Stanisław Leszczyński, titular king of Poland and Duke of Lorraine, at Lunéville, and enjoyed the hospitality at Avignon of the Marquise of Bayreuth, Frederick the Great's sister, to whom he

[30] *Daily Journal*, 9 September 1734.   [31] Gautier, *Médecine à Genève*, pp. 390–2.

[32] Jean Antoine Butini, *Traité de la vérole, communiqué par l'inoculation* (Paris, 1752); Gautier, *Médecine à Genève*, p. 393.

[33] Samuel Auguste Tissot, *L' inoculation justifiée, ou dissertation pratique et apologétique sur cette méthode* (Lausanne, 1754), esp. pp. 8–9; Henry Tronchin, *Un médecin du xviiie siècle. Théodore Tronchin (1709–1781)* (Paris, 1906), p. 105.

[34] [Charles Marie de] La Condamine, *Mémoire sur l'inoculation de la petite vérole* (Paris, 1754), pp. 18–19.

[35] La Condamine, *Mémoire*, pp. 64–5.

dedicated the third edition.[36] On a tour of Italy in 1755, he was pleased to hear that some ladies in the Romagna were inoculating their children without informing their husbands He was informed, too, that 'no theological scruples ... would be opposed at Rome' to 'a practice which tends to the good of mankind', and that learned societies were planning to conduct trials with the Accademia dei Fisiocritici in Siena doing so in autumn 1755.[37]

La Condamine's call to arms fanned sparks of interest across Europe. In Holland, the practice already had some credit in French Huguenot circles. Inspired by Bishop Maddox's sermon of 1753, Charles Chais, pastor of the French Church in The Hague, published a defence of inoculation that was then made available in Dutch by the Haarlem Academy of Sciences.[38] Luisa von Wassenaar, Countess of Athlone, who had been inoculated as a child in London, led the way in 1754 by having her children inoculated in The Hague.[39] Dr Mathieu Maty, a Dutch physician, secretary of the Royal Society in London and editor of the *Journal Britannique*, translated La Condamine's *Mémoire* into English and Dutch, and proved an influential lobbyist for smallpox prophylaxis. La Condamine's *Mémoire* was translated into German, and his second *Mémoire* included a report on the revival of inoculation in Hanover.[40] In 1754 the Medical College in neighbouring Brunswick (Braunschweig) discussed introducing the practice.[41] In Denmark, Count Bernstorff, former ambassador in Paris and friend of La Condamine, was likely responsible for the publication of the *Mémoire* in the *Mercure Danois*.[42] His eighteen-year-old wife Charitas von Buchwald, the first noblewoman to be inoculated in Denmark, emerged from the operation in summer 1754 scarred but applauded for her pluck.[43] In Sweden, Carl Gustaf Tessin, the Chief Minister, wrote to the Crown Prince explaining its value and recommending

---

[36] [Charles Marie de] La Condamine, *Second mémoire sur l'Inoculation de la petite vérole* (Geneve, 1759), p. 12, and *Mémoire sur l'inoculation de la petite verole*, 3rd ed. (Avignon, 1755), pp. i–ii.

[37] [Charles Marie de] La Condamine, *Journal of a Tour to Italy* (Dublin, 1763), pp. 107–9; Francesco Vannozzi, 'La "questione dell'innesto de vajuoli" ovvero la lutta contro il "veleno varioloso"' in Francesco Vannozzi, *Siena. La città laboratorio* (Siena, 1999), pp. 15–16. Reports of early trials of inoculation make up the first volume of the Accademia's published proceedings: *Gli atti dell'Accademia delle Scienze di Siena detta dei Fisiocritici dell'anno 1760*, 1 (1761).

[38] Charles Chais, *Essai apologétique sur la méthode de communiquer la petite vérole par inoculation* (The Hague, 1754); Uta Janssens, 'Mathieu Maty and the adoption of inoculation for smallpox in Holland', *BHM*, 55 (1981), 248–9.

[39] Janssens, 'Maty and inoculation', 248.   [40] La Condamine, *Second mémoire*, pp. 32–3.

[41] Mary Lindemann, *Health and healing in eighteenth-century Germany* (Baltimore, MD, 1996), p. 331.

[42] The *Mercure Danois* was one medium through which the *Mémoire* was known in Spain: Gratton, 'Smallpox prevention in Spain', p. 168.

[43] Julius Petersen, *Kopper og koppeindpodning*, electronic version (1896), p. 63.

trials on condemned prisoners.[44] After sending Dr David Schultz to study the practice in London, the Swedish Medical Board resolved to authorise the practice early in 1756. Tessin commissioned a medal in honour of Katarina de Geer, who had set an example by having her four children inoculated.[45]

The princes of continental Europe were aware of the perils of smallpox, but their physicians hesitated to recommend inoculation. The Empress Maria Theresa spent her life in the shadow of the scourge. Her husband, Francis of Lorraine, had seen four older siblings fall to the disease, and her anxieties for her children increased over the years. Gerard van Swieten, her physician, was inclined to inoculation in 1755, but became more cautious in the 1760s.[46] The prince who came closest to championing inoculation in the early 1750s was Stanisław Leszczyński, titular king of Poland. Installed in Lorraine by his son-in-law Louis XV of France, he cultivated an image of himself as an enlightened ruler. After La Condamine's visit in 1754, he sought advice from the newly established royal medical college at Nancy.[47] In March 1755, Dr Bagard presented the case for inoculation on the college's behalf, arguing the desirability of princes introducing the practice into their states and offering the king an opportunity 'to give an example to the universe that could only be glorious to the realm'.[48] As opposition to inoculation hardened in France in the following years, Bagard's recommendations were shelved.[49] Early in 1755, the political economist Turgot organised the inoculation of several poor children in Paris and allies in government circles received a favourable report from Ambrose Hosty, an Irish-born doctor-regent in the Medical Faculty, who had been sent to London on a fact-finding mission.[50] On 14 May, the Chevalier de Chastellux became the first French nobleman to submit himself to the procedure.[51] Conservatives in the Faculty, however, were staging a counter-offensive. Their cat's-paw was another Irish doctor-regent, Andrew Cantwell, who prepared a thesis attacking inoculation. Claiming long familiarity with the practice in Ireland, England and France, he presented evidence of fatal and other adverse outcomes and reported that medical opinion in Britain had turned against it. In approving the publication of the thesis in July, the royal censor

---

[44] [Carl Gustaf Tessin], *Letters from an old man to a young prince; with the answers. Translated from Swedish*, vol. 3 (London, 1759), pp. 134–48, at p. 147.

[45] Sköld, *Two faces*, p. 260.

[46] Frank T. Brechka, *Gerard van Swieten and his world 1700–1772* (The Hague, 1970), p. 117.

[47] La Condamine, *Second mémoire*, p. 12.

[48] Pierre-Joseph Buc'hoz, *Manuel de médecine pratique, royale et bourgeoise; ou pharmacopée tirée des trois regnes, appliquée aux maladies des habitans des villes* (Paris, 1771), pp. 453 and 489.

[49] Nicolas Louis François, *Éloge historique de M. Gandoger* (Nancy, 1770), pp. 32–5.

[50] [Ambrose Hosty], *Extrait du rapport de M. Hosty* (no place, no date), p. 12.

[51] La Condamine, *Second mémoire*, pp. 15–16.

declared that, given the urgent need to combat favourable representations of inoculation, it could not be published soon enough.[52]

As the controversy broke, the Duke of Orleans was considering inoculating his children. If he hesitated in the face of the assault of the practice, he may have had his resolution strengthened by a clear statement of support from physicians in London. In the Harveian Oration to the College of Physicians in London in autumn 1755, Dr Robert Taylor praised the late Dr Jurin for demonstrating statistically the value of a procedure, 'by which so many thousands of mortals were freed from the fate hanging over them'. In the published text, Taylor reported that twenty of his colleagues, aware that the facts had 'lately been misrepresented among foreigners', had issued a statement that objections to inoculation had 'been refuted by experience', that it was currently 'more generally esteemed and practised in England than ever', and that it was, in their view, 'a practice of the utmost benefit to mankind'.[53] Early in 1756, Orleans made his decision to have his children inoculated, and Tronchin's success in April was a triumph for the practice, the practitioner and the patron. In his poem *L'inoculation*, Poinsinet hailed Orleans as a prince *philosophe*.[54] Describing the change of attitude to inoculation as a 'revolution', one Parisian journal gave credit to La Condamine's *Mémoire*, which was widely read.[55] It was Dr Tronchin, however, who won most celebrity. He was soon called on to inoculate other members of high society, including the Duke of Villequier, the Marchioness of Villeroy and Turgot.[56] Inoculation became a fashion statement with ladies sporting '*bonnets à l'inoculation*', decorated with ribbons with red spots.[57] Dr Kirkpatrick crossed to France to seek a share of the action but, after the declaration of war between Britain and France in May, his time in the sun proved brief. His most illustrious patient, the Count of Gisors, only son of the Duke of Belle-Île, France's War Minister, was killed in action in 1758.[58]

The outbreak of war initially firmed up opposition to inoculation in France. The Diplomatic Revolution of 1756, in which the Catholic powers of France and Austria made common cause against Britain and Prussia, was mirrored by

---

[52] [Andrew Cantwell], *Dissertation sur l'inoculation, pour servir de réponse de M. de la Condamine* (Paris, 1755).

[53] Robert Taylor, *Oratio anniversaria in theatro Collegii regalis medicorum Londinensium ex Harveii instituto festo divi lucæ habita* (London, 1756), pp. 38–9, 50–3.

[54] [Antoine-Alexandre-Henri Poinsinet], *L'inoculation. Poëme à Monseigneur le Duc d'Orleans* (Paris, 1756), p. 10.

[55] Seth, *Les rois aussi en mouraient*, pp. 53, 239–40.

[56] La Condamine, *Second mémoire*, p. 25.

[57] A. H. Rowbotham, 'The "philosophes" and the propaganda for inoculation of smallpox in eighteenth-century France', *University of California Publications in Modern Philology*, 18 (1935), 268.

[58] James Kirkpatrick, *The analysis of inoculation: comprizing the history, theory and practice*, 2nd ed. (London, 1761), pp. 198–200, 405–9.

a conservative axis between medical men in Paris and Vienna. In a short tract against the practice in 1757, Anton de Haen, doyen of the Vienna Medical School, posed four questions – namely whether inoculation was permitted by God, whether it would save more lives than leaving matters to nature, whether everyone must have smallpox, and whether inoculation gave life-long immunity – that set the terms of debate for a decade.[59] De Haen's first question did not prove a sticking point. The theological consensus was that inoculation was not an offence if it could be shown to be a prudential measure that saved lives. The three other questions went to the heart of the matter. They were not easy to answer as a great deal depended on details of cases that were hard to verify and statistical evidence that could be variously interpreted. Given the complexity of the issues and uncertainties of the data, medical men with doubts about the procedure cannot be dismissed as blind reactionaries. Few physicians wished to limit the freedom of parents who had the means to have their children inoculated with minimal risk to their children, but they had good reason to fear the consequences of making inoculation available to the urban poor. Above all, they were reluctant to endorse formally and publicly the safety of a practice about which some had strong reservations.

The Seven Years War saw some marking of time in the controversy. Although it involved the movement of large armies across northern Europe, the conflict was not accompanied by major smallpox epidemics. British military surgeons were practising inoculation and it is likely, too, that many of the combatants – with the exception of the Cossacks, notable for their vulnerability to the disease – had immunity. The war, however, served to focus attention on preventive medicine as a means of saving lives for the state. In 1759, French supporters of inoculation enlisted Daniel Bernoulli, a pioneer of probability theory, to demonstrate the value of smallpox prophylaxis more precisely. He constructed a series of life tables, factored in the risks of natural and inoculated smallpox, and quantified the potential contribution of inoculation to increases in life expectancy and population. Even if one in nine inoculations proved fatal, he informed the Academy of Sciences in 1760, it remains 'geometrically true that the interest of princes is to favour and protect inoculation by all possible means; likewise, the father of a family with regard to his children'.[60] The rationalist approach, of course, left human nature and ethical

---

[59] Anton de Haen, *Quæstiones sæpius motæ super methodo inoculandi variolas, ad quas directa eruditorum responsa hucusque desiderantur; indirecta minus satisfacere videntur: orbi medico denuo propositæ* (Vienna, 1757), pp. 10–11. For La Condamine's and Tissot's responses and De Haen's rejoinder: La Condamine, *Second mémoire*, pp. 42–7; [Samuel A. Tissot], *Lettre à Monsieur de Haen ... en reponse à ses questions sur l'inoculation* (Lausanne, 1759); [Anton de Haen] *Refutation de l'inoculation, servant de reponse à deux pièces qui ont paru cette année 1759* (Vienna, 1759).

[60] Rusnock, *Vital accounts*, ch. 3, at p. 84.

considerations out of the equation. D'Alembert challenged not only Bernoulli's statistics but also his understanding of the psychology of risk. Since it cannot be assumed that children would catch smallpox, he argued, parents might be unwilling to take a present risk for an uncertain future advantage. He was unhappy, too, about Bernoulli's privileging the interests of the state. Observing the war in Europe, he noted that the state would happily sacrifice some lives to advance its larger ends. Intervening in the debate, Diderot professed to be more impressed by D'Alembert's mathematics than his ethics, declaring him 'a fine geometer but a very bad citizen'.[61]

Inoculation continued in aristocratic circles. The old Duke de La Rochefoucauld sponsored trials of inoculation in the French capital and, in March 1760, had his grandchildren immunised. In praising the La Rouchefoucaulds as 'a model of paternal and maternal tenderness', Dr Onglée observed that all parents had as great a cause as grandees to wish to protect their children, and reported, approvingly, that the Duke of Villars had established an inoculation hospital in Aix-en-Provence and was offering a *louis* to each child inoculated.[62] In 1760, a new celebrity inoculator appeared in Paris. Dr Angelo Gatti, a professor at the University of Pisa, used a gentle mode of inoculation that involved raising a blister on the arm into which smallpox matter was injected. Sponsored by the Duke of Choiseul, whose grandchildren he had inoculated in Rome, Gatti was taken up by fashionable society. The *philosophe* Baron d'Holbach, who engaged him to inoculate his three children, became a great admirer. An outbreak of smallpox in Paris in 1762–3 increased the demand for his services, with the Princess of Chimay and the Duchesses of Pecquigny, Boufflers and Sully among his patients.[63] Sadly, Gatti was accident prone. His high-profile mishaps, the mistakes of colleagues and the carelessness of backstreet operators played into the hands of the opponents of the practice. In June 1763, the *Parlement* of Paris imposed a ban on inoculation until it had been explicitly approved by the Faculties of Medicine and Theology.

Voltaire and the *philosophes* lambasted the ban on inoculation. The theologians declined to pronounce on the procedure until their medical colleagues had given their advice. Divided on the issue, the Faculty of Medicine appointed a committee of twelve, six from each side of the debate, to solicit information about the safety and efficacy of the procedure and make recommendations. Questionnaires were sent to physicians across Europe. Many of

[61] Harry M. Marks, 'When the state counts lives: eighteenth-century quarrels over inoculation,' in Gérard Jorland, Annick Opinel and George Weisz (eds.), *Body counts: medical quantification in historical and sociological perspectives* (Montreal, 2005), pp. 51–64, at 57.

[62] *Journal de médecine, chirurgie et pharmacie*, 13 (July–December 1760), 79–85.

[63] [Angelo Gatti], *Lettre ... à M. Roux, Docteur Régent de la Faculté de Médécine de Paris* (1763), pp. 3–7.

the respondents had little direct experience of inoculation but took the trouble to collate the views of colleagues. Although most responses were cautiously favourable, the committee remained divided and issued two reports. In August 1764, Dr Guillaume-Joseph de L'Épine presented a detailed case for continuing the ban on inoculation. A week later, Dr Antoine Petit, physician to the Duke of Orleans, made a pithier case for lifting it. While the Faculty voted around two to one to permit inoculation, the conservative minority argued that a final decision should await further information arising from practice in England and elsewhere. The deadlock was never formally broken. By the late 1760s, the ban was relaxed in practice and then lifted, and attitudes to inoculation in France were becoming decidedly more positive.

The New Inoculation

During the 1760s, the practice of inoculation in Britain was transformed. Two developments proved mutually reinforcing. One was a growing demand for prophylaxis from people who could not afford the money and time associated with the highly-medicalised procedure of the early decades. Some practitioners began to offer a stripped-down version of the procedure. There was naturally concern that country folk were seeking inoculation on market days from 'some operator, too often as crude and thoughtless as themselves'.[64] Still, some surgeons who were hired to inoculate groups of people – charity children, estate-workers, and entire villages – began to find that lighter incisions and simpler regimens delivered better outcomes than deeper cuts and purging. The complementary development, then, was an advance in technique that reduced the risk as well as the cost to the patient. Furthermore, the observation of groups of patients under inoculation showed the benefits of Dr Sydenham's cool regimen in which patients were encouraged to take the air. There were interesting similarities between the new modes of inoculation in Britain and America and the practices of the celebrity inoculators in continental Europe, with both Tronchin and Gatti puncturing the skin rather than making deep incisions and recommending convalescence in well ventilated rooms and strolls in the garden.

In Britain, the new inoculation was supported by an innovative business model. In the mid-1750s Robert Sutton, an apothecary of Kenton, Suffolk, was one among many inoculators offering a simplified procedure at a reduced rate.[65] He and his sons recognised the value of vertical integration and brand marketing. In 1757, he announced that he had set up 'a large commodious

---

[64] Kirkpatrick, *Analysis* (1754), p. 267.
[65] David Van Zwanenberg, 'The Suttons and the business of inoculation', *MH*, 22 (1978), 71–82; Smith, *Speckled monster*, pp. 68–91.

house' for inoculation under the care of 'one of his constant nurses, the well-known Mrs Elizabeth Alexander, widow, of Framlingham'. He offered patients the choice of residential packages ranging between three and seven guineas a month, and a special deal at half a guinea for 'those that can board and nurse themselves'. Over time he leased other houses and inducted eight sons into the business. In 1761–2, he announced an 'improved method' that reduced the severity and expense of the operation.[66] In place of the costly preparation and after care, he offered colour-coded pills to be taken before and after the operation, and recommended a healthy diet and plenty of fresh air. The light incision, painlessly administered, left a minimal scar. The Suttons may have initially derived a good deal of their income from the accommodation they provided wealthier patients and the pills, made up from 'secret' ingredients, supplied to their out-patients. They trained other practitioners in the Suttonian system and sold them franchises in East Anglia and further afield.

The most enterprising of his sons, Daniel Sutton established himself at Ingatestone in Essex and made his mark in 1764 by suppressing smallpox in Maldon by inoculating 487 villagers in a single day.[67] In 1766, he successfully defended himself at the assizes against an indictment that his activities had caused an outbreak in Chelmsford. A clever move was to appoint Oxford graduate Robert Houlton as chaplain to his establishment. Houlton ministered to the patients and published a sermon that justified inoculation and celebrated his work. Sutton made house calls to inoculate the children of local notables like Bamber Gascoigne, who took surreptitious notes on his methods.[68] Around 1767, he set up 'Sutton House' in Kensington Gore, on the outskirts of London, aiming to go up-market. In spring 1769, children of the Duke of Bolton, the Earl of Coventry and Lord Pomfret passed through the house.[69] An empire-builder, Daniel Sutton extended his father's scheme of associates. In 1768, there were sixty-two accredited Suttonian 'artists' in Britain, Ireland, British America, France and the Netherlands. Acquiring a large fortune and the trappings of gentility, including a coat-of-arms, he lacked the breeding and education for social acceptance. Hester Thrale, Samuel Johnson's sharp-tongued patron, recalled him as 'a fellow of very quick parts [but] as ignorant as dirt both with regard to books and the world'.[70]

---

66 Smith, *Speckled monster*, pp. 68–9.
67 Robert Houlton, *Indisputable facts relative to the Suttonian art of inoculation with observations on its discovery, progress, encouragement, opposition* (Dublin, 1768), pp. 16–17.
68 Smith, *Speckled monster*, pp. 73–82. Robert Houlton, *The practice of inoculation justified. A sermon preached at Ingatestone ... 1766* (Chelmsford, 1767), pp. 56–60.
69 *Public Advertiser*, 15 June 1767; *Lloyd's Evening Post*, 13–15 March 1769.
70 Hester Lynch Piozzi, *Dr Johnson by Mrs Thrale. The anecdotes of Mrs Piozzi in their original form* (London, 1984), p. 17.

By the late 1760s, inoculation was a highly competitive business. A jocular piece appeared in newspapers about young boys charging half a penny for the procedure, a range of practitioners from men in greasy caps to men in pompous wigs, and Giles Wilcox the sow-gelder, 'by far the most in vogue', who 'takes pupils at 2s 6d a head, and teaches 'em the true orthodox method'.[71] The Suttons operated on an industrial scale. Between 1760 and 1767, they reportedly had registers documenting 55,000 inoculations, with only six fatalities.[72] Their prowess did not stop a canny estate manager like Thomas Davies, bailiff of the Glynde estate in Sussex, from shopping around. Observing the arrival of smallpox in the district in 1767, he hoped to 'persuade our little parish ... to inoculate all, in order to be clear of it in about a fortnight or three weeks'. He found a local surgeon who had recently inoculated 2,000 people in eastern Sussex, 'with equal success but less physicking and more expedition than Sutton or his people', and agreed to inoculate forty or more villagers for twenty guineas. 'This will spoil Sutton's trade in Pleshut House', Davies observed, where the lowest price was four guineas for people sharing a bed, with eight beds in a room.[73] Some practitioners competed on grounds other than price. Thomas Dimsdale, a Quaker physician, was well educated and appeared less mercenary than the Suttons. He began inoculating in the late 1740s, and drew on his own experience as well as his understanding of the Suttonian method to achieve good results. His book on the 'present method' of inoculation, dedicated to the Royal College of Physicians, helped to give the 'new inoculation' professional respectability.[74]

From the late 1760s inoculation was a familiar practice in Britain and Ireland. Few letter collections in the following decades fail to include some reference to the inoculation of a child, usually presented as an event of shared concern, but not unusual. As the fussy bachelor Horace Walpole reassured his sister, the procedure 'now can scarce be called a hazard'.[75] Even among the elite, though, not all parents inoculated their children proactively in infancy and recourse to inoculation was frequently prompted by perceptions of a threat. In the countryside, there were opportunities to share the expense, inconvenience and anxiety associated with inoculation by hiring a practitioner to inoculate all the children. Young people who had not had smallpox often sought out inoculation. Groups of adolescents had themselves inoculated in

---

[71] *St James's Chronicle or the British Evening Post*, 1–3 March 1768; *Gazetteer and New Daily Advertiser*, 4 March 1768.

[72] Peter Razzell, *The conquest of smallpox. The impact of inoculation on smallpox mortality in eighteenth-century Britain*, 2nd ed. (Firle, 2003), p. 33.

[73] Razzell, *Conquest*, pp. 82–3.

[74] Thomas Dimsdale, *The present method of inoculating for the small-pox ...* (London, 1767).

[75] *Horace Walpole's correspondence with the Countess of Upper Ossory. Vol. 2. 1778–1787*, ed. W. S. Lewis and S. Dayle Wallace (New Haven, 1965), p. 85.

town on market day, sometimes recklessly bringing the contagion back to their villages. Many others, seeking to make their way in the world, did so more purposefully. Arthur Young, whose mother arranged his inoculation behind his father's back, attributed London's rapid growth to smallpox prophylaxis. In 1768, he claimed that, in the past, smallpox 'frighted millions at the idea of London' but within a few years 'there will not be a lout in the country, that has not been inoculated; from which moment all bars are removed, and whip he flies to make his fortune at *London*'.[76] The value of inoculation was well recognised in Scotland and Ireland. After early mishaps, the practice resumed in Scotland in the late 1740s, becoming common from 1753. In his response to the Paris questionnaire in 1763, Alexander Monro, Professor of Anatomy at Glasgow University, reported over 5,500 inoculations across the country.[77] In Ireland, George Cleghorn lectured on 'inoculation, and its advantages' at Trinity College as early as 1756.[78] In his response to the questionnaire, he referred to Irish colleagues whose practice went back to the 1720s and reported that inoculation was offered by surgeons in many towns.[79] Itinerant inoculators may already have been active in the countryside. One of whom, a Gaelic-speaker, told an informant in 1796 that, lacking the means to train as a priest, he had taken lessons on inoculation and made a living from it in County Mayo for the thirty or forty years.[80]

The social range of inoculation in England was extended by paternalism and community-based initiatives. When arranging the inoculation of their own children, landed and professional gentlemen often offered prophylaxis to their servants and dependants. The leaders of village communities saw the advantages of 'general inoculations', in which all the population at risk could go through the procedure together. A collective approach brought down the unit costs to individual villagers and, most important, the co-ordination of activity reduced the dangers of cross-infection and the inconveniences of quarantine. The cost of inoculating the poor, it was often noted, would be less than the expense to the parish that might be necessary to treat smallpox victims and provide for orphans. From the late 1760s, general inoculations became quite common in the southern counties and the midlands. The system worked best in more nucleated settlements with a tradition of activism in poor relief. Even so,

---

[76] [Arthur Young], *The farmer's letters to the people of England* ... 2nd ed. (London, 1768), p. 341.

[77] Alexander Monro senior, *An account of the inoculation of the small pox in Scotland* (Edinburgh, 1765), pp. 4–5, 27–9.

[78] [George Cleghorn], *Index of an annual course of lectures* (Dublin, 1756), p. 3.

[79] *Medical and Philosophical Memoirs*, vol. 2., 1758–68, pp. 377–86, Medico-Philosophical Society, Dublin, ACC/1831/1, Royal College of Physicians of Ireland, Dublin.

[80] [Jacques Louis de Bougrenet, Chevalier de La Tocnaye], *A Frenchman's walk through Ireland 1796–7*, transl. John Stevenson (Belfast, 1917), pp. 175–7.

general inoculations were difficult to arrange. Aristocratic sponsorship could play a role. In 1788 David Stuart, vicar of Luton and grandson of Lady Montagu, funded a 'general inoculation' in Luton and declared his intent to repeat the exercise every few years.[81] Parishes did not always welcome aristocratic largesse and condescension. The parishioners of Shute in Devon pointedly declined to take up an offer by Sir John William de la Pole to sponsor a general inoculation and used their own funds to pay for the inoculation of ninety people.[82]

For the residents of small market towns, smallpox presented more complex challenges. An outbreak of the disease and even rumours of its presence had a deleterious impact on trade. For this reason, there was often opposition to inoculators setting up in town. The city of Oxford threatened anyone found harbouring a smallpox patient with legal action.[83] For the most part, inoculation houses were set up on the outskirts of the city, with two such establishments just outside Bristol.[84] Once smallpox took hold, there were calls for general inoculation, but after the outbreak began to subside the practice would again be disallowed. In many towns in the midlands and the north, however, the newly established infirmaries and dispensaries provided infrastructural support for prophylaxis. Dr John Haygarth, physician at Chester Infirmary, proved an energetic and visionary campaigner against smallpox. In 1778, he founded a Small-Pox Society to gather epidemiological data and to develop plans to eradicate the disease locally. His scheme involved incentives for poor parents to have their children inoculated within a framework of strict reportage and isolation of cases of smallpox.[85] Several other northern towns, notably Carlisle, Leeds, York and Newcastle, offered, usually through the dispensaries, free inoculation to the poor at specified times.[86]

London presented the greatest challenge. Many Londoners acquired immunity casually as children and many newcomers sought inoculation prior to moving to the metropolis. In inoculating several hundred people a year, the Smallpox Hospital (Figure 2.1) made a significant but minor contribution to protecting the population. The Suttons and their rivals set up inoculation

[81] *GM*, 58 (1788), 283–4.
[82] Pamela Sharpe, *Population and society in an east Devon Parish. Reproducing Colyton 1540–1840* (Exeter, 2002), p. 215.
[83] Jessie Parfit, *The health of a city: Oxford 1770–1974* (Oxford, 1987), pp. 3–5.
[84] Mary Elizabeth Fissell, *Patients, power, and the poor in eighteenth-century Bristol* (Cambridge, 1991), pp. 66–7.
[85] Haygarth, *Inquiry*.
[86] Henry Lonsdale, *The life of John Heysham, M.D. and his correspondence with Mr Joshua Milne relative to the Carlisle bills of mortality* (London, 1870), pp. 39–40, 45, 47, 51; *GM*, 60 (1790), 835–7; Katherine A. Webb, *One of the most useful charities in the city: York Dispensary, 1788–1988* (York, 1988), pp. 2, 13; Deborah C. Brunton, 'Pox Britannica: smallpox inoculation in Britain', unpublished PhD thesis, University of Philadelphia, 1990, p. 166.

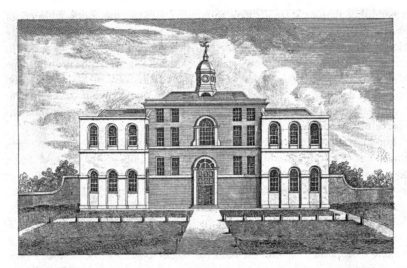

View of the SMALL-POX HOSPITAL *near St Pancras.*

Figure 2.1 View of the Smallpox Hospital near St Pancras, 1771
(Wellcome Collections)

houses in the suburbs and unlicensed practitioners may have been offering their services in the city. In January 1770, Daniel Sutton announced a charitable scheme to inoculate the London poor in their homes.[87] To be funded by subscription, patrons would be able to recommend, for each guinea subscribed, three people for treatment.[88] The plan was that patients would visit Sutton's house twice, first to collect preparatory medicine and then for inoculation, and would go through the infective stage in their homes, where they would be visited by one of Sutton's assistants.[89] The proposal caused some alarm in the city and threats of legal action.[90] The concept, however, gained some traction. The Quaker physician and philanthropist John Coakley Lettsom formed a Society for the Inoculation of the Poor in their own Homes in 1775 and established a Dispensary for General Inoculation in 1777. This well-meaning initiative by no means allayed concerns. Drawing a distinction between 'general inoculations' and 'partial inoculations', Dr Dimsdale denounced the scheme, in which patients would bring the infection to their dwellings 'in close

---

[87] *Public Advertiser*, 9 February 1770; 21 October 1772; 30 December 1772. Cf. *Oxford Magazine*, 4 (1770), 43–6.
[88] *Public Advertiser*, 9 February 1770.   [89] *Lloyd's Evening Post*, 12–14 February 1770.
[90] *Oxford Magazine*, 4 (1770), 43–6.

alleys, courts, and lanes', as 'fraught with very dangerous consequences for the community'.[91] Reportedly flourishing in 1779, Lettsom's Dispensary disappeared soon afterwards.[92]

From the 1760s, the bills of mortality show that smallpox deaths in London were rising numerically and, most importantly, as a proportion of overall mortality.[93] It was argued in some quarters that the use of inoculation in the metropolis was serving to spread the infection.[94] Dr John Watkinson, physician at the London Dispensary, claimed that inoculated smallpox was less infectious than casual smallpox, but the hazard was real enough.[95] The out-sourcing of laundry and the comings and goings of servants meant that even inoculations conducted in the mansions of wealthy Londoners could be a source of contagion.[96] In any case, there was probably more casual inoculation among the lower orders than had been assumed. In seeking to explain the higher proportion of smallpox deaths in London, where inoculation was extensively practised, than in Paris, where it was restricted, Jonas Hanway pointed to 'indiscretion, with regard to the contagion, and the communication arising from inoculation.'[97] Though a decade later, in 1776, he called for measures to encourage inoculation 'among the labouring part of our fellow-subjects', he still acknowledged that the 'poor in the metropolis are very *thoughtless*' and that smallpox was spread by carelessness.[98] In continental Europe, London appeared less a showcase for the success of prophylaxis, and more the site of a failed experiment.

Princes and Bodies Politic

La Condamine's advocacy in 1754 and Orleans's example in 1756 set the scene for the adoption of inoculation among the princely families of continental Europe. The first sovereign prince outside Britain to have a child inoculated was the Duke of Saxe-Gotha in 1759. His wife, Louise-Dorothea, wrote to Voltaire, after the operation, 'You see we are people who are up with the fashion and above prejudice'.[99] In 1760, Frederick V of Denmark arranged the

---

[91] Thomas Dimsdale, *Thoughts on general and partial inoculations* (London, 1776), pp. vi–vii, 36–7.

[92] Brunton, 'Pox Britannica', p. 162.

[93] Jonas Hanway, *Letters on the importance of the rising generation of the laboring part of our fellow-subjects*, vol. 1 (London, 1767), p. 42.

[94] Rusnock, *Vital accounts*, ch. 4.

[95] John Watkinson, *An examination of a charge brought against inoculation by De Haen, Rast, Dimsdale and other writers* (London, 1777), p. 46.

[96] Dimsdale, *Thoughts*, pp. 23–4.   [97] Hanway, *Letters on rising generation*, 1, p. 42.

[98] Jonas Hanway, *Virtue in humble life: containing reflections on relative duties, particularly those of masters and servants*, 2nd ed., 2 vols. (London, 1777), 1, p. vii n.

[99] *Correspondance de Frédéric II avec Louise-Dorothée de Saxe-Gotha (1740–1767)*, ed. Marie-Hélène Cotoni (Oxford, 1999), p. 10.

inoculation of the Crown Prince, the future Christian VII. According to Dr C. F. Rottböll, who presided over and publicised the event, the king showed the Danish people his complete confidence in variolation by submitting to it his dear son, 'the hope of the twin Kingdoms'.[100] At the electoral court of Saxony, Princess Marie-Antonie, widely admired for her intellect and musical talents, was responsible for adopting inoculation in early summer 1763. In a letter to Frederick the Great, she acknowledged his assistance in helping to persuade her husband to accept the practice.[101] The adoption of inoculation at the Catholic court of Parma in 1764 was especially noteworthy. A cadet of the Spanish Bourbons, the Infante-Duke Philip of Parma, was a modernising ruler, who was left bereft by the death of his wife, a French princess, from smallpox. Their daughter, Isabella of Parma, who married the future Joseph II of Austria, believed that she too would fall victim to the scourge. News of her death from smallpox in Vienna in 1763 prompted her thirteen-year-old brother Ferdinand, pupil of the *philosophe* Condillac, to insist on his inoculation.[102] Dr Tronchin was invited to perform the operation and the Infante-Duke issued a letter to the magistrates and churchmen of Parma to explain the operation on his son. Prayers were arranged for the prince's safety and, after a period of some anxiety, his recovery was the occasion of popular rejoicing. A commemorative medal was struck depicting Condamine's image of inoculation as a boat carrying a person safely across a raging torrent and reports of the prince's inoculation were published in Italian and French.[103]

Smallpox made the case for inoculation irrefutable in Austria. Empress Maria Theresa's eldest son, Joseph II, survived smallpox in 1757, allowing him to attend his first wife, Isabella, in her final days. In selecting his second wife, he made the mistake of preferring Josepha of Bavaria, unblemished by smallpox, to a Polish princess who bore its marks.[104] Josepha's death from smallpox in 1767 wreaked havoc in the house of Austria. The Empress herself caught the disease and was left scarred. Maria Josepha, one of her daughters, due to set out for her marriage to the king of Naples, visited her father's resting place in the family vault and caught the disease from her sister-in-law's unsealed tomb. A fortnight later, it was grimly reported, 'the princess-bride became a bride of the Heavenly Bridegroom'. Maria Elisabeth, another daughter, was so badly scarred that she retired to cloistered life. Early in 1768, still raw from the tragic

---

[100] Anne Eriksen, 'A case of exemplarity: C. F. Rottböll's history of smallpox inoculation in Denmark–Norway, 1766', *Scandinavian Journal of History*, 35 (2010), 356.

[101] *Correspondance de Frédéric le Grand roi de Prusse*, vol. 9, ed. J.-D.-E. Preuss (Berlin, 1854), pp. 41–3.

[102] Henri Bédarida, *Parme et la France de 1748 à 1789* (Paris, 1928), pp. 350–3.

[103] *Relation de l'inoculation de Ferdinand, prince héréditaire de Parme* (Paris, 1764).

[104] Derek E. D. Beales, *Joseph II: In the shadow of Maria Theresa, 1741–1780* (Cambridge, 1987), pp. 33, 76–8, 84–5.

events, the Empress met the young Wolfgang Amadeus Mozart, who himself had just recovered from smallpox. In a rare display of emotion, she hugged Mozart's mother, and the pair wept on each other's shoulders.[105] By this stage, the matriarch was ready to set aside the doubts of her physicians and have her surviving family inoculated. Count Seilern, her ambassador in Britain, made enquiries about the 'new inoculation', secured a testimonial from leading British physicians attesting its standing, and recruited for the task Dr Jan Ingenhousz, a Dutch Catholic and pupil of Boerhaave, who gained experience of inoculation with Dr Dimsdale in England.[106] Passing through Brussels, where he demonstrated inoculation, Ingenhousz arrived in Vienna in May.[107] After being introduced to the imperial family, he set to work over summer inoculating groups of charity children in a house near the Schönbrunn Palace. Satisfied with their trials, the Empress and her son, now Emperor Joseph II, authorised the inoculation of two of the Empress's younger sons and the Emperor's eldest daughter in September. Appointed a royal physician with a retainer of 5,000 gilders a year, Ingenhousz inoculated other members of the imperial family, including the young Marie-Antoinette, future queen of France. Many nobles, too, availed themselves of the practice, and a clinic was established at the Archbishop of Vienna's summer palace at Ober-Sankt-Veit.[108]

1768 was an *annus mirabilis* for smallpox inoculation in Europe. Anticipating the inoculations in Vienna, the Anglophile Duke Leopold of Anhalt-Dessau and his wife were inoculated in June and the princes of Holstein-Gottorp, cousins of Catherine the Great, were inoculated in July.[109] Long anxious about smallpox and probably aware of Maria Theresa's resolve to introduce inoculation, Catherine, Empress of all the Russias, likewise instructed her ambassador in London to seek the services of a practitioner to inoculate her and the Tsarevich. Dr Dimsdale, Ingenhousz's mentor, took on the awesome responsibility reluctantly, but his success in St Petersburg in the last months of 1768 set him up for life with a fee of £10,000, a pension of £500 per annum, and a baronage.[110] The imperial inoculations were widely reported. The adoption of

---

[105] Robert W. Gutman, *Mozart: a cultural biography* (Orlando, FL, 2001), pp. 231–4.

[106] Jan Maarten Ingen Housz, Norman Beale, Elaine Beale, 'The life of Dr Jan Ingen Housz (1730–99), private counsellor and personal physician to Emperor Joseph II of Austria [by M. J. Godefroi]', *Journal of Medical Biography*, 13 (2005), 15–21. *Lettre de Monsieur Ingenhousz, Docteur en Médecine, à Monsieur Chais, Pasteur de l'Église Wallonne de la Haye* (Amsterdam, 1768).

[107] Geerdt Magiels, *From sunlight to insight. Jan IngenHousz, the discovery of photosynthesis and science in the light of ecology* (Brussels, 2010), pp. 22–3.

[108] Magiels, *IngenHousz*, pp. 22–3.

[109] Jennifer Penschow, 'Wrestling *der Würgengel*: smallpox and inoculation in German society and culture, 1754–1800', PhD thesis, University of Tasmania, 2016, pp. 67, 71.

[110] Philip H. Clendenning, 'Dr. Thomas Dimsdale and smallpox inoculation in Russia', *JHM*, 28 (1973), 109–25, at 118–23; Simon Dixon, *Catherine the Great* (London, 2009), pp. 188–91.

the practice by the Empress Maria Theresa, a pious and motherly figure, sent a powerful message through Catholic Europe. She arranged for Ingenhousz to go to Florence to inoculate her fourth son, Archduke Leopold of Tuscany, in 1769 and then again to inoculate Leopold's children in 1772.[111] Catherine the Great's inoculation in 1768 achieved even greater celebrity. She was hailed by the *philosophes* across Europe. Voltaire applauded her bravery and German poets celebrated the event in song and verse.[112] Crown Prince Gustav of Sweden, who was inoculated with his wife and brothers in 1769, was probably inspired by her boldness. Travelling home from St Petersburg, Dr Dimsdale anticipated further commissions in northern Germany. In Berlin, however, he was given a brusque reception by Frederick the Great, seemingly peeved by the plaudits for the Russian empress. In 1781 Dimsdale returned to Russia to inoculate the empress's grandchildren.[113]

The French royal family remained unmoved. Although *Parlement* lifted its ban in 1768, smallpox inoculation remained under a cloud.[114] In congratulating Empress Catherine on accepting the procedure, Voltaire quipped: 'You have been inoculated with less fuss than a nun taking an enema ... We French can hardly be inoculated at all, except by decree of the *Parlement*'.[115] Louis XV, who had reputedly had smallpox as a child and turned sixty in 1770, could not be expected to break with past prejudices. When he fell ill in 1773, it was some time before his illness was diagnosed as smallpox. The court physicians were so desperate that they called in Robert Sutton junior, Daniel Sutton's brother, who was running an inoculation house outside Paris. The French king's agonising and undignified death underlined the value of inoculation. His successor, Louis XVI, had himself inoculated shortly after his accession in 1774 and he and Marie Antoinette ensured that their children, born in the early 1780s, were inoculated.[116] After losing family members to smallpox, even the Spanish and Portuguese royal families became cautious converts to inoculation.[117]

The inoculation of princes had a public dimension. The stability of dynastic states depended on an orderly succession that was disrupted by smallpox on many occasions in the seventeenth and eighteenth centuries. Its ravages in the house of Habsburg-Lorraine and among the Romanovs certainly predisposed

---

[111] Magiels, *IngenHousz*, pp. 22–3.

[112] Penschow, 'Wrestling *der Würgengel*', 71–3, 189–90.

[113] Clendenning, 'Dimsdale in Russia', 123–5.

[114] Rowbotham, '"philosophes" and inoculation', 271–3.

[115] *Voltaire and Catherine the Great. Selected correspondence,* ed. Anthony Lentin (Cambridge, 1974), p. 56.

[116] Pierre Darmon, *La variole, les nobles et les princes. La petite vérole mortelle de Louis XV* (Paris, 1989).

[117] Gratton, 'Smallpox prevention in Spain', p. 49, Jennifer Roberts, 'Portugal's mad queen', *History Today*, 57, no. 12 (2007), 32–8, at 33.

the two empresses to adopt the practice in 1768. Maximilian III Joseph, Elector of Bavaria, held the distemper in such dread that he could not bear the thought of being inoculated with it. His death from smallpox at the end of 1777 precipitated the War of the Bavarian Succession, the last of the wars of succession that embroiled Europe.[118] The princes born in the second half of the eighteenth century not only shed the robes of traditional rulership to don the uniforms of soldiers, they also rolled up their sleeves to receive inoculation. In 1780, an enthusiast for inoculation produced an impressive list of contemporary princes protected by the procedure.[119] Even if personal and dynastic concerns were paramount, some princes sought to set an example to their people. Disappointed by the neglect of inoculation, Frederick V of Denmark showed his support for the practice by publicising the Crown Prince's inoculation. Princess Marie-Antonie of Saxony claimed that her example had led to the inoculation of thousands in Saxony.[120] In 1761, Dr Kirkpatrick, who had earlier described George II as the 'political father' of all the British children inoculated after his adoption of the practice, congratulated George III for accepting the title of 'patron of inoculation'.[121] Although Catherine the Great was careful to keep her operation secret until its success was assured, she expected the court nobility to follow her lead and was happy to have her patronage of prophylaxis hailed across Europe.[122]

The rulers of Europe were conscious of the costs of smallpox to their states. It was axiomatic that a large and healthy population was a crucial determinant of power and prosperity and there was a growing interest in the collection and analysis of demographic data to inform policy. Statesmen and bureaucrats often led the way in assessing and acknowledging the advantages of prophylaxis. In the republic of Geneva, the magistrates took the initiative to make enquiries about the practice in 1754 and formally introduce it into state institutions. In the kingdom of Sweden, there was a nexus between close attention to demography – with a National Bureau of Statistics established in 1749 to receive annual reports on births, marriages and deaths from the parish clergy – and the early approval and promotion of the practice.[123] By the 1750s and 1760s, many European statesmen – like Bernstorff in Denmark, Tessin in Sweden, and Turgot in France – adopted inoculation for themselves and their families and explored the possibility of giving it the backing of the state. Most

---

[118] Nathaniel William Wraxall, *Memoirs of the courts of Berlin, Dresden, and Vienna in the years 1777, 1778, and 1779*, 2 vols. (London, 1800), 1, pp. 305–7; Marvin E. Thomas, *Karl Theodor and the Bavarian Succession, 1777–1778* (Lewiston, NY, 1989), p. 49.

[119] Hugues Maret, *Mémoire sur les moyens à employer pour s'opposer aux ravages de la variole* (Paris, 1780), pp. 150n–1n.

[120] Eriksen, 'Case of exemplarity'; *Correspondance de Frédéric le Grand*, 9, pp. 41–3.

[121] Kirkpatrick, *Analysis* (1754), p. iv; Kirkpatrick, *Analysis* (1761), p. iv.   [122] See Chapter 9.

[123] Sköld, *Two faces*, pp. 257–8.

governments, though, regarded inoculation as a matter for parents. Even Frederick the Great, an early advocate of the practice, seems to have taken this view. In 1774–5, he brought an English physician, Dr William Baylies, to Berlin to demonstrate inoculation, ordering each province to send a medical man to receive training, but showed no interest in providing incentives or applying pressure to establish the practice.[124] Catherine the Great was the only ruler with the power and inclination to conscript large numbers of people for inoculation. Even she appears to have limited her role to setting an example at court, introducing the practice in charitable institutions under her patronage, and probably offering inoculation to her serfs. Although Sir Robert Walpole had his children inoculated and Lord Bute, Britain's Prime Minister in the 1760s, was the grandson of Lady Montagu, the British government seemingly showed no interest in Daniel Sutton's offer to divulge his trade secrets in return for a premium or in various proposals to make inoculation more generally available.[125] Despite his celebrity in Europe, Dr Dimsdale called in vain on the British Parliament in 1776 to support a modest scheme for the inoculation to the poor. Just as 'we are the first European nation who received and encouraged inoculation', he declared, 'we may also have the honour of being the first who have generously diffused the benefit of it to the community at large, and transmitted it to posterity'.[126]

Smallpox Prophylaxis outside Europe

In relation to smallpox prophylaxis, Europe learned a good deal from the wider world. Medical men in western Europe adopted a prophylactic practice first observed among Greek women in Istanbul. Travellers like La Condamine and Gatti continued to be impressed by the relatively simple procedure in the Levant. Reference back to the authentic folk practice, even against the grain of learned medical opinion, served to inspire and vindicate the lighter procedures, like Gatti's use of a needle rather than a lancet, that increasingly gained ground in western Europe. There was interest, too, in Chinese prophylaxis. Drawing on reports to the Royal Society, Dr Mead made a trial of smallpox insufflation but found that it produced a severe response in the patient. In 1726, the French Jesuit D'Entrecolles produced a fuller account of the Chinese practice. During the inoculation controversy in the late 1760s, the French minister Turgot sought information and advice about the Chinese experience

---

[124] William Baylies, *Facts and observations relative to inoculation in Berlin, and to the possibility of having smallpox a second time* (Edinburgh, 1781).

[125] Jonas Hanway, *The defects of police: the cause of immorality ... particularly in and about the metropolis* (London, 1775), pp. 89–90; Dimsdale, *Thoughts*, pp. 58–61; GM, 49 (1779), 192–3.

[126] Dimsdale, *Thoughts*, p. 68.

of prophylaxis from the Jesuit mission in Beijing. Father Martial Cibot provided a garbled summary of the information in the *Golden Mirror*, a medical treatise published under imperial auspices in 1749, and observed, a little unhelpfully, that the different modes of reasoning in Chinese and western medicine made it difficult to draw useful lessons.[127] A more promising focus of attention was the practice of inoculation in India. In setting pen to paper in 1767, John Z. Holwell, who had spent many years in Bengal, was keen to present his knowledge of the practice in India to inform discussion in Britain. He challenged the old canard that inoculation was a barbaric practice learned from ignorant women by presenting it as a venerable, precise and well proven procedure in India. He pointed, too, to the success in Bengal of the cooling regime that was still only beginning to gain acceptance in Britain.[128] The European style of inoculation was born and honed in a transnational setting.

The key driver in development, however, was the marketplace. Increasing demand for smallpox prophylaxis provided incentives and opportunities to inoculate more efficiently and improve outcomes for patients. The inoculation of people in groups, as when an outbreak of smallpox led to general inoculation or when inoculation was practised on children in institutions or on slaves, provided the clearest incentives for cost-cutting and the best chance of introducing and testing refinements to the procedure. The crucible of change was again by no means confined to Europe. The 'new inoculation' owed a great deal to experimentation in the colonial world. The early practice in Boston in 1721–2, involving a large socially and ethnically diverse population, proved far more instructive than the small-scale trials in London. In an epidemic in spring 1730, over 2,000 Bostonians defied a ban on the practice to have themselves inoculated.[129] In Philadelphia, inoculation was first used during an outbreak in 1730–1, when over 500 people followed the example of a prominent citizen in seeking inoculation. When smallpox returned in 1735–6, there were 129 inoculations, only one of which proved fatal.[130] During an epidemic in Charleston in 1738, medical men inoculated some 800 people, including many slaves. The thousands of people of all ages, backgrounds and states of health who were inoculated in Boston, Philadelphia and Charleston, many more than in Britain in the 1720s and 1730s, provided important datasets for British assessments of the procedure. Many British surgeons, too, gained experience of the practice through the inoculation of slaves in the Middle

---

[127] Larissa N. Heinrich, *The afterlife of images. Translating the pathological body between ancient China and the West* (Durham NC, 2008), pp. 20, 23–32.
[128] [John Zephania Holwell], *An account of the manner of inoculating the small pox in the East Indies* (1767).
[129] John B. Blake, 'Smallpox inoculation in colonial Boston', *JHM*, 8 (1953), 284–300, at 287–9.
[130] J. M. Toner, *Inoculation in Pennsylvania* (Philadelphia, 1865), pp. 7–8.

Passage and in the plantations of the Caribbean.[131] Since some African slaves would have been familiar with forms of smallpox prophylaxis, they themselves may have helped to shape the practice in the Caribbean. The inoculation of cohorts of slaves provided surgeons with opportunities to assess the value of prophylaxis and to put possible improvements to the test.[132]

Inoculation in the English-speaking world developed as a transatlantic enterprise. Although it was alert to developments in Britain, the medical fraternity in North America needed to be resourceful. Born and educated in Massachusetts, Zabdiel Boylston showed some boldness in inoculating in Boston, was acknowledged as an expert in the practice in London, and was elected to the Royal Society in 1726.[133] The Irish-born James Kirkpatrick, who was living in Charleston when smallpox struck in 1738, could present himself in London in 1743 as the leading expositor of inoculation. In Maryland, Dr Adam Thomson, an Edinburgh graduate, achieved success in treating smallpox with small doses of mercury and antimony. Using this prescription to prepare patients, and prescribing a cool regimen after the procedure, he experienced good results as an inoculator in Scotland in the late 1730s. He helped to establish inoculation as a routine practice in Philadelphia in the 1740s.[134] Benjamin Franklin, who had lost a son to smallpox, published Thomson's lecture on inoculation to the Academy of Philadelphia, and, on a visit to London in 1758–9, reported on the American experience to Dr William Heberden, who prepared a short tract on inoculation for Franklin to publish in America.[135] A new generation of practitioners in British America embraced the 'American method', somewhat anticipating the 'new inoculation' in Britain. According to Benjamin Gale, the method reduced the case fatality rate of inoculated smallpox from one in 100 to around one in 800.[136]

Medical practice in the colonies encouraged a simplification of inoculation and provided scope for adaptation. On Antigua in 1758, Dr Thomas Fraser inoculated forty white people, including twenty-one soldiers, and oversaw the treatment of 270–300 slaves, only two of whom died, almost certainly from prior infection. He felt some unease with the hurried inoculation of the slaves and regretted that the 'scanty allowance' he received did not allow for preparatory medicine. 'Reputation, however, as well as conscience', he declared, 'was always with me a motive to avail myself of every artifice that might secure a happy event.' In any event, his experience soon led him to doubt the value of

[131] *London Evening Post*, 15 July 1738.   [132] Stewart, 'Edge of utility', 54–70.

[133] Boylston, *Defying providence*, pp. 116–23.

[134] Henry Lee Smith, 'Dr Adam Thomson, originator of the American method of inoculation for small-pox: an historical sketch', *The Aesculapian* 1 (3–4) (1909), 151–5.

[135] John Farmer, 'Letter from Dr Franklin to Dr Heberden, 1759, on inoculation for small pox', in *Collections of the Massachusetts Historical Society*, 2nd series, VII (1826), pp. 71–4.

[136] Smith, 'Adam Thomson', 154.

elaborate preparation.[137] Dr Quier, who arrived in Jamaica in 1767, found that the inoculation was well accepted. He heard details of the 'new inoculation' from an acquaintance, recently returned from England, and he soon had to hand a copy of Dr Dimsdale's book.[138] He reported his own findings to his mentor in London. One task was to inoculate a group of slaves, including pregnant women. Since medical men in Britain thought it dangerous to inoculate women during pregnancy, he reported that he had been able to so without any mishaps. When he later conceded that inoculation may have occasioned two miscarriages, he stressed that there was greater danger in leaving them exposed to casual smallpox. In a letter in 1775 he reported observations of immune responses and the use of inoculation to test previous exposure to smallpox.[139]

Inoculation was taken up in French and Spanish colonies in the Americas. Saint-Domingue, with its huge slave population and prosperous colonial elite, led the way in inoculation in the French-speaking world. After early trials in 1745, inoculation on a large-scale became common in the late 1760s. Dr Joubert de la Motte, director of royal botanical gardens at Port-au-Prince, was a great champion of the practice. In 1774 Simeon Worlock, Daniel Sutton's father-in-law, relocated from France to Saint-Domingue to exploit the burgeoning market.[140] From the 1760s onwards there was more interest in inoculation in Spanish America than in metropolitan Spain. During a lethal epidemic in Santiago de Chile in 1765, Pedro Manuel Chaparro inoculated some 5,000 people.[141] His success inspired the use of prophylaxis in Lima the following year and Cosme Bueno published a treatise in 1774 calling for its general adoption in Peru.[142] When major epidemics spread through Spanish America in the late 1770s, the authorities, political and medical, were sufficiently familiar with the value of inoculation to make some effort to promote it. The arrival of smallpox in Mexico City in summer 1779 presented a formidable challenge. An epidemic in the most populous city in the New World generated a 'centrifugal force' that spread the disease far and wide, as is evident from spikes in monthly burial records of parishes and mission stations as far as New Mexico and California.[143] The Viceroy of New Spain wasted little time in authorising inoculation. Despite the increasing death-toll,

---

[137] *Letters and essays on the small-pox and inoculation ... of the West Indies* (London, 1778), pp. 105–12.

[138] *Letters of West Indies*, pp. 6–7.

[139] *Letters of West Indies*, pp. 11–12, 54–6, 67–70 and 89–99.

[140] James E. McClellan III, *Colonialism and science. Saint Domingue in the old regime* (Baltimore, MD, 1992), pp. 144–5; Bennett, 'Curing and inoculating smallpox', 35–6.

[141] Diego Barros Arana, *Historia jeneral de Chile*, vol. 6 (Santiago, 1886), pp. 227–30.

[142] Adam Warren, *Medicine and politics in colonial Peru. Population growth and the Bourbon reforms* (Pittsburgh, 2010), pp. 81–4.

[143] Fenn, *Pox Americana*, p. 142 and ch. 5 passim.

Dr Esteban Morel, who headed the government facility, was disappointed by the lack of response, attributing it to 'the innate repugnance of those who were naturally healthy to voluntarily contract a sickness by artificial means' and who remained hopeful that they would escape the disease.[144] In giving the practice official countenance, however, the authorities proved themselves more pragmatic than their counterparts in Old Spain and laid the foundations for larger and more successful programmes in the 1780s and 1790s.

In British North America, inoculation was widely known, though not generally used except when smallpox threatened. Familiarity with inoculation even led, on at least one notorious occasion, to the attempted use of smallpox as a weapon of war against the Native Americans. During Pontiac's War in 1763, the British commander at Fort Pitt – crowded with civilians and with smallpox breaking out – sent out blankets from the smallpox ward to disperse the warriors conducting a siege.[145] Smallpox and inoculation played a major role in the War of American Independence. Drawing impetus from the movement of armies and refugees, a major epidemic ravaged North America from the mid-1770s to the early 1780s, adding to the distress and death-toll, and ultimately spreading the contagion across the continent. Most of the recruits to the Continental Army had not previously been exposed to smallpox, putting them at a disadvantage to the British soldiers, most of whom had had smallpox casually or by inoculation.[146] The American commanders faced a real dilemma. During the assault on Quebec, where smallpox raged, they prohibited inoculation, although some soldiers risked court martial by inoculating themselves.[147] Although he was desperately short of combat-ready men, and recognised that inoculation would put many of them out of action for two weeks, Washington took the bold decision early in 1777 to make the procedure mandatory for all recruits who had not had smallpox and to conduct a general inoculation in winter quarters at Valley Forge.[148] Efficiently conducted, and involving tens of thousands of men, the inoculation of the Continental Army was the largest and most successful immunisation campaign to date. During this time, too, large numbers of civilians had themselves inoculated.

In the late eighteenth century, the western style of inoculation spread in all directions in the wake of trade and empire. After a terrible epidemic in 1713, the Dutch colony at the Cape of Good Hope sought to keep smallpox at bay through strict quarantine. In Ceylon in 1754–5, however, the Dutch authorities turned to inoculation, with Governor Loten expressing his disappointment that

---

[144] Donald B. Cooper, *Epidemic disease in Mexico City 1761–1831* (Austin, TX, 1965), pp. 64–7.
[145] Elizabeth A. Fenn, 'Biological warfare in eighteenth-century North America: Beyond Jeffery Amhurst', *Journal of American History*, 86 (4) (1999–2000), 1552–80, esp. 1553–7.
[146] Fenn, *Pox Americana*, pp. 49–50.   [147] Fenn, *Pox Americana*, p. 71.
[148] Fenn, *Pox Americana*, pp. 93–102.

the local people were unwilling to accept the 'salutary and universal remedy, which ... has had such happy and certain results in various climates temperate as well as tropical'.[149] In 1756 Governor Magon authorised the inoculation of 400 slaves on the French island colonies of Mauritius and Réunion.[150] Around this time, too, Cape Colony authorised inoculation during a smallpox outbreak, withdrawing permission once it had been staunched. In Bengal and Java, where smallpox was virtually endemic, western style inoculation was practised, largely in the European enclaves and, in Bengal, in competition with the Indian form of inoculation. In Madras and in Ceylon, the governments made inoculation available to the indigenous population in the late 1790s and large numbers were seemingly inoculated. In Mauritius, again, the authorities introduced the practice to staunch an epidemic and then banned it again for fear that it would serve to maintain the infection. The British medical men on the First Fleet to Australia who brought variolous matter for use in inoculation may have been indirectly responsible for a major epidemic among the Aboriginal peoples living near the British settlement early in 1789.[151]

In the last decades of the eighteenth century, the western style of inoculation became familiar in many parts of the world. Prior to 1740, the number of people inoculated in the western world may have been no more than a few thousand, with half that number being in British America. By the 1790s, the total number of people inoculated with smallpox would have been many hundreds of thousands, including large numbers of people of non-European descent. Its success in the wider world helped to establish its reputation in Europe and built up pockets of experience and expertise among colonial officials, soldiers and medical men. Governor Magon's experience of inoculation in Mauritius inspired him, a decade later, to take the lead in having his child inoculated in his home-town of St Malo.[152] French champions of prophylaxis like Dr Louis Valentin gained important experience of inoculation in Saint-Domingue and the United States.[153] British America and the United States offered lessons on the controlled use of inoculation. Philadelphia was unusual in its liberalism with respect to inoculation. In Massachusetts, where inoculation was first introduced, the practice was ironically most closely regulated. Aware of the risks, the robustly independent townships of New England put proposals to inoculate to the vote and mandated quarantine, with red flags, in smallpox cases. Inoculation centres on islands off the Atlantic

---

[149] Alexander J. P. Raat, *The life of Governor Joan Gideon Loten (1710–1789): a personal history of a Dutch virtuoso* (Hilversum, 2010), p. 101.

[150] *Journal de médecine, chirurgie et pharmacie*, 34 (January–June 1770), 135n.

[151] Bennett, 'Smallpox and cowpox', 43, 46–9.

[152] *Journal de médecine, chirurgie et pharmacie*, 34 (January–June 1770), 135n.

[153] François Dezoteux and Louis Valentin, *Traité historique and pratique de l'inoculation* (Paris, An. VIII), pp. 14–15.

coast and in rural New York attracted clients from places where the practice was outlawed. In Virginia, too, a private initiative to inoculate in a country house in 1768–9 provoked riots, a notable court case, and highly restrictive legislation.[154] In letters to Dr Haygarth in England, Dr Benjamin Waterhouse, a Rhode Islander and professor at Harvard, pointed out that, despite the regulation of the practice, a high proportion of Bostonians were inoculated when necessary and that, notwithstanding the prohibition of inoculation, strict quarantine measures proved very effective in controlling smallpox in New England, not least in Rhode Island, where smallpox had been largely eliminated.[155] In response to Haygarth's claim that some of the American measures were unnecessary, he playfully observed that 'we have some pretence of knowing more of the disease than you in Europe'.[156]

The Mirage of Eradication

In the late eighteenth century, the western style of inoculation, stripped down by experiment and experience, was accepted as a prophylactic tool in Britain and elsewhere, and was proving a catalyst for wider changes. In England, the tally of inoculations rose from a few thousand in the 1740s to hundreds of thousands in the 1760s. In 1771, George Baker, doyen of the Royal College of Physicians, observed that among the benefits of the 'modern method of inoculating' was that the practice, 'which was heretofore in a manner confined to people of superior ranks, is now practised even in the meanest cottages, and is almost universally received in every corner of this kingdom' and did not doubt that 'many valuable lives have hence been saved to the community'.[157] The role of inoculation in Britain's rapid population growth in the late eighteenth century has been hard to establish. The decline in infant mortality-rates began before inoculation became widespread in the 1750s, and the London bills of mortality reveal increases in the proportion of smallpox deaths in the capital in subsequent decades. Still, inoculation was evidently important in reducing mortality-rates in many towns and villages.[158] As Baker and other

---

[154] Patrick Henderson, 'Smallpox and patriotism: the Norfolk riots 1768–9', *Virginia Magazine of History and Biography*, 73 (1965), 413–24; Frank L. Dewey, 'Thomas Jefferson's law practice: the Norfolk anti-inoculation riots', *Virginia Magazine of History and Biography*, 91 (1983), 39–53.

[155] Haygarth, *Inquiry*, pp. 138–46.

[156] Philip Cash, *Dr Benjamin Waterhouse. A life in medicine and public service (1754–1846)* (Sagamore Beach, MA, 2006), p. 118.

[157] George Baker, 'Observations on the modern method of inoculating the small-pox', *Medical Transactions*, 2 (1772), 275–324, at 279.

[158] Alex J. Mercer, 'Smallpox and epidemiological-demographic change in Europe: the role of vaccination', *Population Studies*, 39 (1985), 287–307; Razzell, *Conquest*, pp. 187–210; Mary J. Dobson, *Contours of disease in early modern England* (Cambridge, 1997), pp. 481–3.

contemporaries observed, there can be no doubt that it saved 'many valuable lives'. Outside of Britain, the scale of inoculation activity in the late eighteenth century was too small to have a significant demographic impact. Even in Sweden, where there was official commitment to inoculation, the number of people inoculated may have been no more than 35,000.[159]

The impact of the new inoculation needs to be seen in broader terms. The idea of smallpox prophylaxis as the means of protection against an ineluctable scourge, a force of nature and indeed part of a divine plan, was revolutionary in its implications. Initially, it appeared almost blasphemous. As late as 1766, a dissenting minister in Newcastle publicly declined to pray for the recovery from inoculation of George III's eldest son, declaring that 'he was in the hands of Man, not of God since his inoculation'.[160] By this stage, clerical opposition of this sort was not at all common. Across Europe, the major Catholic and Protestant churches generally took the position that, if the practice could be recommended as beneficial by medical men, it raised no ethical concerns and could even be regarded as a blessing. Superstitious unease about tempting fate continued to weigh with some parents but, as many thousands of children went through the procedure with little danger, there was increasing optimism that smallpox could be prevented and controlled. Broad acceptance of the legitimacy and benefits of smallpox inoculation, along with recognition of the hazards of fighting fire with fire, would provide a receptive milieu for the promotion of a novel form of inoculation, cowpox inoculation, that promised to provide the same level of protection without risk either to the individual or the community.

The scale of inoculation activity likewise meant that large numbers of medical practitioners, including university-educated physicians and empirically observant surgeons, made it their business to concern themselves with smallpox prevention. The practice established beyond doubt that smallpox spread by contagion and the insights derived from observing the progress of the disease from the moment of infection made it increasingly possible to isolate cases and make therapeutic interventions in a timely fashion. It was found that improvements associated with the 'new inoculation', especially the use of mild purgatives and a cool regimen for recuperation, were as relevant to cases of casual smallpox as inoculated smallpox.[161] The discovery that the inoculated disease 'outruns and anticipates accidental infection', made it possible to use inoculation to good effect on patients already exposed to the disease, including babies nursed by mothers with smallpox.[162] Among

---

[159] Sköld, *Two faces*, p. 288.   [160] *Newcastle Courant*, 15 March 1766.

[161] Sarah Stidstone Gronim, 'Imagining inoculation: smallpox, the body, and social relations of healing in the eighteenth century', *BHM*, 80 (2006), 247–68, esp. 254–8.

[162] Baker, 'Observations', 310–11.

specialists in inoculation, a major focus of interest was the possibility of attenuating the smallpox by diluting variolous matter, or by using fresh 'humanised' lymph from mild cases. In the late 1780s, Jenner and his friends were intrigued by an outbreak of an unknown disease that was popularly dubbed swinepox, and decided to inoculate with it experimentally. After observing their patients' responses to swinepox and subsequently confirming that they were no longer susceptible to smallpox, they felt it reasonable to assume that swinepox was a mild strain of smallpox.[163] The focus on smallpox was leading to other advances in comparative pathology. The ability to distinguish more clearly between smallpox and chickenpox was a great boon. The interest in pustular diseases, their specificity and cognateness and the use of inoculation as an investigative tool, would make possible the discovery and demonstration of the prophylactic value of cowpox.

Observation of the process of infection and recognition of the role of contagion encouraged new studies of the epidemiology of smallpox that could assist in managing cases and preventing its spread. In his report on an epidemic in Chester that took 202 lives in 1774, Dr Haygarth found a case fatality rate of almost one in six, with a quarter of deaths being infants less than one year old and a concentration in the poorer parishes.[164] He found that smallpox spread almost entirely between people in close proximity and, while he recognised the utility of inoculation, he highlighted the importance of isolating smallpox cases and other sanitary measures. When smallpox struck again in 1777, he organised a Society for the Prevention of Smallpox to promote inoculation but, critically too, 'rules of prevention'. The Society gave sums of money to poor parents who were willing to have their children inoculated and commit to keeping them off the streets during the infective stage.[165] Although he thought that it was less contagious than casual smallpox, he nonetheless recognised that inoculated smallpox could still spread the disease. He solicited information about smallpox cases that could be attributed to particles of variolous matter surviving in clothes and other fomites. Although he found that such cases were very rare, he recognised that smallpox in this form had the capacity to spark a severe outbreak. In the late 1780s, he put forward a scheme for the eradication of smallpox in Britain, district by district, through a combination of strict reportage, isolation of cases, and inoculation of people in contact with them.[166] Although costly and hard to enforce, it seemed feasible in theory. A concern to eliminate future sources of infection gave an added reason to be

---

[163] Baxby, *Jenner's vaccine*, pp. 53, 151.

[164] John Haygarth, 'Observations on the population and diseases of Chester, in the year 1774', *PTRS*, 68 (1778), 131–54.

[165] Haygarth, *Inquiry*; Christopher C. Booth, *John Haygarth, FRS (1740–1827): a physician of the enlightenment* (Philadelphia, 2005), pp. 54–9.

[166] Haygarth, *Sketch of plan*, 1, pp. 113–89.

interested in the length of time that smallpox matter remained infective. His colleague James Currie of Liverpool conducted an experiment in 1792–3 that showed that variolous matter, dried on glass and left at room temperature, remained viable for inoculation purposes for some seventeen months.[167]

The recognition that smallpox was not innate and the use of inoculation and other prophylactic measures made it possible to imagine the eradication of smallpox. In the British colonies of North America, for example, it proved feasible to keep smallpox at bay for periods of time by quarantine measures and then to deploy inoculation whenever it made landfall. It was probably his experience of the use of inoculation to suppress a smallpox epidemic in Charleston, South Carolina, in 1738, that prompted Dr Kirkpatrick to claim in the wake of the epidemic in Britain in 1751–3, when inoculation was used extensively, that the practice has 'very nearly expunged the small pox from the catalogue of mortal diseases'.[168] The stubborn persistence of smallpox in London and the suspicion that inoculation added fuel to the contagion, made this sort of optimism hard to sustain. In Germany, on the other hand, the recognition that smallpox was avoidable appeared to some physicians to offer the promise of expelling smallpox through the sorts of containment and sanitary measures that had assisted in banishing bubonic plague. In a much-discussed work in 1763, Dr F.-C. Medicus of Mannheim included inoculation as another tool to suppress and eradicate smallpox.[169] Medical men in Germany began to collect data on smallpox outbreaks, the advantages of inoculation for individuals and the risks of inoculation for the broader community. In 1797, Dr Juncker launched a bi-annual journal that served as a clearing house for this material. Inspired by Dr Haygarth's plan for smallpox eradication in Britain, he and Dr Faust set forward a scheme in 1798 for the eradication of smallpox in continental Europe, using quarantine measures and inoculation in a network of inoculation houses.[170]

At the close of the eighteenth century, inoculation was more than holding its own in Britain and elsewhere in the European world. Medical men expressed surprise that the practice, well accepted in the upper strata of society, was neglected by most people. There were signs of interest, not least in France before and after the Revolution, in making the practice more available to the population at large. In the 1790s, too, inoculation was put into service on a significant scale in Europe's colonies and on the colonial frontier. In the interstices of the wars that followed the French Revolution, there was some readiness to acknowledge inoculation as one of the beneficial innovations of

---

[167] James Currie, *Medical reports on the effects of water, cold and warm, as a remedy in fever and other diseases . . .* 4th ed., 2 vols. (London, 1805), I, pp. 61–2n.
[168] Kirkpatrick, *Analysis* (1754), p. iv.   [169] Penschow, 'Wrestling *der Würgengel*', 255–7.
[170] Penschow, 'Wrestling *der Würgengel*', 274–91.

the age. In a relatively short time, it was showing some capacity to transform lives for the better. Even in Britain, the transformation had taken place in a single lifetime. Lady Mary Wortley Montagu, who died in 1762, did not live to see the large-scale adoption of the practice and the posthumous celebration of her achievement. The Countess of Bute, her daughter, the first person to be inoculated in Britain, survived until 1794. In 1796, William Woodville, director of the Smallpox and Inoculation Hospital, published the first volume of what might have been the decline and fall of the smallpox empire.[171] In the following year, Drs Faust and Juncker seized the opportunity of a lull in the European war to present to the Congress of Rastatt a plan for the eradication of smallpox on the continent. Practitioners across the world were continuing to seek improvements, technical and organisational, in smallpox inoculation. Very few people had heard about cowpox and still less paid it any heed. Still, it was the remarkable expansion of smallpox inoculation (variolation) that revealed its prophylactic value of cowpox, built the technology, expertise and interest that made inoculating cowpox (vaccination) a viable practice, and provided the impetus for its rapid spread around the world.

[171] William Woodville, *The history of the inoculation of the small-pox in Great Britain*, vol. 1 (London, 1796), p. v.

3 Good Tidings from the Farm

Jenner and the Cowpox Discovery

On 14 May 1796 Edward Jenner was finally able to test a theory that had become an obsession. Spring had seen an outbreak of cowpox on a farm near his home in Berkeley, Gloucestershire. He had examined the cowpox vesicle on the hand of Sarah Nelmes, inspected the lesion on the cow's udder from which she had taken the infection while milking, and chosen a suitable subject for the experiment. He now proceeded to inoculate James Phipps, the eight-year-old son of his gardener, with cowpox matter from Sarah's hand to test whether it would protect him against smallpox. Over the following days, he observed the boy's response. The mildness of the infection inclined him to doubt that the inoculation would serve its purpose. On setting out for his practice in Cheltenham, he left Henry Jenner, his nephew, to conduct the final stage of the experiment. On the next occasion that Henry had some children to inoculate with smallpox, he added Phipps to the list and found him insusceptible. Advised of the outcome, Jenner returned from Cheltenham to see for himself.[1] On 19 July he wrote to his friend Edward Gardner in a state of high excitement. 'I have at length accomplish'd', he wrote, 'what I have been so long waiting for, the passing of the vaccine virus from one human being to another by the ordinary mode of inoculation'. 'But now listen to the most delightful part of my story', he continued, 'The boy has since been inoculated for the small pox which as I ventured to predict produc'd no effect. I shall now pursue my experiments with redoubled ardor'.[2]

Over summer Jenner drafted a paper detailing his findings. It was almost two years, however, before he again found cowpox for further experiments. He later recalled his state of mind as the implications of the new mode of smallpox prophylaxis dawned on him. There was a joy, he wrote, 'at the prospect of being the instrument destined to take away from the world one of its greatest calamities, blended with the fond hope of enjoying independence and domestic peace and happiness', that proved so overwhelming 'that, in pursuing my favourite subject among the meadows, I have sometimes found

---

[1] R. B. Fisher, *Edward Jenner 1749–1823* (London, 1991), p. 67.   [2] MS0016/2/8, RCS.

myself in a kind of reverie'.[3] After publishing the *Inquiry into the causes and effects of the* variolæ vaccinæ in June 1798, in which he set forward evidence that cowpox infection provided protection against smallpox, and his theories as to the origin of cowpox and its relationship with smallpox, he had to wait six months before the reappearance of cowpox and clinical trials in London that provided support for his thesis. In 1799, he found himself on the national stage, struggling to retain leadership in cowpox inoculation, as physicians in the capital made the running in the expansion of the practice. In addition, it was proving more difficult than anticipated to secure good vaccine and achieve a clear vaccine response. During 1800, however, the new prophylaxis gained in repute among medical men. In securing a premium from Parliament in 1802, he had the satisfaction of receiving some recompense for the cowpox discovery and, above all, some endorsement of his claims. The problem remained how it was possible to make a living from the practice and establish it more firmly. The early enthusiasm for vaccination culminated in the establishment of the Royal Jennerian Society in 1803 and an incipient cult of Jenner. A reluctant celebrity, Jenner was first lauded and then reviled, delighted by the advances of vaccination and frustrated by the setbacks. For the rest of his life, he would find himself the servant of a fickle virus and a seductive vision of success in the war on smallpox. Hailed as a humanitarian hero, he would not measure up to the expectations placed on him. To a remarkable degree, he remained, for better and for worse, the chief protagonist in the war against smallpox.

Jenner and the Discovery of Cowpox

Born in Berkeley in 1749, Edward Jenner came from a genteel background. The son of the Rev. Stephen Jenner, vicar of Berkeley, he was orphaned as a child, becoming the ward of his eldest brother, another clergyman. He first went to school in Wotton-under-Edge, where he had his encounter with the old style of inoculation, and later attended the grammar school at Cirencester, where he acquired some enduring friendships. Lacking the aptitude and means to follow his older brothers to Oxford, he was apprenticed at fifteen to Daniel Ludlow, a surgeon in Chipping Sodbury. On completing his apprenticeship in autumn 1770, he went to London to round off his training as house pupil to the brilliantly iconoclastic John Hunter, who claimed that he 'totally rejected books', preferring to consult 'the volume of the animal body'.[4] Jenner attended four terms of Hunter's lectures and participated in his surgical practice and scientific experiments. Sharing his mentor's passion for natural history and

---

[3] Baron, *Life*, 1, p. 140.   [4] Moore, *Knife man*, p. 23.

pathology, he brought to the table acute powers of observation and a strong visual memory. Though he lacked a university education, Jenner never sought to make book learning a virtue, reading widely, though in a dilettante fashion. He had the intellect, the range of knowledge and imagination to describe what he saw, make comparisons and connections with other observed phenomena and boldly theorise.[5]

After his return to Berkeley in 1773, Jenner built a reputation as a skilful practitioner, 'medical philosopher' and naturalist. He corresponded with Hunter, who gave direction to his researches in natural history and medicine. In 1789, he was elected Fellow of the Royal Society for his study of the nesting habits of the cuckoo, not fully verified until the cuckoo's behaviour could be captured on film.[6] By this stage he had taken a wife, Catherine Kingscote, and was starting a family in the handsome house, The Chantry, near Berkeley church that now houses the Jenner Museum. Widely regarded as a kind and genial man, he had good friends in the district who shared his interest in literature, natural history and medicine. Jenner and a group of scientifically-minded medical colleagues, including Dr Caleb Hillier Parry of Bath and Dr John Hickes of Gloucester, held regular meetings at the Fleece Inn at Rodborough to discuss advances in medicine and report on their observations.[7] Describing themselves as the Gloucestershire Medical Society, they presented papers on medical matters, keeping minutes of their proceedings. Jenner was seeking to change the balance of his professional work. Encouraged by Parry and Hickes, who wrote the necessary testimonials, he obtained a doctorate of medicine from the University of St Andrews in 1792.[8] By taking on his nephew as his assistant at Berkeley in 1794, he freed himself of the burden of routine surgical work and in the following year established a practice in the newly fashionable spa-town of Cheltenham. Thenceforward, he divided his time between Berkeley and Cheltenham. If he owed cowpox to his time at Berkeley, Cheltenham proved the ideal place to build his professional reputation and spread the word about cowpox inoculation.

According to Jenner, he first heard about cowpox and the belief that it prevented smallpox from a young woman in Chipping Sodbury in the late 1760s. He reportedly informed John Hunter about the phenomenon in 1770.[9] As an apprentice of Daniel Ludlow, he may have heard the views of Ludlow's colleague John Fewster, whose practice of inoculation disclosed some patients who explained their insusceptibility to smallpox by reference to prior cowpox

---

[5] Michael Bennett, 'Note-taking and data-sharing: Edward Jenner and the global vaccination network', *Intellectual History Review*, 20 (2010), 415–32.
[6] E. L. Scott, 'Edward Jenner, F.R.S. and the cuckoo', *Notes and Records of the Royal Society of London*, 28 (1974), 235–40.
[7] Bennett, 'Note-taking'.   [8] Fisher, *Jenner*, p. 59.   [9] Baron, *Life*, 1, p. 124.

infection. In the 1770s, Fewster 'communicated this fact to a medical society, to which [Jenner] then belonged', almost certainly the informal 'Convivio-Medical Society' that met at the Ship Inn, near Alveston, to which Ludlow and, later, Jenner belonged.[10] Back in Berkeley from 1773, Jenner probably discussed cowpox with Fewster prior to beginning more systematic enquiries in the mid-1770s.[11] A crucial point, though, is that Fewster gave up his own researches. On being asked to comment on Jenner's *Inquiry* in 1798, he reported his earlier interest, his finding that cowpox was unpredictable and the infection quite severe, and his assessment that there would be no advantage to be derived from replacing smallpox inoculation with it.[12] For his part, Jenner retained his obsession with cowpox. The minute-book of the Gloucestershire Medical Society attests his serious interest in pox viruses. In 1789–90, a pustular disease, popularly termed swinepox, spread through the county. Suspecting it to be a mild strain of smallpox, Jenner used it to inoculate his son and two girls in Berkeley, and then confirmed their resistance to smallpox by variolation, with Dr Hickes replicating his findings at the Gloucester Infirmary.[13] In the late 1780s, too, he wrote a paper on cowpox as a preventive of smallpox that Hunter read and reported on to his pupils, and took to London a drawing of cowpox pustules.[14] Given the elusiveness of cowpox, Jenner had limited opportunities to pursue his investigations. He later recalled how he was often discouraged as each stage in research revealed further anomalies. He carefully distinguished between several diseases known as cowpox, some of which had no prophylactic value. Finding that even 'true' cowpox did not always provide protection, he made another breakthrough when he discovered that only infection from a ripe pustule served this end. From the late 1780s, if not earlier, Jenner undoubtedly knew more about cowpox than anyone.

After the publication of Jenner's *Inquiry* in 1798, it emerged that cowpox also had the reputation of a preventive of smallpox in dairy districts in Dorset. Early hints gained in substance in 1802, when a Parliament considered Jenner's petition for a reward for his discovery. Robert Fooks, butcher of Bridport, reportedly inoculated himself with cowpox around

---

[10] George Pearson, *An inquiry concerning the history of the cowpox, principally with a view to supersede and extinguish the smallpox* (London, 1798), pp. 102–4. The misapprehension that Fewster presented a paper to the London Medical Society in 1768 originated with Georg Friedrich Krauß, *Die Schutzpockenimpfung in ihrer endlichen Entscheidung als Angelegenheit des Staats, der Familien und des Einzelnen* (Nürnberg, 1820), p. 223, and was incorporated into English scholarship in C. W. Dixon, *Smallpox* (London, 1962), p. 250.

[11] Edward Jenner, *On the origin of vaccine inoculation* (London, 1801), p. 1.

[12] Pearson, *Inquiry*, pp. 102–4. A contemporary claim that Fewster inoculated with cowpox in April 1796 is muddled or mischievous: cf. George Charles Peachey, 'John Fewster, an unpublished chapter in the history of vaccination', *Annals of Medical History*, 1 (1929), 229–40.

[13] Fisher, *Jenner*, pp. 55–6; Jenner, *Inquiry*, pp. 54–5.

[14] Baron, *Life*, 1, pp. 133–4; Pearson, *Inquiry*, pp. 5–6.

1771, and Benjamin Jesty of Yetminster, a farmer, used a stocking needle to scratch cowpox into the arms of his wife and children in 1774.[15] Dr John Pulteney, a learned physician at Blandford Forum, took an interest in the phenomenon, and Nicholas Bragge, a local surgeon, allegedly attempted to put cowpox to the test as early as 1772, although he seemingly did no more than variolate three women who had caught cowpox to test their resistance to smallpox.[16] This flurry of interest and activity rapidly petered out. When his wife reacted badly to the procedure, Farmer Jesty was reviled for his cruelty and a medical man in Dorset, presumably Bragge, 'was injured in his practice by a prejudice raised unjustly that he intended to substitute the cowpox for the smallpox in inoculation.'[17] Pulteney found that information on cowpox was 'very scanty' as it occurred 'so rarely' and farmers did not wish to advertise its appearance in their dairies. Like Fewster, he doubted the potential value of cowpox in prophylaxis. In addition to cowpox infection often being painful, it would be hard to overcome the natural distaste for inoculating an animal disease.[18]

In the early 1790s, Jenner had a great deal to occupy him.[19] As he built up his new practice in Cheltenham, he had less occasion to visit the dairy farms around Berkeley and observe cowpox lesions on the hands and arms of cottagers. In time, his interest in cowpox may have begun to atrophy. Happily, he did not give up on his ruminations and may have found new audiences in the spa-town for his ideas. A major puzzle for him, still unresolved today, was the identity of 'cowpox'. Although he was aware that it could spread among a herd of cows, he knew that it was not strictly a cattle disease and he surmised that it was spread on the hands of farm workers during the milking process. From long observation, he knew that cowpox was not human smallpox communicated to the cow. While he assumed that smallpox and cowpox were related, he believed that they were distinct diseases. His theory was that the infective agent of cowpox was a pustular disease found on the heels of horses, known colloquially as 'horse-grease', transmitted from the stable to the milking shed on the hands of farm workers. Initially, he must have been very hesitant about inoculating with matter taken directly from an animal. Even if he could find a willing subject, he would risk great opprobrium. Furthermore, he reasoned, on analogy with variolation, in which it was observed that the

---

[15] Williams, *Angel of death*, pp. 165–7; Patrick J. Pead, 'Benjamin Jesty: grandfather of vaccination', *The Historian*, 110 (2011), 27–9.

[16] Pearson, *Inquiry*, pp. 8–11; *MPJ*, 8 (July–December 1802), 155; George Pearson, *An examination of the Report of the Committee of the House of Commons on the claims of remuneration for the vaccine pock inoculation* (London, 1802), pp. 20–1.

[17] Pearson, *Examination*, p. 19.

[18] Pearson, *Inquiry*, pp. 8–11; *MPJ*, 8 (July–December 1802), 155.

[19] Fisher, *Jenner*, pp. 61–5.

severity of the smallpox virus was moderated by its use in successive inoculations, that the severity of the cowpox would be moderated by passage from the
horse through the cow to a human subject. Jenner was evidently waiting for an
opportunity to conduct an experiment with humanised cowpox. He needed a
case of recent cowpox infection and a compliant subject.

In spring 1796, he finally got his chance. After spending winter in
Berkeley, he was preparing to return to Cheltenham, when he heard that
Sarah Nelmes, a local girl, had been infected with cowpox. He knew the
family and inspected the cow, reputedly named Blossom. His subject was
James Phipps, the eight-year-old son of his gardener, who presumably
consented to the procedure. Jenner was trusted locally, but was probably
cavalier in such matters. Frustrated by his inability to experiment in London
in 1803, he informed a colleague, perhaps tongue in cheek, that 'in the
country' he could 'always find little cottagers on whom I can introduce
vaccine virus in any form'.[20] He himself was not averse to experimenting
on his own children, inoculating his first son Edward with swinepox in
1789 and his second son with cowpox in 1798. In any event, the inoculation
of Phipps with cowpox on 14 May went smoothly. A week later the boy had
a slight fever and a headache, but was otherwise well. In describing the
cowpox pustule, Jenner noted the strong colour and the efflorescence which
'died away ... without giving me or my patient the least trouble'.[21] Since the
symptoms were so slight, he was far from confident that the infection would
secure the boy from smallpox. On his departure for Cheltenham, he left the
final stage of the experiment to his nephew. He may have been somewhat
surprised as well as very excited to hear some weeks later that the boy had
been shown to be immune to smallpox.

For Jenner, the breakthrough was not a moment too soon. If he did not find
an early opportunity to make a trial of cowpox someone else might have done
so. In London, Dr George Pearson recalled Hunter's reading from Jenner's
paper on cowpox around 1789 and reported that he subsequently made mention of the theory that cowpox prevented smallpox in his lectures. In his book
on morbid poisons in 1795 Joseph Adams, another of Hunter's pupils, did not
mention Jenner by name, but reported that cowpox, 'well known to the dairy
farmers of Gloucestershire', had the ability, 'as far as facts have hitherto been
ascertained', to render a person 'insensible to the variolous poison'.[22] Jenner
was sufficiently concerned to ask Henry Cline what Adams knew, and may not
have been reassured by his friend's response that Adams only knew what he
had been told by him.[23] Dr William Woodville, Director of the Smallpox and

---

[20] MS. J27, RCP.   [21] Jenner, *Inquiry*, p. 33.

[22] Joseph Adams, *Observations on morbid poisons* (London, 1795), p. 156.

[23] Baron, *Life*, 1, p. 134.

Inoculation Hospital, likewise presumably knew Jenner's ideas when, in his *History of Inoculation* in 1796, he alluded to the conjecture that a person 'having received a certain disorder from handling the teats of cows, is thereby rendered insensible to variolous infection ever afterwards'.[24] Jenner may have been aware of a young rival in his neighbourhood. In a letter on inoculation to Dr Beddoes in 1795, which Beddoes published, Thomas Rolph, an apprentice of Fewster's former partner, referred to a patient infected with cowpox. 'In such cases', he wrote, 'I have learned from my own observation and the testimony of some old practitioners, that susceptibility to the small-pox is destroyed', adding 'some advantage may probably in time be derived from this fact'.[25] After Jenner published his *Inquiry*, Rolph contacted Fewster, who admitted his early interest in cowpox, expressed his doubts about the advantages of inoculating it in preference to smallpox, but conceded that it might 'lead to other improvements'.[26]

Over summer, Jenner began work on his *Inquiry* into cowpox. He begins with reflections on nature and civilisation, and the introduction of new diseases through the domestication of animals. He alludes to the common descent of wild and domesticated animals. After explaining the transmission of cowpox from stable to dairy, he describes the appearance and symptoms of cowpox on human subjects.[27] The main body of his work is a record of cases of people infected with cowpox whose insusceptibility to smallpox he had confirmed. In the first draft, he presents seventeen cases, all but one of whom had acquired cowpox casually, and whose insusceptibility to smallpox was demonstrated by their lack of response to casual or inoculated smallpox. Jenner's only full experiment, then, was James Phipps, case 17, who had been inoculated with cowpox from the hand of Sarah Nelmes.[28] For Jenner, the historical cases and the experiment on Phipps nonetheless served to demonstrate the singular interest of cowpox infection, namely 'that the person who has been thus affected is for ever after secure from the infection of the small pox'.[29] In his final section Jenner can do no more than speculate how cowpox infection prevents smallpox. Given the similarities between smallpox and cowpox, and the assumption that smallpox 'proves a protection against its own future poison',[30] he naturally assumes some family relationship between them. A footnote in which he refers to John Hunter's claim that 'the dog is the wolf in a degenerated state' shows the influence of his mentor's argument that wolves, dogs and jackals were all descended from a wolf-like ancestor and

---

[24] Woodville, *History of inoculation*, p. 3n.

[25] Thomas Beddoes, *A new method of operating for the femoral hernia ... to which are added queries respecting a safer method of performing inoculation* (London, 1795), pp. 63–4 (*recte* 65–6).

[26] Pearson, *Inquiry*, pp. 102–4.   [27] Jenner, *Inquiry*, pp. iii–iv, 1–7.

[28] Jenner, *Inquiry*, pp. 9–34.   [29] Jenner, *Inquiry*, p. 6.   [30] Jenner, *Inquiry*, p. 21.

that jackals were probably descended from dogs that had reverted to the wild.[31] In a somewhat analogous fashion, Jenner seems to be suggesting that smallpox and cowpox (or rather the horse-disease with which it was associated) shared a common ancestor. Assuming a cowpox-like ancestor, he asks, in regard to smallpox, whether it may not 'be reasonably conjectured ... that accidental circumstances may have again and again arisen, still working new changes upon it, until it has acquired the contagious and malignant form under which we commonly see it making its devastations amongst us?'[32]

Aiming to present his paper to the Royal Society, Jenner probably took a draft with him on a visit to London in September.[33] Two drafts of the *Inquiry* show that it was still a work in progress in March 1797, when he enlisted the help of friends to refine and strengthen the argument.[34] By early April, he had sent it to Sir Joseph Banks, who solicited advice from Lord Somerville, president of the Board of Agriculture, and Everard Home, Hunter's brother-in-law. Somerville reported that he had consulted a surgeon who testified to the reputation of cowpox, but was sceptical of the horse-grease theory.[35] For his part, Home pointed to the lack of evidence for Jenner's claim that cowpox provided lifelong security from smallpox. In replying to Jenner, Banks warned of the risk to his reputation in presenting 'anything which appeared so much at variance with established knowledge'.[36] Since there was no cowpox in the local dairies, Jenner saw little prospect of further experimentation in the immediate future. He may have considered publishing the work as it stood. In August 1797, the *Gloucester Journal* announced that *An enquiry into the natural history of a disease known ... by the name of the cow pox*, by Edward Jenner was 'in the press'.[37] Since no publication details were provided, the advertisement was probably a declaration of intent to discourage rivals or to encourage subscribers. The appearance of cowpox in the neighbourhood in spring 1798 provided new opportunities. Three farm workers who had become infected while tending horses had reportedly communicated it to cows while milking. Jenner began by inoculating a boy, case 18, with lymph from one of the workers, but the inoculation failed to elicit the expected response.[38] He then took the risk of inoculating the five-year-old William Summers, case 19, with matter directly from an infected cow, and then took lymph from him to

---

[31] Jenner, *Inquiry*, p. 2n; John Hunter, 'Observations tending to shew that the wolf, jackal, and dog, are all of the same species', *PTRS*, 77 (1787), 253–66, esp. 262–4.

[32] Jenner, *Inquiry*, pp. 2, 52–3.   [33] Fisher, *Jenner*, p. 69.

[34] Derrick Baxby, 'The genesis of Edward Jenner's Inquiry of 1798: a comparison of the two unpublished manuscripts and the published version', *MH*, 29 (1985), 193–99.

[35] Jenner, *Inquiry*, pp. 45–6.

[36] Derrick Baxby, 'Edward Jenner's unpublished cowpox inquiry and the Royal Society: Everard Home's report to Sir Joseph Banks', *MH*, 43 (1999), 108–10; Baron, *Life*, 2, p. 168.

[37] *Gloucester Journal*, 14 and 21 August 1797; Fisher, *Jenner*, p. 71.

[38] Jenner, *Inquiry*, pp. 35–7.

inoculate William Pead, case 20.[39] This boy provided matter for case 21, a group of seven adults and children inoculated on 5 April. Describing the case of Hannah Excell, Jenner stressed similarities with smallpox inoculation, the main difference being that the liquid in the pustules remained clear rather than 'becoming purulent'.[40] On 12 April, case 22, he inoculated four children with cowpox lymph drawn from the vesicle on her arm, including, unsuccessfully, his eleven-month-old son, and in some cases applied a 'mild caustic' to inhibit inflammation.[41] In his last experiment, case 23, he inoculated a boy called Barge with vaccine matter from one of the girls. He then demonstrated the insuceptibility of Summers and Barge to smallpox by variolation. His special concern was to demonstrate the continuing virtue of cowpox virus, describing Barge as 'the fifth who received the infection successively' from Summers 'to whom it had been communicated from the cow'.[42]

Resolved to publish his *Inquiry* privately in London, Jenner set out for the capital at the end of April. In dating the foreword 'Berkeley, 21 June 1798', he presumably acknowledges his home town as the place where his book was conceived and largely written, but probably records the date on which the final proofs went to print. The dedication to Caleb Hillier Parry, an old friend and medical scientist, and the preface, in which he professes surprise that 'in the present age of scientific investigation' cowpox 'should have escaped particular attention', bear witness to his sense of himself as involved in a scientific enterprise, who after finding 'the prevailing notions of the subject ... so extremely vague and indeterminate, and conceiving the facts might appear at once both curious and useful', began 'as strict an enquiry into the causes and consequences' of the disease 'as local circumstances would admit'.[43] Given his powers of observation and analysis, his readiness to theorise by making inferences from knowledge of the natural world, and his commitment to putting theories to the test of experiment, he has good claims to be considered a scientist. A valuable feature of his book is its two plates, 'coloured from Nature', depicting the soon-to-be iconic image of the pustule on the hand of Sarah Nelmes and the picture of the progress of the cowpox vesicle after inoculation on the arm. Still, the *Inquiry* is open to criticism. Although his ideas about the origins and nature of cowpox and the processes of infection and resistance are richly intuitive, they are not always well formulated. His decision, late in the piece, to translate cowpox as *variolæ vaccinæ*, literally cow-smallpox, and to include it in the title of his study, was ill considered and misleading His experiments were quite limited and conducted and recorded in a hurried and careless manner. In exoneration, his personal and professional life left him little time for his researches and experiments. He himself asked his readers to bear in mind that

---

[39] Jenner, *Inquiry*, pp. 37–8.   [40] Jenner, *Inquiry*, pp. 39–40.   [41] Jenner, *Inquiry*, pp. 40–2.
[42] Jenner, *Inquiry*, pp. 42–4.   [43] Jenner, *Inquiry*, pp. iii–iv.

his professional obligations prevented him from conducting experiments that were entirely satisfactory considering 'the coincidence of circumstances necessary for their being managed so as to prove perfectly decisive'.[44] It is certainly hard to imagine an experiment so dependent on a 'coincidence of circumstances' as one that brought together a busy physician, a girl with a ripe cowpox pustule and a boy ready to be inoculated from it.

Jenner did not claim originality in stating that cowpox infection gave protection from smallpox. Far from concealing the traditional lore, he presented it as a basic axiom of his thesis. His claim that mass inoculation 'first occasioned the discovery' is historically insightful and an implicit acknowledgement of the attention given to cowpox by inoculators from the late 1760s. Still, he seems not to have known anyone who had used cowpox purposefully to protect their families, and there is no evidence that anyone attempted to make it the basis of a serious experiment. The few medical men familiar with cowpox appear to have regarded it as a quite severe disease and a not wholly reliable protection against smallpox. By the late 1780s, Jenner was moving, slowly, to a new stage of investigation, writing a paper on the topic and making a drawing of the cowpox pustule to take to London. By examining the infection on animals and humans, taking note of cases in which cowpox infection did and did not give protection from smallpox, and distinguishing different forms and states of 'cowpox', he was slowly beginning to convert popular beliefs about cowpox into a formal body of knowledge. He certainly went further than his colleagues in Gloucestershire and Dorset in documenting the diversity of cowpox infections and, in 1796, in inoculating cowpox experimentally. He was original, too, in his decision to conduct his first inoculation experiment with fresh lymph from a human case of cowpox infection. Given the distaste for inoculating a child with an animal disease, he had no practical alternative, but he also believed that humanised lymph would be less severe. In addition, he probably recognised that the viability of the new practice would depend on the inoculation of the patients to propagate the rare virus. In the *Inquiry*, Jenner does not labour such claims to originality. Given his primary audience of medical men and gentlemen of science, he had reason to regard his priority in respect of his observations, experiments and publication as a matter of fact. He was pleased, too, by the advances he was able to make since his vaccination of Phipps, especially his successful use of cowpox from the cow, his propagation of humanised cowpox for further inoculation and his success in maintaining the virus through five generations. Overall, Jenner was somewhat reticent about the significance of his findings. After referring to the risks and anxieties associated with smallpox inoculation, and to the mildness of

---

[44] Jenner, *Inquiry*, p. 46.

cowpox and the fact that it could only be communicated by direct contact, not through 'effluvia', he did no more than suggest that 'inoculation with this disease may be preferable to the variolous inoculation'.[45] He did not draw attention to the progress he had made in establishing a means by which cowpox could be used reliably and effectively and could be made generally available. The only hint of the larger vision is his statement in the final sentence that he intends to 'continue to prosecute this inquiry, encouraged by the hope of its becoming essentially beneficial to mankind'.[46]

Cowpox in the Frame

Jenner's *Inquiry* was published in late June 1798.[47] Apart from advertisements, it was not noticed in the press for some time. His basic thesis, of course, was already percolating through medical and other networks linking Gloucestershire and London. In spring 1796, the surgeon of the North Gloucester Militia learned about the value of cowpox from the colonel of the regiment, who relayed to him what he had often heard from Jenner.[48] With its seasonal concourse of notables from across Britain, Cheltenham was becoming an important centre for the dissemination of news of the cowpox discovery or, as the poet Robert Bloomfield proclaimed it, the 'good tidings from the farm'.[49] In autumn 1796, Joseph Farington, the London-based painter, met Jenner socially in both Cheltenham and the capital and reported his claims about cowpox in his diary.[50] In London, a number of medical men knew the gist of Jenner's thesis, including his friend Henry Cline, Everard Hume, who reviewed the first draft of the work, and William Woodville at the Smallpox Hospital at St Pancras. Dr George Pearson, physician of St George's Hospital, who had heard about Jenner's ideas from Hunter ten years earlier, described the *Inquiry* as 'long-expected'.[51] Soon after its publication, Pearson sent out a questionnaire on cowpox to colleagues across England. The responses, from as early as 7 July, show that Jenner's book was read over summer by a range of physicians, including the professors of medicine in Oxford and Cambridge.[52] Dr Bartholomew Parr of Exeter, who read it with some care, was critical of some of Jenner's 'gratuitous suppositions', especially the supposed role of

---

[45] Jenner, *Inquiry*, pp. 66–71.   [46] Jenner, *Inquiry*, pp. 46, 66–9, 74–5.

[47] *Evening Mail*, 29 June 1798; *Morning Chronicle*, 30 June 1798; Baron, *Life*, 1, p. 145. Cf. Fisher, *Jenner*, p. 75.

[48] Edward Jenner, *Further observations on the variolæ vaccinæ, or cow pox* (London, 1799), pp. 50–1.

[49] Robert Bloomfield, 'Good tidings; or, news from the farm,' in *The poems of Robert Bloomfield* (London, 1814), 1, pp. 101–25.

[50] *The diary of Joseph Farington*, vol. 3, 1796–1798, ed. Kenneth Garlick and Angus Macintyre (New Haven, 1979), pp. 660–3.

[51] Pearson, *Inquiry*, p. 1.   [52] Pearson, *Inquiry*, pp. 7, 34, 83.

farm workers in infecting the cows with horse-grease, which he felt was a 'libel' on the farms in Jenner's district.[53] Dr Jan Ingenhousz, who won fame for his inoculation of the imperial family in Vienna in 1768, read the *Inquiry* during an autumn visit to Bowood House, the seat of the Marquis of Lansdowne, and consulted with local practitioners and farmers. After hearing reports that cowpox did not provide security against smallpox, he wrote to Jenner advising him to withdraw his claims. In blustering fashion, Jenner held his ground, reiterating his findings about the need to use the right sort of cowpox at the right time.[54]

Jenner was disappointed by the apparent lack of interest in London. Anticipating a demand for the new prophylaxis, he had brought cowpox with him, but found no one prepared to have their children inoculated with it. On leaving the capital, he left a sample with Henry Cline, who used it on a young boy in July, ostensibly as a 'counter-irritation' for a diseased hip. After confirming the boy's resistance to smallpox, he became a convert to cowpox inoculation, but was unable to replicate his experiment.[55]   Back in Gloucestershire, Jenner anticipated having access to cowpox and opportunities to make progress in establishing the practice. His earlier experiments, in which he had passed vaccine lymph through a series of children, appeared to relieve his dependence on the availability of cowpox on a local farm. Aware that cowpox lymph would not survive long, he had taken care to dry samples on quills and store them in corked vials for transport to London. Back in Gloucestershire, he was frustrated to find that he had no vaccine in an active state. He had to accept the prospect that, after announcing cowpox's potential to the world, he would have to wait until winter or spring, the seasons associated with cowpox, to resume his experiments and extend the practice more broadly. While he took some consolation from Cline's success with dried vaccine that was three months old, he took no pleasure in having to inform practitioners who, after reading his book, were eager to make a trial of cowpox that he had 'not an atom' to send them.[56]   One of his correspondents, William Simmons, who had secured permission from the Manchester Infirmary to experiment with cowpox, decided to inoculate horse-grease in its place, causing reputational damage for the new prophylaxis locally.[57]

---

[53] Pearson, *Inquiry*, pp. 84–5.

[54] Norman Beale and Elaine Beale, 'Evidence-based medicine in the eighteenth century: the Ingen Housz–Jenner correspondence revisited', *MH*, 49 (2005), 79–98.

[55] John Ring, *A treatise on the cow-pox; containing the history of vaccine inoculation*, 2 parts (London, 1801 and 1803), 1, pp. 369–73; Baron, *Life*, 1, pp. 150–3.

[56] *Letters of Edward Jenner, and other documents concerning the early history of vaccination*, ed. Geneviève Miller (Baltimore, 1983), pp. 8–9.

[57] William Simmons, *Reflections on the propriety of performing the Caesarian operation, to which are added ... experiments on the supposed origin of the cow-pox* (Manchester, 1798), pp. 93–4.

In the meantime, Jenner followed from a distance the progress of Dr Pearson's inquiry into the history of cowpox. Some of Pearson's informants in the western counties of England reported that they had heard of cowpox and were familiar with the popular belief that it was a preventive of smallpox. There was even some reference to a few medical men who, for a time at least, took the belief seriously. Overall, though, it was clear that cowpox and its alleged properties were not widely known, still less credited by medical men elsewhere in England.[58] In autumn 1798, Pearson presented his findings in a lecture and, on being shown a copy, Jenner encouraged him to publish it. Though he met him in London and appreciated his support, Jenner became anxious that Pearson aspired to take over the management of vaccination. In his *Inquiry concerning the history of the cow-pox*, published in November, Pearson felt the need to defend himself against insinuations that he was seeking to usurp Jenner and declared that he 'would not pluck a sprig of laurel from the wreath that decorates his brow'.[59] In building on Jenner's work, though, Pearson was inevitably raising himself above it. He criticised Jenner's use of the term *variolæ vaccinæ* and publicised scepticism about his 'gratuitous suppositions'. Even testimonies supporting Jenner's claims about cowpox had the capacity to undermine perceptions of his priority in the field. Initially, Jenner could be confident about his leadership in vaccination given his unrivalled knowledge of cowpox and his assumption that he would be better placed than his rivals to secure a supply of fresh lymph from the dairy districts of Gloucestershire. At the onset of winter, he obtained some cowpox from a farm at Stonehouse not far from his home but, though he used it to inoculate the children of his friend Henry Hicks of Eastington, he proved unable to build up a supply of vaccine.[60] Over the winter, he waited anxiously for the appearance of the distemper in other local dairy farms. To his surprise and perhaps consternation, it was milkmen on the doorsteps of London who delivered.

Early in January 1799, Thomas Tanner, a Gloucestershire-born veterinary surgeon, discovered cowpox in a dairy in Gray's Inn Lane in London. He brought it to the attention of Dr Woodville at the Smallpox and Inoculation Hospital, who contacted Dr Pearson and other interested parties. In a remarkable scene, Sir Joseph Banks and Lord Somerville accompanied Woodville, Pearson and other gentlemen to the dairy, inspected the pustule on the arm of a dairy-maid, Sarah Rice, and confirmed its correspondence to the coloured plate in Jenner's *Inquiry*.[61] Shortly afterwards, Pearson received 'the agreeable

---

[58] Pearson, *Inquiry*, pp. 63–4.   [59] Pearson, *Inquiry*, p. 3.

[60] Jenner, *Further observations*, pp. 57–61.

[61] William Woodville, *Reports of a series of inoculations for the variolæ vaccinæ, or cow-pox, with remarks and observations on this disease, considered as a substitute for the small-pox* (London, 1799), pp. 9–13.

intelligence' that cowpox had appeared in a large dairy near Paddington, to which 'no one could obtain admittance but myself'.[62] The focus of research on cowpox shifted decidedly to the capital when Woodville immediately began large-scale trials at the hospital at St Pancras. Within a week or so, he and Mr Wachsel, the house apothecary, had inoculated more people with cowpox than Jenner had ever done. Advising Jenner of the trials in February, Woodville informed him in April of the inoculation of 200 patients with cowpox and their resistance to casual and inoculated smallpox. In his *Reports of a series of inoculations for the cow-pox*, published in May, he provided strong statistical support for Jenner's claims regarding the safety and value of cowpox inoculation.[63] In February, Pearson also wrote to Jenner, sending him a sample of cowpox and a report on the trials, including the troubling observation of generalised eruptions on some patients. In his response in March, Jenner expressed concern about the smallpox-like symptoms, but reported his satisfaction with the results of the vaccine sent him, adding poignantly: 'No cowpox yet in the country!'[64] If he trusted Pearson at this stage, Jenner soon had cause for suspicion. Shortly afterwards he received a letter from his nephew, the Rev. George Jenner, urging him not to delay 'coming to [London] to wear the laurels you have gained, or to prevent their being placed on the brows of another'.[65] Without informing Jenner, Pearson had made it his business to disseminate cowpox and promote the new prophylaxis across Britain. On 12 March, he sent a printed letter to some 200 physicians, in which he reported on the trials in London, enclosed samples of 'vaccine virus' for their use, and invited them to report back on the outcomes.[66] Already planning to go to London to publish his *Further Observations*, Jenner arrived in the capital within a week of receiving his nephew's letter. In a meeting with Dr Woodville on 23 March, he raised his concern about the smallpox-like eruptions appearing on patients inoculated with cowpox at the Smallpox Hospital.[67] Reluctant to impugn Woodville's professionalism or the validity of the experiments that provided strong support for his thesis, he accepted his assurances that great care had been taken to avoid cross-contamination with smallpox matter and was relieved to learn that the proportion of cases with generalised eruptions was on the decline. Since he himself had found no problem with the vaccine sent from London, Jenner speculated for a time that the vaccine virus behaved a little differently in town and country.

During 1799, cowpox became better known. Jenner's *Inquiry* was widely read and its plates proved valuable in identifying cowpox and confirming a genuine vaccine response. In his *Further Observations*, Jenner elaborated his

---

[62] Pearson, *Examination*, pp. 43–4.   [63] Woodville, *Reports,* esp. pp. 147–55.
[64] Baron, *Life*, 1, pp. 313–17.   [65] Baron, *Life*, 1, pp. 318–20.
[66] *MPJ*, 1 (March–July 1799), 113–14.   [67] Baron, *Life*, 1, p. 322.

advice regarding 'spurious' cowpox and the need to use only translucent lymph taken from the vesicle on or before the eighth day of infection. He also noted cases in which smallpox inoculation had also failed to provide continuing protection. In this work, however, he was only able to add reports of a dozen or so cowpox inoculations that he had conducted in the previous year.[68] In contrast, Dr Woodville's *Reports of inoculations* documented a clinical trial of unprecedented scale. Dedicated to Sir Joseph Banks, it included a great deal of solid information on cowpox inoculation and added significantly to the credibility of the new practice. Newspapers and periodicals were likewise beginning to play a major role in the dissemination of knowledge and interest in cowpox. The Edinburgh-based *Annals of Medicine* was first in the field with a summary of Jenner's *Inquiry* and a notice of Pearson's survey.[69] The *Medical and Physical Journal*, launched in London in spring 1799, proved a timely forum for the new prophylaxis. In the first issue the editors offered the 'physiological facts ... evinced in the inoculation for the cow-pox' as the chief example of the new discoveries it would report and discuss, and its first substantive article was a review of Jenner's and Pearson's books accompanied by an engraving of the cowpox pustule.[70] After reading the article in Cork and making enquiries locally, Dr John Milner Barry reported that cowpox was known in western Ireland as *shinach* and, though it had not been observed recently, several women recalled being infected as children to prevent smallpox.[71]

In establishing and extending cowpox inoculation in 1799, Jenner played a somewhat subsidiary role. Pearson and Woodville supplied most of the vaccine put into service in Britain and provided the bulk of the data on which the reputation of the practice was built. The two physicians held positions of influence in London and had access to institutional networks that Jenner largely lacked. A Quaker and philanthropist, Woodville cannot be dismissed as an opportunist. His prior commitment to smallpox inoculation might have inclined him to regard cowpox as a distraction. A medical scientist of some standing, Pearson likewise had much to lose from committing himself too early and decisively to Jenner's cowpox theory. A man of ability and ambition, he had the vision and drive to translate what he subsequently termed the 'Gloucestershire bubble' into a serious and sustainable national programme. In sending out the questionnaire in 1798 and the circular letter in 1799, he assumed some centrality in the development of vaccine inoculation. Jenner was being marginalised. When publishing his circular letter in the *Medical and Physical Journal*, Pearson added the somewhat patronising postscript that

---

[68] Jenner, *Further observations*.   [69] *Annals of Medicine*, 3 (1799), 77–90, 447, 494.
[70] *MPJ*, 1 (March–July 1799), i, 1–11.   [71] *MPJ*, 4 (July–December 1800), 428.

Jenner was continuing his trials 'with vaccine matter sent from London with good success'.[72] In fact, Jenner was in danger of losing his position of leadership. Far from producing vaccine for national distribution, he depended on supply from London to inoculate his nephew's son and some boys employed in a factory at Eastington. On his visit to London, he obtained some cowpox from a dairy in Kentish Town, but again was not able to propagate it on any scale. From the outset, he had anticipated practical difficulties in achieving consistent outcomes. The use of cowpox of the wrong sort left patients unaware that they were still susceptible to smallpox. The use of lymph from doubtful cases in further inoculations compounded the problems. Jenner's concern about his loss of control of the practice, then, was not wholly selfish. Fortunately, his nephew and other colleagues succeeded in maintaining the practice in Gloucestershire. Dr Joseph Marshall, who had taken up residence in Eastington, initially sought vaccine for his own family but, finding the 'minds of the people in general' disposed to the new practice, vaccinated 100 people in April and 300 more over the following six months.[73]

Jenner was poorly placed to champion the new prophylaxis. His lack of cowpox and the opportunity for experiment hindered his ability to refine his thinking about the vaccine virus and is relationship with smallpox. His basic premise was that the infective agents of the two poxes were distinct and readily distinguishable by their effects on a person but that they were related in some fashion. Furthermore, although the cowpox virus had the power to override the smallpox virus, it was gentler on the human constitution, as evidenced by a slight fever and a single pustule at the inoculation site, and by the fact that it presented little or no danger of infection other than through inoculation. For many people, professional and lay, it was the evident mildness of the vaccine disease that made the claim that it rendered a person permanently insusceptible to smallpox hard to credit.[74] It is somewhat ironic, then, that the first major problem arising from the new practice was that many of the patients inoculated with cowpox at St Pancras manifested generalised eruptions that appeared all too like smallpox. Instructively, Jenner's first thought, and his final position, was that some patients had been exposed to smallpox prior to cowpox inoculation or that some contamination had occurred in the inoculation process. By August, he was relieved to hear that the 'variolous appearance' was 'more retiring' among patients while cowpox 'maintains its ground'. He found in the report some support for his belief that smallpox was 'a malignant variety' of cowpox, its 'parental root'.[75] By this stage, though, the problem in London was being translated to the national

---

[72] *MPJ*, 1 (March–July 1799), 114.   [73] Fisher, *Jenner*, pp. 89–90.
[74] Fisher, *Jenner*, pp. 92–3.   [75] Baron, *Life*, 1, pp. 355–7.

stage by the dissemination of vaccine from St Pancras.[76] Exasperated by this development, Jenner pointed to the folly of conducting a trial of cowpox in a smallpox hospital and Pearson's recklessness in distributing the contaminated vaccine. In October, an unfortunate occurrence on the Earl of Egremont's estate at Petworth, Sussex, prompted him to go on the offensive. In preparation for a general inoculation, Egremont's surgeon had obtained lymph from children in Brighthelmstone (Brighton) inoculated with cowpox supplied by Pearson. He used it to vaccinate fourteen children at Petworth, all of whom had severe variolous symptoms and one of whom died. Billeting the children in his own house 'to prevent the disorder spreading', Egremont wrote to Jenner, who supplied his surgeon with fresh vaccine. In his response, Jenner explained his concerns about the conduct of the trials at St Pancras, and the 'error and confusion' caused as the contaminated virus 'became the source of future inoculations'.[77]

The identity of much of the cowpox in circulation in 1799 is obscure and a matter of controversy. Some of the early patients in the trials at St Pancras were doubtless exposed to smallpox prior to being inoculated cowpox. The problem was perhaps inevitable in the Smallpox and Inoculation Hospital but proved more general and persistent because many people only sought prophylaxis when smallpox was already in the vicinity and many practitioners continued to offer variolation as well as vaccination. In seeking to explain some of the 'error and confusion', Peter Razzell advanced the bold claim that much of the cowpox disseminated from St Pancras was attenuated smallpox.[78] As an expert in smallpox inoculation, Woodville knew that using lymph from patients whose symptoms were least severe increased the chances of a mild response, applied this strategy to reduce the variolous eruptions that appeared in early cases and, according to Razzell, propagated an attenuated form of smallpox without realising it. Given the wide distribution of matter from St Pancras, it might then follow that the greater part of the cowpox in circulation was attenuated smallpox. After all, Jenner himself resumed inoculating cowpox in spring 1799 with matter taken from Anne Bumpus, one of Woodville's patients, on whom 300 pustules were counted, and presumably supplied cowpox from this stock to his nephew and Dr Marshall.[79] Quite a number of medical men reported variolous responses with cowpox from St Pancras, and it is likely enough that some of the 'cowpox' they used was indeed smallpox. Still, the theory does not explain Jenner's acceptance of samples from this stock as entirely conformable to cowpox and the rarity of occasions when the matter in circulation occasioned an outbreak of smallpox.

[76] Simmons, *Reflections*, pp. 91–7; *MPJ*, 2 (August–December 1799), 134–9.
[77] Baron, *Life*, 1, pp. 341–5.   [78] Razzell, *Jenner's cowpox*.
[79] Razzell, *Jenner's cowpox*, pp. 30–7.

In reviewing the evidence, Derrick Baxby has argued against the likelihood that Woodville managed in such a short time to attenuate smallpox sufficiently for it to pass muster as cowpox, and to eliminate, almost entirely, reversions to type.[80] His hypothesis is that Bumpus and others had concurrent cowpox and smallpox, though with the former moderating the latter's severity. In such cases, Woodville and his team can be assumed to have generally taken lymph from the vaccine pustule at the inoculation site rather than the pustular eruptions elsewhere. In the specific case of Bumpus, the lymph was assuredly taken from the vaccine vesicle which developed a week before the generalised eruption took place.[81] As both Razzell and Baxby show, the relationship of cowpox and smallpox remained a matter of uncertainty and debate for over a century, with some influential physicians, including John Baron, Jenner's friend and biographer, claiming that cowpox was a modified strain of smallpox. Jenner and most medical men in the early nineteenth century, however, believed them to be clearly distinct, though related infective agents, a line that has been largely corroborated by the genetic analysis of *variola* and nineteenth-century strains of *vaccinia*.[82]

Jenner would have been astonished by the proposition that he was inoculating with smallpox. In stressing some similarities between inoculated cowpox and smallpox, he was seeking to reassure people who, familiar with the old practice, found the idea of substituting an animal disease repugnant or unconvincing. Cowpox was represented as doing the same work as smallpox but in a gentler fashion, allowing the inoculation of infants and pregnant women safely, the immunisation of children and adults without disrupting their routines and the extension of prophylaxis to the urban poor without risk to the community. A countryman at heart, Jenner himself had no qualms about inoculating a virus transmitted by unwashed hands from the lesions of horses' heels to the udders of cows, but he presumably anticipated some concern about infecting a healthy infant with it. In one of the earliest responses to cowpox inoculation, Dr James Sims, president of the London Medical Society, acknowledged the public interest of the research but raised questions about the ethics of experimentally infecting human subjects with animal diseases.[83] In a treatise on the natural history of sugar published in July 1799, Dr Benjamin Moseley added a section satirising the 'cow-mania' of the time.

---

[80] Baxby, *Jenner's vaccine*, ch. 7.   [81] Baxby, *Jenner's vaccine*, ch. 8.

[82] Li Qin, Min Liang and David H. Evans, 'Genomic analysis of vaccinia virus strain TianTan provides new insights into the evolution and evolutionary relationships between orthopoxviruses', *Virology*, 442 (2013), 59–66. A sample of *vaccinia* from the 1840s has been shown not to be smallpox: Kathryn M. Weston, Wendy C. Gallagher and James M. Branley, 'Smallpox vaccination, colonial Sydney and serendipity', *Medical Journal of Australia*, 200 (2014), 295–7.

[83] *MPJ*, 1 (March–July 1799), 11–12.

'The Cow-Pox has lately appeared in England', he wrote facetiously, 'This is a new star in the Æsculapian system. It was first observed from the Provinces. It is so luminous there, that the greasy-heeled hind feet of Pegasus are visible to the naked eye'. The question that he posed would reappear in the following years. 'Can any person say what may be the consequences of introducing a bestial humour ... into the human frame, after a long lapse of years?' he asked, not entirely rhetorically.[84]

Establishing Cowpox Inoculation

Jenner was eager to share his interest in unravelling the mysteries of cowpox, and his presentation of his paper to the Royal Society suggests that he never contemplated keeping his observations and ideas secret. A conscientious doctor, he had strong charitable and humanitarian instincts. Aware of the horrors and the distress caused by smallpox, he placed some priority on seeking to make cowpox inoculation a practicable option for as many people as possible. As he later recalled, the immense significance of the new prophylaxis only gradually dawned on him and was accompanied by a sense of the providential nature of the discovery and his responsibility to make it available to the world. His reverie, though, included some thought as to the benefits to himself. By the standards of the time, Jenner was comfortably positioned, but not especially rich. He was advancing in years and his wife and children needed provision. His move to Cheltenham, partly for reasons of health, involved some expense. He could not afford to give up his general medical practice and initially at least the attention he gave to cowpox involved some reputational risk. As he contemplated its wondrous potential, he can perhaps be forgiven for entertaining some hope that it might give him and his family financial security.

In the 1760s and 1770s, smallpox inoculation brought a few practitioners fame and fortune and many others a solid source of income. By the late 1770s, however, even the Suttons, who developed a strong business model with income streams from inoculation, patent medicines, accommodation and franchise arrangements, found it hard to hold their ground in a marketplace in which the elite had their children inoculated by their own doctors and the poor were immunised cheaply or charitably in towns and villages across the land. In any case, Jenner would not have wished to model himself on Daniel Sutton. He saw himself as a gentleman of science and perhaps assumed no more than that his discovery would bring him the means to make it available to Britain and the world. He certainly had reason to anticipate that his priority

---

[84] Benjamin Moseley, *A treatise on sugar* (London, 1799), pp. 162, 165.

in the field and his access to cowpox in Gloucestershire would give him the time to introduce, refine, establish and expand the practice on his own terms. After setting out for London in 1798, however, events rather conspired against him. In addition to the outlay in publishing the *Inquiry*, his stay in the capital was costly and his hopes of demonstrating the safety and effectiveness of the new prophylaxis were dashed by the unwillingness of parents to accept it for their children. Back in Gloucestershire, he found himself bereft of cowpox and unable to respond to the interest that his book began to arouse. Around November, he wrote a despondent letter to Gardner about his situation, adding that he was 'touched hard with the reigning epidemic – impecuniosity'.[85] In spring 1799, he was warned that Dr Pearson was making a bid to be 'the chief person known in the business'.[86] When he set out again for London, he left the cowpox business in the hands of his nephew and Dr Marshall. In autumn, Henry Jenner advertised his availability to inoculate cowpox in Bath and Bristol.[87] He and Dr Marshall may have conducted the business in Gloucestershire in a manner that led to a later allegation that Jenner sought to profit from cornering the supply of cowpox.[88] Jenner certainly sought potentially lucrative opportunities for Henry Jenner. In letters over winter, he offered his nephew's services to the Earl of Egremont to complete the general vaccination at Petworth and to Louisa of Prussia, niece of Frederick the Great, to vaccinate in Berlin.[89]

The new prophylaxis ideally required institutional support. Practitioners ready to embrace cowpox inoculation needed training, access to a supply of genuine cowpox, and advice in complex cases. Even if he were better organised, Jenner could not do it all himself. In contrast, Dr George Pearson proved an effective operator. He secured exclusive access to cowpox in Paddington and, in spring 1799, took the opportunity to use cowpox in a general inoculation on the Oatlands estate of another Prussian princess, Frederica, Duchess of York.[90] He had a network of friends and colleagues, alumni of Edinburgh University, and members of professional associations. A native of Gloucestershire, Dr William Turton turned to his 'friend' Pearson to obtain advice and vaccine to begin the new practice in Swansea.[91] Over summer 1799, Pearson began planning a charitable institute for cowpox inoculation in London. Securing the Duke of York as patron and promises of subscriptions, he had

[85] Baron, *Life*, 1, p. 297.   [86] Baron, *Life*, 1, pp. 319–20.
[87] *Bath Chronicle and Weekly Gazette*, 22 August 1799, p. 4; 5 September, p. 1; 31 October, p. 1.
[88] Fisher, *Jenner*, pp. 199–200.   [89] Baron, *Life*, 1, pp. 345, 348–9.
[90] William Turton, *A treatise on cold and hot baths … To which is added a letter to … the Jennerian Society, on the introduction and success of the cow pock in the principality of Wales* (Swansea, 1803), p. 57.
[91] Turton, *Treatise*, pp. 57–62.

gone a long way to establishing the London Institute for the Inoculation for the Cow-Pock by November when he invited Jenner to serve as its 'extraordinary consulting physician'. Offended by the effrontery, Jenner wrote coolly: 'For the present, I must beg leave to decline the *honour* intended me'.[92] Despite the withdrawal of the Duke of York when he learned that Jenner was not associated with the initiative, the Cow-Pock Institute in Golden Square opened its doors at the beginning of 1800.[93] Funded by subscription, it offered free inoculation on the recommendation of subscribers; maintained a supply of cowpox, certified under its own seal, for purchase by practitioners; investigated alleged failures and conducted experiments; and issued regular reports on the practice. On the medical side, Pearson was supported by several physicians, surgeons and apothecaries. The Institute's secretary and public face between 1800 and 1807 was the book-seller William Sancho, son of Ignatius Sancho, a former African slave, author and composer.[94] Renamed the Original Vaccine Institute in 1803, it contributed a lot to the early spread of the practice. It immunised a thousand or so children in London and distributed vaccine widely in Britain and overseas. In 1804 it claimed credit, directly and indirectly, for some 60,000 inoculations.[95]

Jenner relied on a smaller circle of relatives and friends, some quite well connected. His nephews, Henry in Berkeley and George in London, assisted in practical and promotional matters. It is likely, too, that his medical friends in London and some influential people whom he had met in Cheltenham took his side against Pearson. Dr John Lettsom, a Quaker physician who had earlier established a charity for the inoculation of the poor, inoculated his grandson with cowpox, and became an ardent champion of the new prophylaxis. Jenner was fortunate, too, in the support given him by John Ring, a young surgeon who beat a path to his door in August 1799. Classically educated as well as surgically trained, he was a passionate man in search of a cause. Based in the capital, he rapidly became one of Britain's most experienced vaccinators, compiled a history of the spread of the new practice, served as a one-man vaccination institute and was a stout defender of the Jennerian line. In summer 1800, Lettsom and Ring drafted a testimonial supporting cowpox inoculation and secured the signatures of thirty-six leading London physicians and surgeons.[96] Published in the nation's newspapers, its statement that cowpox was milder than smallpox and rendered people 'perfectly secure' proved widely influential. In its wake, medical men across Britain issued similar statements

---

[92] Baron, *Life*, 1, p. 362.   [93] *Times*, 25 January 1800.
[94] *Morning Chronicle*, 29 July 1806; *Norfolk Chronicle*, 5 May 1810.
[95] *MPJ*, 11 (January–June 1804), 573–6.
[96] *GM*, 70 (1800), 640, 1203; *Gloucester Journal*, 28 July 1800.

and hospitals, dispensaries and other institutions began to provide infrastructural support for the practice.[97]

In the first quarter of 1799 the number of inoculations with cowpox rose from scores to hundreds, and then, over the course of the year, from hundreds to thousands. By early 1800 Jenner believed that at least 5,000 people had already been inoculated with cowpox.[98] In the last year of the old century, the new practice expanded dramatically. Robert Willan, a pioneering dermatologist, estimated that by the end of 1800 some 10,000 medical men, clergymen and gentle folk, exclusive of 'very many illiterate persons', had made a trial of inoculating cowpox.[99] If that number of people were inoculating cowpox, the number of people immunised in the new mode in England may already have been over a hundred thousand. As will be discussed in Chapter 4, this broad-based mobilisation on behalf of cowpox inoculation was driven by personal and professional networks, supported by a growing number of books, pamphlets, journal articles and newspaper reports that informed and promoted a nationwide conversation, and not a little argument, about cowpox. The degree to which the theory and practice of the new prophylaxis was developed in the public sphere rather than universities and medical colleges is quite remarkable. The pooling of experience and insight added significantly to an understanding of the practical and technical aspects of the new prophylaxis. Through the chatter and clamour, new concepts and terms gained traction. Though comfortable with the term 'cowpox', Jenner used the terms 'vaccine virus' and 'vaccine inoculation' as early as 1796. Though critical of the term *vaccinæ variolæ*, Pearson too generally referred to 'vaccine virus', but insisted that since infection produced only one pustule, the correct term for the procedure was 'inoculation for the cow-pock', using the singular form in the title of his institute.[100] Early in 1800 Richard Dunning, surgeon of Plymouth Dock, coined the term 'vaccination'.[101] The trend towards the more euphonious 'vaccine' may have been encouraged by the decision of medical men in the French-speaking world to use it to denote cowpox instead of *'la petite vérole des vaches'*. Though 'cowpox' remained in use for some time in Britain, and some people referred to 'Jennerian inoculation', the terms 'vaccine inoculation' and 'vaccination' steadily gained ascendancy. At least one medical man expressed his indignation at the 'new-adopted term of vaccine disease' and 'all inoculation of foreign language on old sound

---

[97] *GM*, 70 (1800), 1203.   [98] *Letters of Jenner*, ed. Miller, p. 11.

[99] Robert Willan, *On vaccine inoculation* (London, 1806), p. 47.

[100] *Philosophical Magazine*, 23 (October–January 1805–6), 81–5.

[101] Richard Dunning, *Some observations on vaccination or the inoculated cow-pox* (London, 1800), p. 4.

English'.[102] For his part, Jenner welcomed the new terminology, using it as early as 1801.[103]

Jennerian Inoculation

By the end of 1799, Jenner was a celebrity, receiving an invitation to be presented to King George III and Queen Charlotte. Over winter, he completed *Continuation of facts and observations*, the third and final instalment of his *Inquiry*. Evidently believing that his basic thesis was generally accepted, he was magnanimous to the sceptics, acknowledging that his ideas were so at odds with accepted science that they did need to be carefully assessed. For the first time, he indulged in print a vision of a world without smallpox: since it has been found 'that the human frame, when once it has felt the influence of the genuine Cow Pox ... is never afterwards ... assailable by the Small Pox, may I not with perfect confidence congratulate my country and my society at large on their beholding, in the mild form of the Cow Pox, an antidote that is capable of extirpating from the earth ... a disease that has ever been considered as the severest scourge of the human race'.[104] Growing interest in cowpox inoculation led to the publication of a new edition of the *Inquiry* that incorporated the *Further observations* and the *Continuation*. Presented at court in March 1800, Jenner obtained permission to include a dedication to George III.

It is not easy to explain Jenner's success in reasserting himself. Acknowledging the wisdom and knowledge of human nature that Jenner brought to the task of advancing vaccination, John Fosbroke, a younger friend, observed that 'envy would have stung him to death and more powerful ambition would have seized and appropriated his laurels', if he had not '*fortune, fame* and *high alliance*' to assist him.[105] Jenner certainly had some money behind him. He had the means to spend two years as John Hunter's pupil in London, live comfortably at Berkeley and indulge his interests in natural history, set himself up in Cheltenham, go to London to publish his *Inquiry* and stand his ground in defence of his discovery. While he owed somewhat to his connections, however, it was his personal qualities and the merits of his cause that turned them to good account. His celebrity arose from his identification with the cowpox discovery in a milieu that valorised individual genius, personal

---

[102] *GM*, 70 (1800), 214.   [103] Baron, *Life*, 1, p. 448; 2, p. 336.

[104] Edward Jenner, *A continuation of facts and observations relative to the* variolæ vaccinæ, *or cow pox* (London, 1800), pp. 41–2.

[105] Thomas Dudley Fosbroke, *A picturesque and topographical account of Cheltenham, and its vicinity* (Cheltenham, 1826), p. 294; Paul Saunders, *Edward Jenner: the Cheltenham years, 1795–1823, being a chronicle of the vaccination campaign* (Hanover, NH, 1982), p. 51.

authenticity and the countryside. It was assisted by Jenner's engaging persona as a country doctor, the appealing narrative of cows and dairymaids and the grand vision of philanthropy and medical progress. Around 1800, Jenner sat for a portrait, in which John Raphael Smith depicted him as leaning against a tree, with a milkmaid, carrying a pail on her head, emerging from a group of cows at pasture in the background (Figure 3.1).[106] From June 1801, the iconic portrait was widely available as a mezzotint print.[107] John Lettsom, president of the Medical Society, used his position to champion cowpox and lionise Jenner.[108] In his *Observations on the cow-pock* (1801), with a silhouette of Jenner as its frontispiece and an engraving of a sacred cow on the title page, Lettsom presented Jenner as a man whose claim to the honours accorded heroes 'is that of having multiplied the human race, and happily invoked the goddess of health, to arrest the arm that scatters pestilence and death over the creation.'[109]

The new prophylaxis became linked more directly with Jenner's name. Dr Joseph Marshall, whose success with cowpox in Gloucestershire provided some counterpoise to the activity in London in 1799, was keen to ensure that the laurels remained with his mentor. In his mission to introduce vaccination in the Mediterranean in 1800–1, he set up 'Jennerian' institutes in Gibraltar and Malta, referred to the new practice as 'Jennerian inoculation', and encouraged the local people to see Jenner as a secular hero.[110] This terminology and thinking may have had its origins in naval circles. Dr Trotter, chief physician in the Channel Fleet, referred to 'Jennerian inoculation' in a letter of May 1800, several months before Marshall set sail from Plymouth on a royal navy supply ship. The naval physicians and surgeons at Plymouth, who had their own medical society, were already strongly supportive of cowpox and early in 1801 lent their name and purses to present Jenner with a testimonial and gold medal that depicts Apollo presenting a vaccinated sailor to Britannia 'who, in return, extends a civic crown on which is written JENNER'. In the accompanying letter, Trotter expressed the hope that 'the present age have the justice and public spirit to remunerate what posterity will be glad to appreciate'.[111] In 1802, the medical fraternity at Plymouth even commissioned James Northcote to paint a portrait of Jenner to hang in their meeting room.[112]

---

[106] Ludmilla Jordanova, 'Remembrance of science past', *British Journal for the History of Science*, 33 (2000), 387–406, at 400–2.

[107] *Morning Chronicle*, 26 June 1801. A copy was sent to Boston, Massachusetts in November 1801: H MS c 16. 1; Countway Library of Medicine, Boston, MA.

[108] *MPJ*, 4 (July–December 1800), 567.

[109] John Coakley Lettsom, *Observations on the cow-pock* (London, 1801), also published as 'Hints respecting the cow-pock,' in *Hints designed to promote beneficence, temperance and medical science*, 3 vols. (London, 1801), 3, pp. 1–80.

[110] See Chapter 5.   [111] Baron, *Life*, 1, pp. 404–7; 2, p. 449.

[112] Jordanova, 'Remembrance', 402–3.

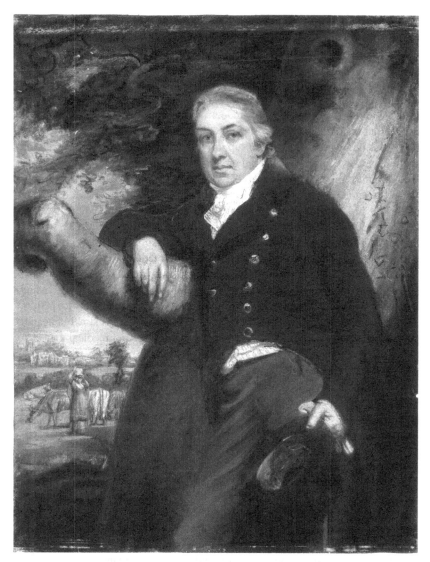

Figure 3.1 Portrait of Edward Jenner. Pastel on vellum by John Raphael
Smith, 1800
(Wellcome Collections)

Around this time 'Jennerian' began to be used quite often as an
adjective to refer to Jenner's doctrine, his system and, perhaps most
significant, his discovery. In his *Observations on the cow-pock*, Lettsom
used the expression 'Jennerian discovery' and invited readers to consider

how great the reward should be to match 'the national good that must result from [it]'.[113]

Declarations as to the value of the new prophylaxis were increasingly linked with assertions that Jenner was worthy of honour and reward as a man who had established the key facts of the most beneficial innovation of the age and who, without seeking to profit from it by keeping it secret, brought it to the attention of the world. Furthermore, it was evident that Jenner had been for some time engaged at his own expense in seeking to establish and refine the practice and that it was in the public interest to support him in this role. Jenner's patrons and friends were aware of his financial circumstances and active on his behalf. By the beginning of 1801, Lady Berkeley was already involved in plans to raise funds for Jenner.[114] In a letter to his brother-in-law shortly afterwards, Jenner expressed his pleasure at the gold medal from Plymouth and cheekily asked 'Should not the ladies of Gloucestershire, over the beauty of whose children I have placed so strong a shield, shew me . . . some similar mark of gratitude?', cheekily adding that he did not 'exactly mean a medal'.[115] During 1801, the Berkeleys led a list of Gloucestershire notables in raising a subscription in appreciation of Jenner's discovery.[116] Aware of the precedent by which inventors and others who had contributed to the common good to petition Parliament for recompense and reward, Jenner and his friends slowly began to gather evidence and testimonials from medical societies and medical men as to the value of Jenner's discovery.[117] In his treatise, published in 1802, Dr Robert Thornton offered an emotionally charged endorsement. After describing his own child's suffering and death following smallpox inoculation, he stressed the point that 'cow-pox never destroys life'. 'Glorious tidings! – Happy annunciation! –', he declared, 'I who have lost by variolous inoculation my first-born child . . . have a right to exult in the present fortunate discovery of Dr Jenner'.[118]

Early in 1802 Jenner returned to London to finalise his claim to have 'discovered' that cowpox can be inoculated from the cow to man with the 'beneficial effect of rendering through life the persons so inoculated perfectly secure from' smallpox and that, far from keeping it secret, he had 'immediately disclosed' his discovery.[119] In March, Henry Addington, the Prime Minister, informed the House of Commons that the king approved the petition in principle. A committee was set up under the chairmanship of Admiral Berkeley, well-disposed to Jenner, to examine the claim. Presenting his case

---

[113] Lettsom, *Observations*, pp. 4, 12.   [114] MS0016/2/10, RCS.

[115] K. Bryn Thomas, 'A Jenner letter', *JHM*, 12 (157), 450–2.

[116] *Letters of Jenner*, ed. Miller, pp. 14–16.   [117] Fisher, *Jenner*, p. 130.

[118] Robert John Thornton, *Facts decisive in favour of the cow-pock* (London, 1802), p. 129.

[119] Fisher, *Jenner*, pp. 123–4.

in person, Jenner was embarrassed and tongue-tied, but he was followed by a line of eminent doctors who testified to the inestimable value of vaccination and his role in its discovery. Sir Walter Farquhar, physician of the Prince of Wales, described it as 'the greatest discovery that has been made for many years' and stated his belief that, if he had kept the secret to himself, Jenner could have earned £10,000 a year from it.[120] Dr Moseley and John Birch, a London surgeon, were isolated voices in expressing concerns about the safety of cowpox and the security it provided.[121] Though professing support for Jenner, Dr Pearson noted the prior knowledge of cowpox and the role of other people in the dissemination of the practice.[122] As Richard Fisher, Jenner's best biographer, observed, it would have been more accurate for Jenner to claim that he had simply discovered that inoculation of cowpox from person to person was a preventative of smallpox.[123] Such a claim, though, would rather have understated the achievement. After all, Farmer Jesty's earlier inoculation of cowpox was not conducted as a scientific experiment and went undocumented until after Jenner's publication. Furthermore, it overlooks Jenner's achievement in identifying the right sort of cowpox and establishing the conditions in which it could be used safely and effectively. Given that few medical men in England had heard of cowpox before this time and almost all were initially sceptical of its value, Jenner's claim to the discovery of cowpox inoculation is entirely supportable. When the committee's report was discussed in Parliament only one member questioned his priority in the discovery.[124] The focus of discussion was the size of the premium.[125] As the committee had proposed that it should be no less than £10,000, a motion to award Jenner this sum was put. Several speakers proposed an amendment doubling this amount, pointing out the value in terms of lives saved and noting, too, Jenner's claim that his work in promoting the new prophylaxis had cost him £6,000 directly and through loss of income.[126] The amendment to double the grant was narrowly defeated. Addington's intervention was probably decisive: in addition to stressing the dire fiscal situation, he observed that Jenner was now well placed to gain financially from the new prophylaxis.

Parliamentary recognition of Jenner's discovery marked an important stage in the acceptance of the new prophylaxis. Although he was gratified by the terms in which his discovery and philanthropic endeavours had been presented, Jenner believed that the premium did little more than compensate

---

[120] *Evidence at large, as laid before the committee of the House of Commons, respecting Dr Jenner's discovery of vaccine inoculation*, ed. G. C. Jenner (London, 1805), p. 13.
[121] *Evidence*, ed. Jenner, pp. 39–42, 56–62, 115–18.
[122] *Evidence*, ed. Jenner, pp. 104–6, 128–34.   [123] Fisher, *Jenner*, p. 123.
[124] *The parliamentary register; or, history of the proceedings and debates of the Houses of Lords and Commons*, 18 (London, 1802), pp. 592–600.
[125] Fisher, *Jenner*, p. 124.   [126] *Parliamentary Register*, 18, pp. 596–9.

him for his outlays and losses. Acting on the advice that he could make a good living in the capital, he moved to London, at significant cost, only to find that few people were willing to pay his fees for a seemingly simple procedure that was becoming available more cheaply. The parliamentary premium itself created a burden of expectation. It was a matter of envy and resentment in some circles: Pearson published misgivings about Jenner's claims.[127] Still, Jenner had admirers who pressed for further recognition and reward. At the end of 1802, he was selected as one of the 'public characters' of the year and his genius and humanitarianism were affirmed in the brief biographical essay. Presenting vaccine inoculation, which 'annihilates a disease ... the most dreadful scourge of mankind', as 'the most valuable, and most important discovery ever made', the anonymous author stresses the meagreness of the premium: 'when we consider how small a surplus will remain, after deducting all [Jenner's expenses], we should be rather inclined to suppose it is meant for the redemption of the town of Berkeley, than that of the whole human race, from the ravages of small-pox.'[128]

There were soon moves afoot to establish a philanthropic foundation to support vaccination and honour Dr Jenner. In two public meetings in London in January 1803, the latter a dinner attended by royalty and aristocracy as well as bankers, lawyers and medical men, a new vaccination society was formed. Once the king and queen had agreed to be patron and patroness, it was denominated the Royal Jennerian Society [RJS] for the Extermination of Smallpox. The Prince of Wales and four other princes were named as vice-patrons, two daughters-in-law and three daughters as vice-patronesses, and several dozen lords and ladies as sub-patrons and sub-patronesses.[129] The Society brought together medical and non-medical supporters of vaccination. Its medical council assumed responsibility for making vaccine available, staffing the vaccine stations in London, and overseeing the integrity of the practice. The broader membership, it was hoped, would provide financial support and political influence to assist in the practice's expansion. The constitution made provision for an annual festival and dinner on Jenner's birthday on 17 May.[130] Over the next few years, it served as the focus of an informal cult of Jenner. At the first anniversary dinner in 1803, Jenner received 'the tumultuous plaudits' of some 300 members and guests.[131] Nathaniel Bloomfield, who had lost his father and two children to smallpox, penned a lyric address to Jenner that was probably presented then.[132] His brother, Robert Bloomfield,

---

[127] Pearson, *Examination, passim.*
[128] Alexander Stephens, *Public characters of 1802–1803* (London, 1803), pp. 17–48, at 18, 43.
[129] *Address of the Royal Jennerian Society for the extermination of the small-pox* (London, 1803), pp. 5–8.
[130] *Address of RJS*, p. 29.   [131] Fisher, *Jenner*, p. 145.
[132] *Bury and Norwich Post*, 4 May 1803; Shuttleton, *Smallpox and literary imagination*, p. 192.

author of the acclaimed *Farmer's boy* (1800), was already at work on a more ambitious poem on vaccination, extracts of which were read at the second RJS anniversary dinner in 1804.[133] In *Good tidings; or news from the farm*, he presented the grandeur of Jenner's discovery: 'The great, the conscious power of doing good / The power to will, and wishes to embrace / Th' emancipation of the human race; / A joy that must all mortal praise outlive, / A wealth that grateful nations cannot give'.[134] In 1804, Christopher Anstey published a Latin ode to Jenner, assigning the proceeds of a translation to the RJS. Unable to be in London for the second anniversary, Jenner attended the third anniversary dinner in 1805 and, addressing the company 'with that artless simplicity and dignity of manner, which equally distinguish his language in speaking and writing', he declared that he met them 'with a heart exulting at the rapid manner in which I perceive vaccination is spreading over the earth'.[135] There were congratulatory speeches and eulogies in verse and song. Dr Lettsom, vice-president of the medical council, brought a ballad to be sung at the festival about a boy blinded by smallpox.[136] Two clergymen were fulsome in Jenner's praise. After describing his own efforts with the lancet, the Rev. Rowland Hill turned to Jenner and asked, 'What avails this little boast, when I stand by my very respectable friend [who] has been the preserver of the lives of millions?' The Rev. Booker, who travelled from Staffordshire to pay tribute, asked rhetorically: 'If a Roman, who preserved the life of *one* citizen, was rewarded with a civic crown, what reward shall be presented to *him* who preserves the lives of *millions*?'[137]

---

[133] Bloomfield, 'Good tidings'; *MPJ*, 11 (January–July 1804), 572.

[134] *Poems of Bloomfield*, 1, pp. 109–10.

[135] *MPJ*, 11 (January–June 1804), 572–3; *GM*, 75 (1805), 521–6.

[136] *Memoirs of the life and writings of the late John Coakley Lettsom, with a selection from his correspondence*, ed. Thomas Joseph Pettigrew, 3 vols. (London, 1817), 2, pp. 109, 128, 589–90.

[137] *GM*, 75, (1805), 524–5.

4 National Mobilisation

Vaccination in Britain and Ireland

In July 1800, James Veiten, surgeon on HMS *Magnificent*, made plans to use cowpox in inoculating men on board. Engaged in the blockade of Brest, his ship had recently been in contact with smallpox. Learning about cowpox on his return from the Caribbean, he observed the practice in London and obtained samples of vaccine. In his letter requesting permission to use cowpox, he pointed out that it could be safely used on a crowded ship, with the men under inoculation continuing their duties. In addition, he felt that the adoption of cowpox inoculation in the navy would prove exemplary as men in the service 'are drawn from all, and a great many from the remotest, parts of the three kingdoms, where the prejudices of education, religion, and ignorance, operate as injuries to society'. It was, then, 'a national and material point to gain an accession of opinion in favour of this mild form of inoculating' since it 'would prove the means of disseminating its advantages widely amongst the descendants of those who have served', who would become 'the bulwark of our country'. He saw the breaking down of the barriers of prejudice against the new practice as 'a revolution' of great importance.[1] Though he would not be the first to introduce cowpox into the senior service, he would have the satisfaction of seeing its spread through the British Isles. He was right to regard the adoption of the new practice as a 'revolution' and associate it with the nation's mobilisation in the war against France.

The spread of vaccination through Britain was faster than Veiten anticipated. After an uncertain start, the practice expanded rapidly in 1800. According to Dr Lettsom's estimates, the number of vaccinations rose from around 60,000 in Britain in the middle of 1801 to 1,400,000 in the British empire by the end of 1805.[2] The proportion of children vaccinated was quite high in some districts. The number of vaccinations in Liverpool between 1802 and 1806 represented almost half the number of live births.[3] Given the

---

[1] *MPJ*, 4 (July–December 1800), 307–8.
[2] Lettsom, 'Hints respecting cow-pock', 5–6; John Coakley Lettsom, *Expositions on the inoculation of the small pox and the cow pock*, 2nd ed. (London, 1806), p. 16.
[3] Willan, *Vaccine inoculation*, appendix, p. xvi.

technical and logistical challenges, the anxieties about inoculating children with an animal disease and the apathy of many people, the vaccination of hundreds of thousands of Britons in a few years was no mean feat. Veiten's 'revolution' involved mobilisation on a massive scale. Medical men generally took the lead in making the practice available across the three kingdoms, but they could have done little without the concurrence of broader sections of the community. Members of the landed, professional and business elites were quick to see the value of the new practice and encourage its use in their spheres of influence. Far from opposing cowpox inoculation, most clergymen presented cowpox as a providential blessing. Parental love was a great driver of the new prophylaxis, with mothers often taking the initiative in appraising it. Aware that vaccination needed to take root to realise its full potential, its advocates looked to public authorities and civil society to provide support.

For all its phenomenal success, vaccination suffered many setbacks. Early enthusiasm gave way to apathy, and the lack of expertise among practitioners led to mishaps. Reports of smallpox after vaccination undermined confidence in assurances of lifelong security. From around 1805, cowpox inoculation came under serious attack and, in London at least, smallpox inoculation came back into use. Though it retained the strong support of the medical profession, its benefits were less easy to see as smallpox itself became less common. The debate over vaccination brought to the fore issues of public health, still understated, especially the status of medical authority and the role of the state. To understand the rapid expansion of vaccination, the responses it demanded, and the changes it brought in its wake, it is necessary first to consider broader developments in this revolutionary age.

Britain in Convulsion

Britain around 1800 was a hospitable site for the vaccine revolution. Long familiarity with smallpox inoculation made it easier for medical men to recognise cowpox's potential and put it in service. The existence of a tradition of smallpox prophylaxis presented some problems. The old-style inoculators stood to lose a profitable line of business and, given their success in reducing the dangers and costs of the practice, some of them had doubts about the advantages of the new prophylaxis. Despite its being less remunerative than smallpox inoculation, however, most medical men moved relatively quickly to embrace cowpox. The rapid adoption of vaccination can be associated with broader developments in medicine and in the groupings that provided health services. Though physicians, surgeons and apothecaries remained formally distinct, there was increasing overlap in their knowledge and skills and, especially outside London, some merging of their practices and identities.

Academically educated, many physicians sought clinical training and were becoming more open to new therapies. Conversely, many surgeons and apothecaries were seeking to advance themselves by more formal training and incorporating improvements into their practice. At the interface of medicine and surgery, the new prophylaxis provided physicians, surgeons and apothecaries opportunities to show themselves to be socially relevant and at the cutting edge of scientific medicine, and opened doors to family-focused general practice.

The broader transformation of Britain set the scene for and drove the vaccination revolution. The massive increase in population, mobility and urbanisation associated with agricultural change and the beginnings of industrialisation made for a more challenging disease environment. For the more mobile sections of the population, especially young people moving from the countryside into the conurbations, smallpox prophylaxis was especially valuable. Unlike variolation, vaccination could be made available to the urban poor without risk to the wider community. The Society for the Condition and Increasing the Comforts of the Poor, founded in 1796, rapidly saw the value of the new prophylaxis.[4] The expansion of the periodical press, including regional newspapers and medical journals, fed broad lay interest in the cowpox discovery and the progress of vaccination. Culturally, the environment was congenial for cowpox. Jenner's discovery could be presented as a fruit of the enlightenment, the product of observation and experiment, but also as a special and surprising gift of God. The mainstream churches were uniformly supportive of vaccination. The highly personalised religious revival of the late eighteenth century, especially the Methodist insistence on free will and the possibility of salvation for all, found space for the cowpox gospel. If vaccination raised the spectre of bestialisation, it conjured up, too, images of the beneficent cow, the clear-complexioned milkmaid and a rural idyll. Jenner was a poet and a friend of poets, especially the celebrants of Nature and the countryside. The parents who first secured their children by inoculating cowpox were the contemporaries of Wordsworth and Turner.[5]

The political context was less obviously consequential. The British government did not regard the health of its subjects as its responsibility, the royal colleges of medicine and surgery had far less power than equivalent bodies in continental Europe, and there was a general disposition to allow new remedies

---

[4] *The twenty-ninth report of the Society for Bettering the Condition and Increasing the Comforts of the Poor* (London, 1807), pp. 196–203.

[5] Fulford, Lee and Kitson, *Literature, science and exploration*, ch. 9. Richard Holmes, *The age of wonder: how the romantic generation discovered the beauty and terror of science* (London, 2009).

to compete in the medical marketplace. In the 1720s, smallpox inoculation had been associated with the Whigs and opposed by the Tories. By the late eighteenth century, prophylaxis was broadly accepted and, in any case, the political landscape had changed. Though a Tory, Jenner disliked Prime Minister William Pitt and had friends across the political divide. The period of ministerial instability following Pitt's resignation in 1801 allowed more scope for the success of a non-government measure like the proposal for a premium for Jenner. After the Truce of Amiens in 1802–3, the focus on national unity, defence and mobilisation helped to make vaccination a patriotic cause. The growth of empire during the Revolutionary and Napoleonic wars likewise encouraged authoritarian approaches. The cause of vaccination found most support in 1806–7 in the two ministries of 'All the Talents', whose leading lights were keen on administrative reform, science and technology, and evidence-based interventions to strengthen the nation.[6] Overall, though, the British government played a much more limited role in supporting vaccination than its European counterparts.

More significant in its impact was Britain's war against France. Jenner's discovery was announced at a climactic moment in the Revolutionary Wars. The conflict variously facilitated and hindered the spread of news about the new prophylaxis and the distribution of vaccine. In Britain itself, the war certainly assisted the expansion of vaccination. Military recruitment in the late 1790s involved the variolation of many soldiers, opportunely disclosing more cases in which resistance to smallpox was explained by prior cowpox infection. From 1800, the potential of cowpox was increasingly realised in the armed forces. Soldiers and sailors could be immunised without impeding the discharge of their duties or posing a danger to their comrades. The rapid expansion of vaccination coincided with unprecedented mobilisation of the nation for war. By chance, the inauguration of the Royal Jennerian Society in May 1803 took place the evening before the return to war after the Truce of Amiens. Legislation two months later set the scene for the expansion of the armed forces, including militia and volunteer regiments, to some 600,000 men by early 1804, over 11 per cent of the adult male population.[7] The marshalling of the nation's manpower, civilian as well as military, heightened recognition of the importance of preventive medicine. The imperatives of defending Britain against invasion and defeating Napoleon seemingly encouraged Jenner and his colleagues to champion the new prophylaxis in military metaphors.

---

[6] Joe Bord, 'Whiggery, science and administration: Grenville and Lord Henry Petty in the Ministry of All the Talents, 1806–7', *Historical Research*, 76 (2003), 108–27, esp. 121–3.

[7] Roger Knight, *Britain against Napoleon. The organization of victory 1793–1815* (London, 2013), pp. 260–2.

Medical Mobilisation

Jenner cannot have assumed that the medical world would respond positively to cowpox inoculation. Even friends and colleagues familiar with cowpox remained somewhat aloof. Dr Caleb Hillier Parry, the dedicatee of the *Inquiry*, did not champion the new prophylaxis in print and Charles Brandon Trye, chief surgeon at Gloucester Infirmary, had reservations about it until 1804.[8] Given the hesitancy in the western counties, it is not surprising that medical men in parts of Britain where cowpox was wholly unknown were incredulous. 'When the cow-pox was first named here', recalled Dr Wood of Newcastle upon Tyne, 'I believe it was only with a smile, as in many other places'.[9] The early interest in cowpox from Dr Pearson and Dr Woodville obviously played a critical role in publicising and corroborating Jenner's work and in translating the 'Gloucestershire bubble' into a national enterprise.[10] Jenner had his own credit in medical and scientific circles in the national capital, however, and would probably have been able to build the reputation of the new prophylaxis, if more slowly, without them. Dr Lettsom was an early and influential champion of Jenner's discovery. His exuberant praise – 'What is the *Georgium Sidus* [Uranus, first observed in 1781], in competition with the Jennerian discovery!' – was probably doing the rounds in London before it appeared in print. His enthusiasm may have been the prompt for Dr Moseley's mockery. Cowpox 'is a new star in the Æsculapian firmament … first observed in the Provinces', Moseley declared in 1800, 'It is so luminous there, that the greasy-healed hind feet of Pegasus are visible to the naked eye'.[11]

The most decisive event in establishing vaccination nationally was the testimonial in support of cowpox inoculation in July 1800 by thirty-six of the leading physicians and surgeons in the capital, including Dr James Sims, president of the Medical Society. Organised by Dr Lettsom and John Ring, Pearson and Woodville are notably absent from the group.[12] The testimonial rather signalled a collective commitment to the new prophylaxis under Jenner's aegis. Among the signatories was Dr Robert Thornton, physician and botanist, who, after losing his own son through smallpox inoculation, received instruction in the new prophylaxis from Jenner, began to offer the procedure at the Marylebone Dispensary and during an autumn visit to the Lake District introduced the practice in Westmorland.[13] Reprinted in provincial newspapers, the testimonial galvanised groups of physicians and surgeons in Leeds and

---

[8] *MPJ*, 12 (July–December 1804), 395–8.   [9] *MPJ*, 13 (January–June 1805), 52–65, at 52.
[10] Pearson, *Examination*, pp. 168–9.
[11] Moseley, *Treatise on sugar*, p. 162; Lettsom, *Observations*, p. 11.
[12] *GM*, 70 (1800), 640; *Gloucester Journal*, 28 July 1800.
[13] Thornton, *Facts decisive*, pp. 129, 189–232.

other towns to announce their commitment to cowpox inoculation and advertise its availability.[14] In the *Hull Packet*, a group of medical men informed the townsmen that 'physicians of the highest eminence in London' had declared cowpox to be 'a certain preventive against the small-pox', and 'perfectly safe, mild and not infectious'. After acknowledging mankind's debt to 'the illustrious Jenner', it advertised the assistance given by other 'men of liberal opinions, science and principle', including Hull's own Dr Alderson, who after using cowpox on his own child persuaded the trustees of the Hull Infirmary to allow him and his colleagues to make the new procedure available to the poor of the town.[15] As British newspapers began to notice the spread of vaccination overseas in the second half of 1800, medical men were rising to the challenge of establishing the new prophylaxis across the British Isles. In Scotland, Thomas Anderson, surgeon of Leith, led the way in May 1799 with cowpox supplied by Jenner. Encouraged by his success, his Edinburgh colleagues conducted their own tests and, early in 1800, offered vaccination charitably in the city's dispensary. In the meantime, Anderson was seeding the practice in other towns in Scotland.[16] In Dublin, John Creighton, surgeon at the Dispensary for the Infant Poor, made a trial of cowpox inoculation in 1799 and offered it routinely from March 1800.[17] After obtaining vaccine from London in June 1800, Dr Barry vaccinated 250 people in Cork and began to extend the practice in Kerry.[18] In November, Dr Halliday secured vaccine for use in a trial in the poor house and infirmary in Belfast.[19]

The cowpox bandwagon left casualties in its wake. Charles Brown was a young surgeon in a hurry to make a name for himself in London. His book on scrofulous diseases, however, was panned in a review.[20] In May 1800, he published an intemperate letter warning families not to allow surgeons 'infected with the Cow-pox mania' to inoculate their children with 'such a hideous disease'.[21] Two months later, he was dining with friends when, after a creditor arrived to call in a debt, he shot himself with a pistol.[22] In a letter to a friend on 15 July, Jenner coldly informed a friend that Brown, after having 'made a variety of efforts to write [the practice] down', shot himself on 'finding himself deserted by every medical man of respectability'.[23] The tale of Mr Thomas, who bought an inoculation practice in Northamptonshire in

---

[14] *MPJ*, 4 (July–December 1800), 570–1.   [15] *Hull Packet*, 16 September 1800.
[16] *Annals of Medicine, 1800*, 5 (1801), 450–3.   [17] Additional MS. 35745, fos. 154r, 156r, BL.
[18] *MPJ*, 4 (July–December 1800), 146, 425–9; John Milner Barry, *An account of the nature and effects of the cow-pock* (Cork, 1800).
[19] R. W. M. Strain, *Belfast and its charitable society. A story of urban social development* (London, 1961), p. 80.
[20] Charles Brown, *A treatise on scrophulous diseases* (London, 1798); *Critical Review*, 24 (1798), 465.
[21] Smith, *Speckled monster*, p. 96.   [22] *European Magazine*, 38 (July–December 1800), 79.
[23] Baron, *Life*, 2, pp. 324–5.

1796 and planned to write a book publicising his mode of inoculating, is also not lacking in poignancy. Sceptical of the claims made for cowpox, he vaccinated sixty people and, after finding them insusceptible to smallpox, immediately saw that his business was doomed. Although he advertised cowpox inoculation in December 1800, he could not make the new practice pay. In a letter in support of vaccination two years later, he declared that 'no one has greater reason to lament the introduction of vaccine' than he himself as it had 'not only been the means of depriving me of a very comfortable support for my family, but absolutely compelled me to leave a place and connection I much valued'.[24] Medical men who made a specialism of smallpox prophylaxis certainly faced challenges to their business model. The standard fee for vaccination, five shillings, was less than half the standard fee for variolation, half a guinea.[25] Announcing the 'fortunate commencement' of vaccination in a northern town, it was declared that 'the only losers' would be members of the 'faculty' as, once the practice becomes general, 'a lucrative branch of the profession will be cut off'.[26] Itinerant inoculators in the countryside experienced a dramatic collapse in the demand for their services. Of the 'smallpox doctors' who had plied their trade in Cambridgeshire, it was said in 1806 that 'Jenner has nearly ruined this class of beings'.[27]

Some medical men welcomed vaccination as a less stressful procedure for themselves as well as their patients. In the early years, however, it was not at all easy to secure reliable vaccine, use it in a manner that inspired confidence among patients and achieve consistent outcomes. Richard Weekes, a London-trained surgeon at Hurstpierpoint, Sussex, saw himself as a man of science and his son, Hampton, was a medical student in London in 1801–2 in the heady days of cowpox. In a letter to his father in January 1802, Hampton reported a meeting of the Physical Society of Guy's Hospital at which Jenner was the guest of honour and Hampton had been called to report on horse-grease in Sussex. Although Richard made a trial of cowpox, he was not able to obtain a secure supply and continued inoculating with smallpox.[28] In his letters home, Hampton described the problem of spurious cowpox, his own vaccination failures and the shortage of good vaccine in London. In July 1802, Richard received a sample of vaccine on glass purchased from the Cow Pock Institute in London at the set rate of half a guinea. In the following year, he decided to pay the guinea subscription to the Institute to secure a continuing supply.[29]

[24] MPJ, 8 (July–December 1802), 165–9; Northampton Mercury, 13 December 1800.
[25] Irvine Loudon, Medical care and the general practitioner, 1750–1850 (Oxford, 1986), p. 144; Smith, Speckled monster, p. 112.
[26] Hull Advertiser, 7 June 1800.   [27] Loudon, Medical care, pp. 81, 250.
[28] A medical student at St Thomas's Hospital, 1801–1802. The Weekes family letters, ed. John M. T. Ford (London, 1987), pp. 90, 107–8, 112–13.
[29] Weekes family letters, ed. Ford, pp. 136, 140–1, 151, 152, 192, 197–9, 244, 249.

Given the problems that medical men were experiencing with vaccine, it is little wonder that many patients settled for smallpox inoculation. The allegation that doctors who continued to variolate were motivated by avarice was not entirely just. In 'general inoculations' conducted in Essex, for example, many parish vestries only offered variolation, while some others offered a choice between variolation and vaccination, with many parents opting for the old practice.[30] Given the practical difficulties, and the reports of mishaps and failures, some doctors lost their enthusiasm for vaccination. Still, the overwhelming majority of medical men, whether through conviction or a desire to conform, remained remarkably firm in their commitment to the new prophylaxis. At the height of the vaccination controversy in 1805–6, a reviewer observed that for each of the anti-vaccinists in the capital there were at least ten medical men 'of higher name' who supported the new prophylaxis, and that 'in the country at large, we believe [the anti-vaccinists] have not one respectable practitioner on their side in five hundred'.[31]

Overall, vaccination probably served the medical fraternity well. The expansion of the practice significantly increased the number of people who were immunised in one form or the other. For younger medical men, seeking to position themselves in a competitive professional market, the adoption of new prophylaxis was a means of showing themselves up-to-date, scientifically minded and socially aware. 'Every young doctor', wrote one caustic observer of the phenomenon, 'who can descend, for the sake of notoriety, to obtrude himself on the public in plumage not his own, writes upon the cowpox'.[32] Many older physicians, revered in their localities for their dedication, learning and support for smallpox prophylaxis, gave their blessing to the new practice. Dr Langslow, a Suffolk physician, gave up 'a *favourite* theory on a *peculiar* mode of treating the inoculated smallpox' that he had 'indulged' since 1775 when, around 1800, 'he *experimentally* discovered the *grand* superiority of the vaccine inoculation'.[33] The new prophylaxis encouraged networking, with vaccine samples and practical advice traded back and forth. In June 1800, when smallpox appeared in Pittenweem, Fifeshire, Alexander Williamson obtained cowpox from a medical friend in Liverpool, probably Dr James Currie, biographer of Robbie Burns.[34] Medical men collaborated in maintaining local supplies of vaccine, often by offering free vaccination at set times in dispensaries or clinics. At the dispensary in York, a subscription society was formed to provide vaccine to rural practitioners who often found themselves using matter that had lost 'its active powers by being transported

---

[30] Smith, *Speckled monster*, pp. 112–14.
[31] *Edinburgh Review*, 9 (October 1806–January 1807), 32–66, at 40.
[32] *Medical Observer*, 2 (1808), 170–1.   [33] *MPJ*, 8 (June 1802–January 1803), 164–5.
[34] *Annals of Medicine, 1800*, 5 (1801), 440–6.

to the distance of several hundred miles'.[35] In May 1801, the Faculty of Physicians and Surgeons in Glasgow established an institute to serve as a vaccine depot for western Scotland and vaccinated thousands of children in its own right.[36] In 1804, a Cowpock Institute was established in Dublin to support the practice countrywide. Dr Samuel Bell Labatt, its energetic secretary, wrote *An address to the medical practitioners of Ireland*, that was described in London as 'the best compendium of vaccination we have yet met with'.[37] If vaccination made few fortunes, it helped build reputations and solid practices. It brought physicians, surgeons and apothecaries together in shows of solidarity in the public interest. The medical men best placed to benefit were practitioners who combined surgical skills, broad medical knowledge and a sense of service. Many of them found vaccination a useful point of entry into family medicine.

The Cowpox Gospel: Parents, Preachers and Patrons

Early vaccination owed almost as much to conscription as mobilisation. James Phipps had no real choice in the matter. His father was presumably inclined to trust Jenner in return for free treatment. The adults and children who were inoculated in the trials of cowpox at the Smallpox and Inoculation Hospital in London in 1799 probably did not know that they were part of an experiment. William Wilberforce later observed that most of the people vaccinated at St Pancras would not have accepted cowpox if they had known.[38] Jenner and most of the pioneers of the practice were ready enough to inoculate their own children with cowpox, both to set an example of others and to secure a supply of vaccine for their use. In the early years of the practice, it was difficult to extend the practice beyond a narrow circle of family and friends. The 'first gentleman that submitted his own children to the new practice', in November 1798, was Jenner's old friend Henry Hicks of Eastington.[39] The maintenance of a supply of vaccine often depended on the vaccination of groups of charity children. The system could be justified, in terms of the medical ethics of the time, by reference to the benefit provided to the children and the belief that the poor 'being the most numerous class of society, are the greatest beneficiaries of the healing art'.[40] To its credit, the Foundling Hospital in London did not make

[35] *MPJ*, 4 (July–December 1800), 429–31.
[36] Fiona A. Macdonald, 'Vaccination policy of the Faculty of Physicians and Surgeons of Glasgow, 1801–1863', *MH*, 41 (1997), 291–321, esp. 297–8, 318.
[37] *MPJ*, 14 (June–December 1805), 84–5.   [38] Smith, *Speckled monster*, p. 106.
[39] Baron, *Life*, 1, pp. 303–4.
[40] L. Haakonssen, *Medicine and enlightenment: John Gregory, Thomas Percival and Benjamin Rush* (Amsterdam, 1997), p. 151.

itself available as a showcase, moving cautiously and quietly to replace smallpox inoculation with cowpox in 1801.[41]

Popular responses to cowpox were mixed. In districts where the association between cowpox and insusceptibility to smallpox was known, there was some readiness to see cowpox inoculation in a positive light. In regions where the cattle disease was unknown, the bovine origin of vaccine may not have been apparent or a matter of great concern. In 1800, though, John Attenburrow only overcame violent opposition in Nottingham by vaccinating his own son.[42] For people familiar with smallpox inoculation, the fact that cowpox inoculation was often available at little or no cost was a commendation. According to Dr Stokes in Chesterfield in 1800, the 'common people, as far as I have observed, receive it with gladness, as it comes to them free of expense', and some speak of it as a blessing sent from God. They do not 'express any more repugnance to the insertion of pellucid lymph from the arm of a neighbour's child into that of their own offspring, because originally taken from a vesicle on the nipple of a cow, than they do to feed them with the milk or flesh of that animal'.[43] Conversely, Dr Harrison of Kirkbymoorside found the mothers preferred the old mode, one insisting on 'the true Christian Small-pox' and another opining that cowpox was 'fitted for Calves'. Many soon revised their views in the light of experience. In Harrison's practice, the mothers did so during a smallpox outbreak, when all were inoculated with smallpox, except for a pregnant woman who accepted vaccination and did well. Conversely, a pregnant woman in a nearby town who insisted on variolation had a miscarriage, recovering only 'after a month of undescribable torture and suffering'.[44]

For most people, it was a matter of accepting cowpox on trust. A great deal doubtless depended on their character, local standing and approach of the practitioner. Dr William Turton, who introduced cowpox in Swansea in 1799, inoculated his infant daughter with cowpox as an example to the community, announcing his intention to name her 'Vaccinia'.[45] In spreading the practice westwards from Plymouth in spring 1800, Dr Huggan was depicted by his colleague as an evangelist. 'Like the early propagation of Christianity, by its Divine Leader', it was reported, the new prophylaxis 'was first *preached to the poor*. The children of poor soldiers and poor fishermen first partook of its blessings: publicans and sinners have since embraced it; and the purity of its doctrine and practice is making proselytes to the very land's end in Cornwall'.[46] Dr Thornton presented the introduction

[41] *MPJ*, 14 (June–December 1805), 506–8.
[42] William Howie Rylie, *Old and new Nottingham* (London, 1853), p. 239.
[43] *MPJ*, 5 (January–June 1801), 17.
[44] *York Herald*, 21 February 1801; *MPJ*, 13 (January–June 1805), 331–6.
[45] Turton, *Treatise*, pp. 56–60.   [46] *MPJ*, 3 (January–June 1800), 525–6.

of cowpox in the Lake District as a humanitarian enterprise. He described the Earl of Lonsdale underwriting the vaccination of his tenants and workers at Lowther; his apothecary joining in the work of humanity by disseminating cowpox to neighbouring towns; the operator of the local turnpike, benefiting from the concourse of people seeking vaccination at Lowther, declining to charge Thornton himself; and the young girl who was vaccinated and then carried on horseback twenty-six miles across the moors so that children in Carlisle could be vaccinated from the pustule on her arm.[47]

The adoption of cowpox inoculation by the elite eased its acceptance among the population at large. 'Fortunately for us in this district', Dr Harrison observed in north Yorkshire, 'a few in the superior classes of life have subjected their offspring to the new practice, with the happiest success, and those in a lower sphere, perhaps more through fashion than conviction, have been insensibly led to follow their example'.[48] A more down-to-earth endorsement from a person of a similar background could be more compelling. During a smallpox outbreak in autumn 1801, a farmer at Eastfield, Northumberland, wrote to his agent in County Durham: 'I would recommend to you and your wife to inoculate yours with the cow pox, if not already done, which is by much the safest way and least sickness to the poor children. Many have been inoculated with the cow pox in this part, and have all done well.'[49] Convinced of the benefits of the new method, many people made shift to avail themselves of it. According to a report from Derbyshire in 1800, Mrs Wasse of Astwith, 'a very intelligent woman', inoculated her five-year-old daughter with cowpox brought by her husband from a patient inoculated by a cabinet-maker in a neighbouring village.[50] The spirit of self-help is likewise well illustrated in west Yorkshire in 1807 when villagers vaccinated over a thousand children using needles and pen-knives. 'If every parent would imitate this example', wrote the reporter, 'the small-pox would soon be unknown'.[51]

The parish clergy played their part in promoting the new prophylaxis, organising vaccinations and sometimes taking up the lancet themselves. Robert Holt, rector of Finmere, Oxfordshire, began inoculating cowpox in autumn 1799 and forwarded vaccine to a colleague in his native Lancashire. The Rev. Finch of St Helens used it to inoculate the son of a clog-maker, recording the event in the parish register as the first vaccination 'in these parts', and vaccinated some 714 people over the following year.[52] Fearing that labourers working on the Grand Junction Canal might bring smallpox to

---

[47] Thornton, *Facts decisive*, pp. 201–4, 217–25.   [48] *MPJ*, 13 (January–June 1805), 334–5.
[49] *Matthew and George Culley, farming letters 1798–1804*, ed. Anne Orde (Woodbridge, 2006), p. 194.
[50] *MPJ*, 5 (January–June 1801), 18, 22.   [51] *Leeds Intelligencer*, 24 August 1807.
[52] *MPJ*, 2 (August–December 1799), 401–4.

his parish, J. T. A. Reed, rector of Leckhamstead, set about inoculating his flock with cowpox in March 1800.[53] Around this time, too, Joseph Berington, a Catholic priest ministering to Sir John Throckmorton at Buckland, Oxfordshire, sought instruction in vaccination from Jenner in Cheltenham. On his return, he vaccinated 400 people in six weeks, and declared his resolve to vaccinate the new born each year.[54] Clerical supporters of the new practice spread the cowpox gospel by a range of means. The Rev. Luke Booker, vicar of Dudley, prevailed on local surgeons to 'inoculate the poor, gratis, with the vaccine', and penned and printed a leaflet on vaccination to present to 'every person who brings a child to be baptised'.[55] Thomas Alston Warren, curate of Kensworth, Bedfordshire, who assisted in a general vaccination of the parish in 1802, prepared a charming sermon to allay the concerns of his parishioners, placing some emphasis on the cleanliness and beneficence of the cow.[56] The Rev. Rowland Hill, who divided his time between his pulpit at Surrey Chapel, London, and Wotton-under-Edge, not far from Berkeley, offered vaccination on his preaching tours, not least in southwest Wales, where he vaccinated over a thousand people in summer 1805.[57] 'Next to the great Salvation', he wrote to a colleague, 'this discovery is by far the most beneficial, because the most easy'.[58]

The aristocracy and gentry proved responsive to vaccination. The Berkeleys were stalwart supporters of their family physician. Lady Berkeley 'surmounted every prepossession in favour of the old practice, and ... ardently recommended and adopted the new'.[59] At Cheltenham, Jenner promoted the new prophylaxis among the chattering classes. Eager to hear about the latest wonder cures, the ladies and gentlemen who came for the season were perhaps more intrigued than disgusted by the cowpox remedy. After all, some of them went to the Pneumatic Institution, just outside Bristol, where Dr Beddoes offered the inhalation of the breath of a cow as a treatment for tuberculosis. In 1797, Anna Barbauld described the cows being 'brought into the lady's chamber', where they 'stand all night with their heads within the curtains', and reported her companion's observation that 'the benefit cannot be mutual' and that 'if the fashion takes, we shall eat diseased beef'.[60] There was some need, of course, to present a wholesome image of cowpox to ease its acceptance in

---

[53] *GM*, 77 (1807), 104.

[54] Joseph Berington, 'A plan for more effectually carrying into execution the design of the Jennerian Society for the extermination of the smallpox' [1804], MS. 1139, WLL.

[55] Baron, *Life*, 1, pp. 592–3.

[56] Thomas Alston Warren, *An address from a country minister to his parishioners on the subject of the cow-pox, or vaccine inoculation* (London, 1803).

[57] William Jones, *Memoirs of the life, ministry, and writings of the Rev. Rowland Hill* (London, 1834), pp. 353–4.

[58] *GM*, 76 (1806), 27–8.   [59] Baron, *Life*, 1, p. 304n.

[60] *The works of Anna Lætitia Barbauld*, 2 vols. (London, 1825), 2, pp. 118–19.

polite society. In a succinct address commending the practice in 1799, Henry Jenner hit the right buttons, presenting cows as 'the most cleanly of our domestic animals', making reference to the healthiness of dairy maids and the alleged 'salubrious effects' of the cow's breath, noting the wholesomeness of milk and even suggesting that cheese 'may very frequently contain a sufficient quantity of vaccine matter for the inoculation of thousands'.[61] In his *Observations on the cow-pock*, Dr Lettsom specifically addresses writers, pastors, parents and mothers. Expressing regret that 'his friend' Dr Moseley had complained about 'cow-mania', he humorously presents himself as a panegyrist of the cow, waxing lyrical about the animal 'whose lactarious fountains afford in our infancy a substitute for that of our parent and from which we draw, through life, a considerable portion of our nutriment' and which is now destined 'to protect the [human] species from the most loathsome and noxious disease to which it is subjected'.[62]

Women of all classes played a prominent part in appraising and promoting the new prophylaxis.[63] According to Jenner, the first person of rank 'who broke through the chains of prejudice' to have her child vaccinated was Lady Frances Morton, later Lady Ducie.[64] In 1800, Selina Mills, wife of Zachary Macaulay, informed her husband, that she was 'rationally convinced' of the value of cowpox. In 1802, Elizabeth Fry likewise researched the practice herself before deciding on vaccinating her firstborn.[65] Older women took the trouble to inform themselves of the new prophylaxis and pass on what they learned to their daughters and daughters-in-law. In March 1802, Lady Jerningham told her daughter that as cowpox was 'in universal practice' and was receiving general professional sanction 'I give up my first prejudice against it and hope that it is a blessing Almighty God has permitted shall be now discovered'.[66] A significant number of women took up the practice themselves. Mrs Bayley of Hope Hall, one of a number of women active around Manchester, vaccinated some 2,500 people and offered 5s. to any of them who subsequently caught smallpox.[67] In reporting on female activism,

---

[61] Henry Jenner, *An address to the public on the advantages of vaccine inoculation: with the objections to it refuted* (Bristol, 1799). pp. 6–7.

[62] Lettsom, *Observations*, p. 2.

[63] Michael Bennett, 'Jenner's ladies: women and vaccination against smallpox in early nineteenth-century Britain', *History*, 93 (2008), 497–513.

[64] Baron, *Life*, 1, p. 304n.

[65] [Margaret Jean Trevelyan], Viscountess Knutsford, *Life and letters of Zachary Macaulay* (London, 1900), p. 247; Journal of Elizabeth Fry, 3 November 1801: Additional MS. 47456, f. 132 v. BL.

[66] *The Jerningham Letters (1780–1843), being excerpts from the correspondence and diaries of the Honourable Lady Jerningham and of her daughter Lady Bedingfield*, 2 vols. (1896), 1, p. 240.

[67] Baron, *Life*, 2, pp. 100–1.

John Ring wondered facetiously whether 'the Lancashire witches' might 'kill more by their charms, than they save by their practice', but expressed the hope that, if his male colleagues declined to offer free vaccination to the poor, 'the ladies will everywhere rise in a mass, and repel that rude invader of the health, peace and happiness of mankind, the small-pox'.[68] Jenner was more positive in his encouragement and commendation of women to take up the lancet, beginning with Lady Peyton, his wife's sister-in-law. Mrs Lefroy, Jane Austen's mentor, took up vaccination in her last years and, before her death in 1804, 'communicated the important benefits of vaccine inoculation to upwards of 800 with her own hand'.[69]

Aristocrats, businessmen and even men of more modest means saw it in their interest or found a vocation in actively assisting the vaccination cause. The Earl of Egremont sponsored a general cowpox inoculation on his estates in Sussex in autumn 1799. After meeting Jenner in Cheltenham in spring 1800, William Fermor, a wealthy landowner 'addicted, not to fashionable pleasures, but to philosophical pursuits, and actuated by motives of humanity', organised a large-scale trial of vaccination on his estates in Oxfordshire and Buckinghamshire and published the results to promote the practice more widely.[70] The Earl of Lonsdale, who had not hitherto sponsored general inoculations because of the danger of infecting people who did not wish to be inoculated, was keen to offer vaccination to his servants, tenant farmers and the workers in the linen mills he had established in Westmorland. William Simmons of Manchester, who recognised its potential among slaves in the West Indies,[71] presumably also promoted its use in local cotton-mills. Since the beginnings of vaccination coincided with a period of dearth and unemployment among working people, its promotion by gentry and businessmen may have sometimes been viewed with suspicion. Though some radicals were hostile to vaccination, some actively promoted the cause. Dr James Currie, who helped to establish vaccination in Liverpool, was regarded as a British Jacobin. William Jaffray, a weaver of Cambusburn, near Stirling, was a member of the illegal Society of United Scotsmen. He took up smallpox inoculation in the spirit of universal brotherhood and, after experimenting on his son, enthusiastically embraced the new prophylaxis. Known as Citizen Jaffray, he vaccinated 13,000 children in his district prior to 1815. Tradition has it that he was then alarmed by the arrival of an official letter from London, expecting to be charged as a political agitator. The letter was from the National Vaccine Establishment advising him that he was

---

[68] Ring, *Treatise*, 1, pp. 262–3.   [69] *GM*, 74 (1804), p. 1178.
[70] William Fermor, *Reflections on the cow-pox* (Oxford, 1800), p. 3; Ring, *Treatise*, 1, p. 274.
[71] *MPJ*, 5 (January–June 1801), 137.

being awarded a silver cup in recognition of 'his exertions in promoting vaccination'.[72]

The armed forces were in the vanguard of vaccination. Most soldiers and sailors were smallpox-survivors, but efforts had traditionally been made to identify the non-immune and encourage variolation. For the army and navy, the potential of vaccination was not hard to see. Service men undergoing the old mode of inoculation needed to be relieved of their duties and to be quarantined during the infective stage. The 'grand old Duke of York', commander-in-chief of the British army, showed leadership in introducing cowpox in the regiments under his direct command and invited Jenner to Colchester in spring 1800 to oversee the vaccination of men still susceptible to smallpox.[73] To the frustration of Jenner's admirers in the senior service, the royal navy moved more slowly. In September 1800, the Admiralty finally issued a general order approving voluntary vaccination and, in the following month, sailors in the Mediterranean Fleet were being offered the new procedure. By this time, Dr Trotter fumed, 'there [was] scarcely a village that has not shared its blessing'.[74] Admiral Nelson proved oddly indecisive in respect of cowpox. In writing to Emma Hamilton about immunising their daughter Horatia in 1801, he observed that one of his colleagues spoke well of cowpox but left the choice of prophylaxis to her. Accepting the advice of Dr Moseley, Emma opted for variolation and Horatia suffered greatly.[75]

Royal and aristocratic support helped to make vaccination a national cause. The establishment of the Royal Jennerian Society (RJS), under the patronage of the royal family, set the seal of social approval on the new practice The Duke of Bedford, a leading Whig aristocrat, became president, but the twenty-two dukes, marquises, earls and viscounts named as sub-patrons came from across the political divide. Interestingly, the sub-patronesses were named ahead of the sub-patrons. They included four duchesses, four marchionesses, eleven countesses and two viscountesses.[76] While six of the twenty-one titled ladies were married to vice-patrons, fifteen of them were independently involved. Several of them, like the Duchess of Devonshire's daughter Georgiana ('Little G'), Countess of Carlisle, had infant children. The rank-and-file of the membership, of course, included statesmen, businessmen and churchmen as well as medical men. The RJS was well placed, on paper, to have oversight of vaccination and to champion it nationally. An early initiative was to approach the major churches to request their assistance

---

[72] *Chambers's Edinburgh Journal*, 4 (1836), 301–2; *Caledonian Mercury* (7 December 1815).

[73] Baron, *Life*, 1, pp. 379–81.

[74] C. Lloyd and J. L. S. Coulter, *Medicine and the navy 1200–1900. Vol. III. 1714–1815* (Edinburgh, 1961), p. 350.

[75] *Memoirs of Lady Hamilton* (New York, 1815), p. 157.   [76] *Address of RJS*, pp. 5–8.

in promoting vaccination.[77] In March 1803, Jenner was a member of a small group that waited on John Moore, Archbishop of Canterbury, asking him whether he might instruct the parish clergy to commend the practice from the pulpit and hand out leaflets to parents arranging the baptism of their children. While the Archbishop expressed his support for 'the great and benevolent object' in view, he regarded it as improper to address the clergy on behalf of a private society. The Presbyterians, Congregationalists and the Baptists took a similar line.[78] Since the churches had no objection to ministers being approaching individually, the RJS printed and distributed, through informal channels, 5,000 copies of the Rev. Warren's *Address on vaccine inoculation*.[79] In practice, the RJS's core business was to offer free vaccination in London, promote vaccination nationally and have oversight of the reputation of the practice, investigating claims of mishaps and failures. Despite its distinguished patronage, it was poorly funded for 'a national undertaking'. At the third anniversary meeting in 1805, Benjamin Travers, the acting chairman, saw the need for a clearer vision. In a business-like speech, he drew attention to the vaccination societies formed in France and elsewhere and reminded the gathering of the RJS of its national remit, 'that everyone who wished well to his country ought to step forward in its support; that, if an increase of children was a nation's strength, an axiom never to be forgotten, the rescue of children from an untimely grave produced the same effect, and was entitled to the same support!'[80]

Vaccination under Siege: Cowpox Controversies

After a hesitant start, vaccination prospered in the first years of the new century. The establishment of the practice in Britain and its spread through Europe and across the Atlantic were well underway by the time of the Truce of Amiens, when the magnitude of its progress became more evident. Dr Ash reported the 'reception' of 'highly favourable' opinions of vaccination in Europe to the parliamentary committee assessing Jenner's claim for reward and Dr Marshall returned from his vaccine expedition to Naples just in time to testify on Jenner's behalf.[81] During the truce, thousands of Britons, unable to visit France for a decade, flocked to see the sights of Paris. Dr Marshall was among them, seeking to establish himself in practice in the French capital. He was joined by the Rev. George Jenner and the pair met with the French society promoting vaccination. At a celebratory dinner toasts were drunk to 'the immortal Jenner', whose portrait was adorned with laurels.[82] One English

[77] Minutes of the Board of Directors of the RJS, MS. 4302, pp. 61–80, 95–6, WLL.
[78] MS. 4302, pp. 106, 114–15, WLL.   [79] MS. 4302, p. 84, WLL.   [80] *GM*, 75 (1805), 524–5.
[81] *Evidence*, ed. Jenner, pp. 7–8, 63–9.   [82] Baron, *Life*, 1, p. 526.

visitor reported seeing Jenner's nephew vaccinating from the window of the house in which he was staying.[83] No one expected the truce to last for long. By May 1803, Britain and France were back at war and, over the next two years, a large French army was poised to invade England. Against the background of the larger conflict, which would last until 1814–15, Jenner found himself fighting to defend the cause of vaccination against popular ignorance and apathy, the growth of anti-vaccination sentiment and debates and divisions in his own ranks. In London, the heart of the British empire and cowpox's first colony, vaccination was under siege.

It was perhaps inevitable that London would see vaccination's first major stumble. Its practitioners were often unable to find reliable cowpox or recognise a true vaccine response, and the circulation of contaminated and 'spurious' matter in the city was the source of many mishaps. Londoners were familiar with smallpox, knew the risks of variolation, and had been prepared to take them. They were rightly angry when, after being assured their children were secure, they took the infection. For some, too, the inoculation of animal disease inspired a natural repugnance. Dr Moseley's warnings about 'introducing the bestial humour into the human frame' added to the anxieties of parents who were disposed to attribute to cowpox any severe reactions to the procedure or any subsequent illness. John Ring recounted the story of a woman who complained that her recently vaccinated daughter 'coughs like a cow' and is 'grown hairy all over her body'.[84] Published in June 1802, James Gillray's print, 'Cow-pock – or – the wonderful effects of the new inoculation!' presents a pompous physician inoculating cowpox as, around him, patients sprout horns, rough hair and tails.[85] An anonymous second print, simply entitled Vaccination, is decidedly more savage. It depicts Jenner, Pearson and Woodville shovelling children into the maw of a hybrid monster (see Figure 4.1).[86] Since it depicts a copy of the parliamentary grant sticking out of Jenner's pocket, it may also reflect some popular resentment at the government's rewarding him.

In the first years of vaccination, Jenner and his colleagues could point to a decline in smallpox deaths in London and present the practitioners who continued to offer smallpox inoculation as being supine or mercenary.[87] In the campaign against smallpox, London was a crucial battle ground, not just symbolically but because, in Jenner's words, 'the metropolis is the very focus of the infection' and 'destroying the disease' there was crucial in limiting its spread through the country.[88] The RJS offered the prospect of setting the

[83] William Gardiner, Music and friends: or pleasant recollections of a dilettante, 3 vols. (London, 1838, 1853), 1, p. 268n.
[84] Ring, Treatise, 1, p. 83.   [85] Satires 9924, BM.   [86] Satires 9925, BM.
[87] Letters of Jenner, ed. Miller, pp. 16, 18.   [88] Letters of Jenner, ed. Miller, pp. 19–20.

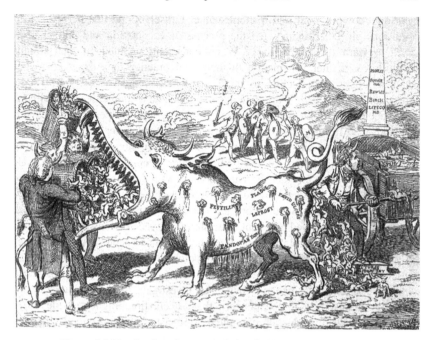

Figure 4.1 Vaccination. A monster being fed baskets of infants and excreting
them with horns; symbolising vaccination and its effects. Etching by
C. Williams, 1805
(Wellcome Collections)

practice on a firm foundation in the capital. Dr John Walker, its first resident
inoculator, was energetic in the cause. The twelve vaccine stations, some
located in chapels and mission halls, and posters advertising vaccination gave
the RJS visibility.   Dr Pearson's Institute, now denominated the Original
Vaccine Institute, was likewise active in vaccinating in the city and supplying
vaccine to country practitioners. Even as the new prophylaxis appeared to be
established on a firmer institutional footing, however, smallpox returned in
virulent form to London and environs in 1804–5. The number of smallpox
deaths, which had fallen in previous years, rose alarmingly. Jenner raged
against the inoculators whose trade in the city was increasing the contagion.[89]

If most vaccinated people escaped smallpox, some did not. In alleged cases
of smallpox after vaccination, medical men often found that the disease was
not smallpox or that a complete vaccination had not taken place, a common
problem when many practitioners lacked expertise and the circulation of

---

[89] R. J. Colyer, 'A letter of Edward Jenner (1749–1823)', *MH*, 21 (1977), 88–9.

'spurious' cowpox confused matters. Jenner himself found that herpetic skin conditions on patients disrupted the process of vaccination and published a paper to warn his colleagues.[90] When conscientious medical men found smallpox cases after vaccination in their own practice they expected to be taken seriously. In a lecture to the Portsmouth Medical Society in 1804, subsequently published, William Goldson documented eight cases of smallpox after vaccination. John Ring published a lengthy and vituperative attack on Goldson, who in turn crafted a careful and cogent rejoinder.[91] Neither could prove, in retrospect, that the cases in question were smallpox, and that, if they were smallpox, they had followed a complete vaccination. Many impartial observers, however, felt that the champions of vaccination were too hasty to slap down anyone who raised doubts. Dr Pearson seized the opportunity to take the moral high ground. From the outset, his institute had labelled the vaccine it had distributed and kept a register of its vaccinations. In November 1804, it contacted some 250 parents whose children had been vaccinated in the early years to allow them to participate in a clinical trial. All the sixty children participating were found to be insusceptible to smallpox.[92] The medical committee of the RJS likewise began to investigate alleged failures more carefully. In response to the concern that vaccination might provide only temporary protection, Jenner continued to insist that it provided lifetime security. In addition to collecting reports of cases of smallpox after variolation, he began to see the need to clarify his position in a crucial respect, increasingly taking the line that cowpox provided no less security from smallpox infection as smallpox itself.[93]

In 1805, Jenner came to London to attend the anniversary dinner and discuss with supporters what could be done to advance the cause. There was outrage in vaccination circles that the Smallpox and Inoculation Hospital had, in response to popular demand, resumed offering smallpox inoculation. Obliged to offer smallpox to out-patients, Dr Adams, Dr Woodville's successor, had managed, through selection, to produce a relatively mild strain of smallpox that took on the gentler aspect of cowpox.[94] This initiative, interesting from a scientific point of view, appeased neither the vaccination lobby nor the parents who wanted their children to be inoculated with smallpox. Jenner wrote to one of the governors at the Hospital expressing his hope that the 'mischievous practice' would be discontinued and that Parliament would give 'its sanction

[90] Edward Jenner, 'On the effects of cutaneous eruptions on modifications of the vaccine vesicle', *MPJ*, 12 (July–December 1804), 97–102.

[91] Fisher, *Jenner*, pp. 158–9.   [92] Willan, *Vaccine Inoculation*, p. 17.

[93] Baron, *Life*, 2, p. 342.

[94] Joseph Adams, *A popular view of the vaccine inoculation, with the mode of conducting it, shewing the analogy between the small pox and cow pox, and the advantages of the latter* (London, 1807); Baxby, *Jenner's vaccine*, pp. 150–2.

to a plan for staying this horrid pestilence in our country'.[95] Though the vast majority of vaccinated children continued to resist smallpox, the scale of vaccination since 1800 meant that the number of reports of mishaps and failures continued to rise. The members of the medical committee of the RJS found themselves busy in investigating claims that threatened to erode confidence in the practice. At the Original Vaccine Institute, Pearson continued to pursue opportunities to upstage the Jennerians. After Jenner left London in early August, Pearson contacted the Dorset farmer, Benjamin Jesty, who had inoculated his family with cowpox in 1774 and paid for him and his son Robert to come to London. In early September, the institute inoculated the son with smallpox, found him insusceptible of infection, and issued a testimonial to the 'antivariolous efficacy' of cowpox after thirty-one years. Farmer Jesty sat for his portrait at the institute's expense and was fêted as the true pioneer of cowpox inoculation.[96]

Anti-vaccination was becoming a significant force in London. Early in 1805, Benjamin Moseley returned to the fray. In a new book he presented cowpox as a dangerous disease, '*lues bovilla*' or bovine syphilis, reporting cases in which vaccination had been followed by serious illness. The publication elicited reports of further cases, almost all doubtful, that he included in a second edition. He denounced cowpox inoculation as 'a medical experiment, commenced without due discrimination, extended by a rash transgression over the bounds of reason, and, after the fullest conviction of its inutility, obstinately continued by the most degrading relapse of philosophy that ever disgraced the civilized world'.[97] Under the pseudonym 'R. Squirrell, MD', John Gale Jones, an apothecary and political radical, published a work arguing that the old method of inoculation was largely problem-free and wholly effective and that inoculated cowpox was scrofula.[98] The authors of a third tract, presenting themselves as surgeons at St Thomas's Hospital, presented more alleged problems, including three cases in which patients had died following septicemia at the vaccination site and the case of a baby who developed large purple nodules on her forehead within a year of vaccination.[99] In a fourth book, Dr William Rowley detailed 128 cases in which vaccination failed to prevent smallpox or had an adverse impact of the child's health. A subsequent edition added significantly to the number. The most

---

[95] Colyer, 'Letter of Jenner', 88–9.
[96] *Philosophical Magazine*, 22 (June–September 1805), 282–3, 367–8.
[97] Notices of Benjamin Moseley, *Treatise on the lues bovilla, or cow-pox* (1805), first and second editions in *GM*, 75 (1805), 152, 555.
[98] R. Squirrell [John Gale Jones], *Observations addressed to the public in general on the cow-pox* (London, 1805).
[99] [W. R. Rogers], *An examination of that part of the evidence relative to cow-pox, which was delivered to the committee of the House of Commons*, 2nd ed. (London, 1805).

striking feature of the work was its inclusion of engravings of an 'ox-faced boy' and a 'mange girl', whose sufferings were attributed, on no clear grounds, to vaccination.[100]

The opponents of vaccination took the battle to the streets. Handbills published in the name of the 'anti-vaccinarian society' were posted in every urinal in the city.[101] Many parents became insistent in their demand for the old prophylaxis. At the Smallpox and Inoculation Hospital, Dr Adams abandoned his experiment in attenuating smallpox because anti-vaccinists 'excited so great a clamour, that every mother was suspicious lest her child should be clandestinely inoculated with the cow-pox' and had to be satisfied that her children had 'unequivocal symptoms of small-pox'.[102] Fear of bestialisation was not the major concern. Many mothers were simply seeking security in a medical marketplace in which bluff, bluster and blatant mendacity were all too common. Some of them had considerable expertise in diagnosing childhood ailments. When Dr Pearson inspected two children who caught smallpox after vaccination, their mother, Mrs Gould, told him 'that both children, as far as she could observe, were alike affected with cow-pock, and that matter was taken from each of them at the hospital'. When Pearson's colleagues expressed the view that the pustules on the second child suggested chickenpox, she insisted that 'the child had already gone through chickenpox since the cow-pock'.[103] Sophia Vantandillo, who ran a fruit stall to support her family in Paddington, made informed decisions about prophylaxis. She had her first child and four others vaccinated, all of whom suffered eruptions, tumours and swellings. Since her second child had been inoculated with smallpox without mishap, she resolved in 1814 to have her sixth immunised in the old mode.[104]

By autumn 1805 the anti-vaccination forces were exultant. Daniel Sutton, the veteran inoculator, hailed Dr Moseley for his 'early, open, and manly attitude' in the struggle against cowpox and congratulated him 'on the prospect of [his] Herculean labours being at an end'. In response, Moseley called to mind his 'first three campaigns' against the 'cow poxers' and declared that, even though 'the press, at the commencement, was so cow pox mad', he 'knew that time would bring them to justice.'[105] In early December, he replied to another admirer: 'I believe I can flatter myself, that I stopped the progress

---

[100] William Rowley, *Cow-pox inoculation, no security against small-pox infection* (London, 1805).

[101] Robert John Thornton, *Vaccinæ vindicia: or, defence of vaccination* ... (London, 1806), p. 161.

[102] Adams, *Popular view*, esp. 28–36, at 34.

[103] John Thomson, *Historical sketch of the opinions of medical men respecting the varieties and the secondary occurrence of small-pox* (London, 1822), pp. 187–8.

[104] KB 1/399/1/1/34, TNA.   [105] *GM*, 75 (July–December 1805), 898–901.

of the widely-spreading calamity; and, by giving the world warning against its mischiefs, created a pause in the public mind'.[106] Over winter 1805–6, the opponents of vaccination maintained their offensive. Dr Rowley saw through the press another edition 'with above 500 proofs of failure' before his death in March 1806.[107] Public confidence in vaccination in London was badly dented. At one vaccine station, demand for the new prophylaxis dropped away completely. At the Smallpox and Inoculation Hospital, some 2,338 people opted for varolation in 1805. As the number of smallpox deaths rose from 622 in 1804 to 1,685 in 1805, Jenner and his allies declared that Moseley, Rowley and their associates had blood on their hands. In October, a 'senior physician', probably Dr Lettsom, estimated that in London 'one child is killed by smallpox every three hours, reckoning day and night, and these murders go unpunished!'[108]

The larger sense of Britain at bay added some intensity to the debate over smallpox prophylaxis. Between 1803 and 1805 Britain had every reason to fear and steel itself against invasion by Napoleon's formidable military machine. The mobilisation of the nation, the close attention to reports of campaigns and battles and the militarisation of British culture encouraged the increasing use of military metaphors in relation to smallpox prevention and the vaccination debate. In congratulating Richard Dunning, a naval surgeon, for his rejoinder to Goldson's pamphlet, Jenner wrote: 'It affords me pleasure to see with what alacrity my troops fly to arms, and rally around me at the approach of an enemy'.[109] In October 1804 he joshed again with Dunning: 'Vaccination calls imperiously for my attention, and to that … all my other worldly concerns shall yield. But while I am fighting the enemy of mankind, it will be vexatious to see my aides-de-camp turn shy'. He then chided his friend because on one matter he 'almost [gives] up the field to the anti-vaccinists'.[110] As the debate heated up between the rival camps in 1805, military metaphors and bellicose language abounded. In a pro-vaccination tract, 'Aculeus' mockingly describes Dr Rowley as 'a true hero, who rallies his vanquishing troops' against the advance of the 'Jennerian forces', and as 'the Commander-in-Chief', who leads resistance to the 'Vaccinating invaders'.[111]

---

[106] *GM*, 76 (January–June 1806), 25–7.
[107] *Monthly Review*, 52 (January–April 1807), 103–5.
[108] *MPJ*, 14 (July–December 1805), 509–10.   [109] Baron, *Life*, 2, pp. 338–9.
[110] Baron, *Life*, 2, pp. 340–4.
[111] 'Aculeus', *Letters to Dr. Rowley, on his late pamphlet entitled 'Cow-pox inoculation, no security against small-pox infection'* (London, 1805), pp. 9, 26–7. For a not wholly persuasive suggestion that Jenner was the author, see Rob Boddice, *Edward Jenner* (Stroud, 2015), pp. 71–3.

Vindications and Vexations

The victory at Trafalgar in October 1805 secured Britain from the threat of invasion, but Admiral Nelson's death brought national mourning. In January 1806, hundreds of thousands lined the streets to pay their respects as Nelson's body was brought by barge to Whitehall and through London to St Paul's. Aware that 401 children had died of smallpox in the previous month,[112] Dr Lettsom must have observed the concourse with some anxiety. From the frontline of the war against smallpox, he wrote to a friend in December: 'I have now under observation, a young woman, who will be lame through life', and two children with smallpox pustules pushing eyes out of their sockets, with one 'blind in both eyes, with a face so disfigured, as scarcely to resemble the human'.[113] As a Quaker physician, he would have regarded the commemoration of Nelson as a 'perfect English hero' with ambivalence. In earlier praising Jenner, he had referred to the 'high honours' accorded to heroes 'who have desolated provinces by the destruction of their fellow creatures', but stressed that Jenner's altar 'is not consecrated by hecatombs of the slain' but by his arresting 'the arm that scatters pestilence and death over the creation!'[114] The terms in which Nelson was described – 'a man whose exalted merit was only equalled by his retreating simplicity, a simplicity so without any visible promise ... that the hero was unknown till seen in his acts, and then, by his unequalled modesty ... considering himself, in his best successes, as an humble instrument of his God' – may have seemed to Lettsom more justly applicable to Jenner.[115]

If Trafalgar secured British mastery of the sea, the battle of Austerlitz several months earlier entrenched French dominance in Europe, setting the stage for a decade-long war of attrition. In the war against smallpox, vaccination's progress in Britain and overseas was matched by a significant reverse in its heartland. As he signed off on a second edition of his work on smallpox mortality in London on the last day of 1805, contemplating the three-fold increase on the previous year, Lettsom could do no more than stress, reasonably but hardly resoundingly, how much greater the loss of life would have been without the new prophylaxis.[116] The struggle against the opponents of vaccination continued. If the anti-vaccinists never looked like prevailing among the educated classes, there was some danger that the assault on its reputation in London would encourage apathy and prejudice in the provinces. In Leicester, 'the windows of booksellers were reportedly filled with pictures

---

[112] Lettsom, *Expositions* (2nd ed.), p. 19.   [113] *Letters of Jenner*, ed. Miller, p. 122.
[114] Lettsom, *Observations*, p. 8.   [115] *Monthly Mirror*, 21 (1806), 69.
[116] Lettsom, *Hints respecting cow-pock*, p. 8; Lettsom, *Expositions* (2nd ed.), pp. 17–19.

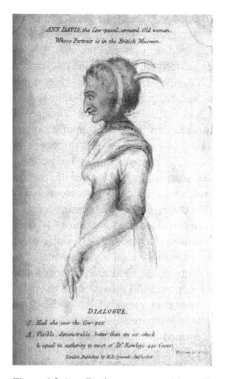

Figure 4.2 Ann Davis, a woman with smallpox and horns growing out of her head. Stipple engraving by T. Woolnoth, 1806
(Wellcome Collections)

of men and women with horns growing out of their heads' (see Figure 4.2).[117] Anti-vaccinist sentiment even found expression in Cheltenham. According to William Perry, the print of the ox-faced boy so alarmed the townspeople that many would rather 'see their children perish by the small pox as risk (as they suppose) their being transformed into beasts by the vaccine inoculation'.[118] Seeking to remain above the fray, Jenner urged his allies to take up their pens. In February 1806, he congratulated the *Monthly Review* on its critique of the tracts of 'that mad animal M[oseley]', and in autumn was delighted to see the 'complete overthrow' of the anti-vaccinists in the *Edinburgh Review*.[119]

The stresses of the time, however, took their toll on the vaccination lobby. Despite its exalted patronage, the RJS lacked the resources to deliver on its

---

[117] Gardiner, *Music and friends*, 3, p. 317.
[118] Vaccination Committee, Letters 71 and 94, MS. 2320, RCP.
[119] *Letters of Jenner*, ed. Miller, pp. 28–9, 31–2.

mission and was falling apart. Dr John Walker, the resident inoculator, was passionate about his work and, though his abrupt manner and brio with the lancet alarmed mothers at the vaccine stations, he evidently won their respect.[120] The problem was that he declined to follow the rules and guidelines that were necessary to defend the integrity of the practice. Over summer 1806, the RJS divided into factions over his performance. Following a move to dismiss him, Walker resigned and set up the London Vaccine Institution, leaching patients and patrons from the RJS. With the supporters of vaccination at cross purposes, confidence in the practice continued to decline in London and elsewhere through 1806–7. In the first editions of his popular *Medical Guide*, for example, Richard Reece had accepted the value of cowpox. Adding some reservations in 1805, he presented a decidedly negative assessment in the edition that he sent to press in December 1806.[121] The anti-vaccination party, however, was becoming increasingly strident and incoherent in its claims and assertions. John Birch raised eyebrows by asking, in print, 'why is it not remembered, that in the populous parts of the metropolis, where the abundance of children exceed the means of providing food and raiment for them, this pestilential disease is considered as a merciful provision on the part of Providence, to lessen the burden of a poor man's family?'[122]

During this time, developments in Parliament proved favourable to vaccination. The coalition government formed in 1806, the so-called Ministry of All the Talents, included Lord Henry Petty as Chancellor of the Exchequer, who was well-disposed to the new prophylaxis. Wishing for more to be done to support vaccination, but recognising that a necessary preliminary was the final settlement of all doubts about it, Petty proposed that the Royal College of Physicians be asked to conduct an enquiry into the current standing of the practice and report back to Parliament. Aware of Petty's interest, Dr Robert Willan, a leading authority on skin diseases, entered the field with a book endorsing vaccination's value as a preventative of smallpox and effectively refuting claims that it occasioned other skin diseases.[123] Over winter and spring 1806–7, a committee of the College canvassed the fellowship, received scores of submissions from Britain and overseas, and conducted a series of interviews, including with Jenner himself, John Birch, who exhibited prints of the 'ox-faced boy' and the 'mange girl', and old Daniel Sutton. Almost all the medical men who gave their views, many of whom provided details of their own and their colleagues' experience, attested the immense success of

---

[120] John Epps, *The Life of John Walker, M.D.* (London, 1831), pp. 119–23.
[121] Richard Reece, *The medical guide, for the use of families, young practitioners of medicine and surgery, being a complete system of modern domestic medicine*, 4th ed. (London, 1807), pp. 247–56.
[122] *Monthly Review*, 52 (January–April 1807), 103–5.   [123] Willan, *Vaccine inoculation*.

vaccination in England and overseas.[124] The College collated subsidiary reports from the College of Surgeons, a little cool in its approbation, and from the respective colleges in Dublin and Edinburgh, which were highly positive.[125] Intellectually sharp and not easily impressed by English fashions, the medical fraternity in Scotland provided the most impressive support, with the physicians finding evidence in favour of vaccination being 'so strong and decisive' that the fellows 'spontaneously and unanimously' elected Jenner as an honorary fellow.[126] European physicians found it hard to understand the need for an enquiry. As John Ring observed, Spain 'has carried the blessings of vaccination round the globe' before Britain 'has determined whether it is worthwhile to adopt the practice at home'.[127] In the final Report, published in April 1807, the College found that vaccination was 'in general perfectly safe' and that 'the security derived from vaccination against the small-pox, if not absolutely perfect, is as nearly so as can perhaps be expected from any human discovery'.[128] Based on a larger and more consistent body of opinion than had ever been 'collected upon any medical question', it was a resounding endorsement of the new prophylaxis.[129] In July 1807, Prime Minister Spencer Percival moved a motion in Parliament to make Jenner a further grant for his discovery, making it public and promoting vaccination. With only one dissenter, the members voted to grant Jenner, in addition to the £10,000 awarded in 1802, the princely sum of £20,000.[130]

In Britain, vaccination, vindicated in theory, continued to flounder in practice. The parliamentary endorsement and generosity to Jenner enraged the anti-vaccinists. Around this time John Gale Jones, alias 'Dr Squirrell', warned Jenner 'to immediately quit London, for there was no knowing what an enraged populace might do'.[131] In May 1808, a bill to curtail smallpox inoculation by requiring practitioners to hold a licence, notify the neighbourhood of inoculation activity and take steps to ensure that patients did not spread the infection failed in parliament, largely because it was seen as an infringement of people's rights. Rather than suppress variolation, the Parliament sought to provide solid support for vaccination. In 1808, it voted to fund a National Vaccine Establishment in London. Given the government's traditional reluctance to fund welfare provision, it was a remarkable innovation.

---

[124] Fisher, *Jenner*, pp. 180–1.
[125] 'Report of the Royal College of Physicians on vaccination ...', *MPJ*, 18 (July–December 1807), 97–111.
[126] 'Report of RCP', 105–6.   [127] *MPJ*, 17 (January–June 1807), 57.
[128] 'Report of RCP', 98.   [129] 'Report of RCP', 100.
[130] Charles Murray, *Debates in Parliament respecting the Jennerian discovery, including the late debate on the further grant of twenty thousand pounds to Dr Jenner* (London, 1808), pp. 55–135.
[131] Baron, *Life*, 2, pp. 367–8.

The title itself – one of the first uses of the term 'national' to describe an institution in Britain – reflects the spirit of the revolutionary age. It was proposed that the institute would be governed by a medical council, whose members would be nominated from and by the Royal Colleges, with Jenner as director. When the names of the council members and the vaccinators were announced early in 1809, Jenner was dismayed to learn that the position of principal vaccinator went not to his nominee, John Ring, but to an associate of Dr Pearson.[132] Recognising that the directorship was wholly honorary, Jenner promptly disassociated himself from the new institution. The key point was that the NVE was designed to supersede the rival vaccine societies and institutes as a national body, to assume an independent role in supporting best practice and investigating alleged failures, and to assure the progress of vaccination nationally. According to a later source, Lord Petty was frustrated by Jenner's stance, declaring that it 'was absurd for [him] to pretend' not to know that 'one of the objects of the establishment would be investigation', and that 'unless completely blinded by conceit, he must have recognised that the general faith in vaccination exhibited in 1801 had been much shaken by the experience of the succeeding seven years'.[133]

In truth, Jenner lacked the time and temperament to provide national leadership. He was strongly attached to his home and family in Berkeley, where his invalid wife and his eldest son, who died in 1810, were sources of anxiety. As he confessed to a colleague, he had a lifelong problem of alternating episodes of vitality and depression.[134] His condition cannot have been helped by the vicissitudes of fortune, with advances in the practice constantly followed by setbacks. After all the trials and reports, the proposition that vaccination was still on trial and needed impartial oversight exasperated him. He had a deep emotional investment in its reputation, seeing himself as having a providential role in bringing the prophylactic value of cowpox to light. Admirers around the world hailed him as 'immortal Jenner' and associated vaccination with his name.[135] Conversely, critics of the practice held him personally responsible for its alleged failings. William Howard, whose wife died of smallpox after vaccination, published an open letter in which he called on him to 'yield to conviction' about 'the direful effects of that disorder you have introduced among the human race'.[136] Although cases of secondary smallpox were being noted, the growing number of cases of smallpox after vaccination seemed increasingly less explicable as exceptions proving rules.

---

[132] Fisher, *Jenner*, p. 199.

[133] William White, *The story of a great delusion in a series of matter-of-fact chapters* (London, 1885), pp. 257–8.

[134] Jenner Letters, First Folder, no 23, History-Medicine Collections, Library, Duke University, Durham NC, USA.

[135] *Evidence*, ed. Jenner, pp. 7–8.   [136] *Morning Advertiser*, 17 March 1808.

In 1811, when Lord Robert Grosvenor became severely ill with smallpox, Jenner faced considerable embarrassment as he had vaccinated him ten years earlier. After consulting his notes, he found that he had not been entirely happy with the result of the vaccination. He pointed out, too, that Robert had been ill with whooping cough prior to coming down with smallpox; his elder brother, who had also been vaccinated by him, had not been infected; he had subsequently recovered fully; and, if vaccination had failed to provide absolute security, it had provided some protection.[137] In writing to a lady whose faith was shaken, Jenner advised her to take 'a comprehensive view' in which a case of this sort was 'a mere microscopic speck on the page which contains the history of the vaccine discovery'.[138] Still, the 'noise and confusion' arising from the Grosvenor case brought vaccination to a temporary halt. 'The vaccine lancet is sheathed; and the long concealed variolous blade ordered to come forth', Jenner wrote, 'The Town is a fool, – an idiot, and will continue in this red-hot, – hissing-hot state about this affair, till something else starts up to draw aside its attention', adding, 'I am determined to lock up my brains, and think no more *pro bono publico*.'[139]

---

[137] Baron, *Life*, 2, pp. 156–8.   [138] Baron, *Life*, 2, pp. 158–60.   [139] Baron, *Life*, 2, p. 161.

5   Vaccine Diaspora

Medical Networks in a World at War

After publishing his *Inquiry* in 1798, Jenner was probably disappointed by the lack of immediate interest in his work. Although it would be some time before he became aware of its wider reception, he would have been pleased to learn that it was soon finding a keen readership in continental Europe. Even before Dr Ingenhousz, resident in England, found time to read Jenner's work, a copy of the *Inquiry* was in the hands of Dr William Batt in Genoa. A graduate of Oxford and Montpellier, Batt was a prominent member of the medical and scientific fraternity in Genoa, connected by correspondence with physicians and scientists in Britain and western Europe. By September, he had formed a positive view of Jenner's thesis, was eager to make a trial of cowpox inoculation and wrote to Jenner for a sample of vaccine.[1] Around this time, too, a copy of the *Inquiry* was attracting interest in Geneva. Marc-Auguste Pictet, the editor of the *Bibliothèque britannique*, a journal reporting on British science and letters for the Francophone world, purchased a copy in London to pass on to Dr Louis Odier, an Edinburgh graduate and leading light among Geneva's more philosophically minded and socially engaged medical men. After announcing the cowpox discovery in Pictet's journal in October 1798, Odier contributed a full summary of the *Inquiry* in successive issues.[2] Like Batt, he sought an early opportunity to make a trial of the practice.

In the two years between Jenner's first experiment and the publication of the *Inquiry*, the war in Europe moved through several phases. French military success in the Low Countries, the Rhineland and Italy had delivered a body-blow to the ramshackle Holy Roman Empire in Germany and the dynastic empire of the Austrian Habsburgs. The treaty of Campo Formio in October 1797 confirmed French rule over Belgium, accepted French expansion to the Rhine and recognised the French client republics in northern Italy. In the following month, French delegates were invited to a meeting of the German princes at Rastatt in Baden to confirm the terms of the treaty and resolve

[1] William Batt, *Giustificazione dell'innesto della vaccina di Jenner* (Genoa, 1801), p. 6.
[2] *BB, S&A*, 9 (1798), 195–6, 258–84, 367–99.

related issues. Two German physicians, Dr Juncker and Dr Faust, sought an opportunity at Rastatt to present a scheme for the eradication of smallpox in Europe involving strict reporting, isolation of cases of inoculated as well as casual smallpox and quarantine. European collaboration in addressing the scourge was an alluring vision. Given the geo-political challenges facing the congress, it is unlikely that there was any formal discussion of the scheme. General Napoleon, who was keenly interested in smallpox prophylaxis, made only a fleeting appearance at Rastatt as he headed north to take command of the army massing at Boulogne for the invasion of England. In a sensational move, however, he shifted his focus from the English Channel to the Mediterranean, easing tensions in northwest Europe. Travel became easier and numerous copies of Jenner's *Inquiry* found their way to continental Europe. By late autumn 1798, it was being translated into French, and was also attracting attention in the German-speaking world. Only too aware of the impracticality of their scheme, Faust and Juncker were disposed to see the potential of cowpox. A copy of the *Inquiry* informed the first vaccinations in Vienna in May 1799. In the meantime, Napoleon's capture of Malta prompted a British focus on the western Mediterranean. In Genoa, Dr Batt may have owed his early receipt of Jenner's *Inquiry* to briefly improved lines of communication.

The idea of cowpox inoculation spread more rapidly than vaccine itself. After his experiments in spring 1798, Jenner himself lacked a supply of the elusive virus for over six months. Almost from the outset, vaccination depended almost entirely on cowpox propagated through the procedure itself. In 1799, Dr George Pearson, with access to the cowpox being propagated in London, led the way in the distribution of dried vaccine. Even in England, medical men found it a struggle to achieve success in vaccination, with the progress of the infection matching Jenner's depiction of the progress of the genuine vaccine vesicle. Often enough, the inoculation of the matter produced no or an equivocal response, with the latter being very problematic if success was wrongly assumed and the patient was given a false sense of security and the practitioner compounded the error by circulating 'spurious' cowpox. For doctors overseas, there was the greater challenge of achieving a vaccine response using dried vaccine that had been on the road for some time. The standard method for storing vaccine, as with smallpox matter for use in inoculation, was to run a cotton thread through the vesicle and to wrap the vaccine-imbued thread in paper. Vaccine, however, proved less durable than smallpox matter in both limpid or even dried form. The vaccine sent to Genoa in response to Dr Batt's request was over a year in transit and predictably useless on arrival. The intense diplomatic activity between Britain and Austria in spring 1799, with couriers making the journey in three weeks, helps to explain the remarkable circumstance that the first vaccine sent to Vienna proved serviceable.[3] As well as sending samples in profusion hoping for a lucky strike, medical men experimented with methods of packing samples of dried vaccine for transmission, including in corked vials or between glass plates sealed with wax. It was soon found, too, that a simple way of delivering fresh vaccine was to escort a child vaccinated in one town to a place where it was lacking. Familiarity with this arrangement made it easy to imagine, if difficult to organise, a system by which a series of people, vaccinated at intervals, could carry the virus over greater distances. As will be seen, the system was used on board ship in 1800 to deliver English cowpox to Gibraltar and Malta, with British sailors and soldiers serving in the vaccination chain. Early in 1801, it was put more systematically into service in Sicily and Naples, with children vaccinated in one town going arm-to-arm with children in the next.

Doctors without Borders

News of the cowpox discovery and samples of vaccine was carried through Europe by medical networks. Prior to 1798, Jenner himself had few connections on the continent. He was not a university graduate, knew no foreign languages and did not travel outside England. If his election as a Fellow of the Royal Society gave him opportunities for networking, he lacked the temperament and means to take them. Dr Pearson, an Edinburgh alumnus and London correspondent for the Edinburgh-based *Annals of Medicine*, was more confident in exploiting his contacts. Elite medical schools like Montpellier, Leiden, Vienna and Edinburgh drew students from across Europe. Literate in Latin and other European languages, the alumni of universities acquired friends and contacts that they maintained through travel and correspondence. Although it lacked a university, London had the population base, the hospitals, clinics, societies and lectures to draw medical men from northwest Europe and further afield. The Smallpox and Inoculation Hospital at St Pancras served for sixty years as a one-stop shop for the latest ideas about smallpox therapy, practical instruction in smallpox inoculation, and samples of smallpox matter. Among the European medical men visiting, studying or working in Britain, the Genevans were especially prominent.[4] As Protestants, they naturally looked to Leiden and Edinburgh for training and sought employment in northern Europe. The French-backed revolution in Geneva and its annexation by France in 1798 gave further stimulus to this diaspora. Dr Alexandre Marcet, a Genevan refugee resident in London, had a Europe-wide correspondence

---

[3] John Ehrman, *The Younger Pitt: the consuming struggle* (Stanford, CA, 1996), pp. 211–14.
[4] Bercé, *Chaudron et lancette*, pp. 16–20.

network. A friend of Jenner, he played a quiet but consequential role in the spread of cowpox inoculation.[5]

For medical men in continental Europe intrigued by Jenner's discovery, the interval between hearing about cowpox and obtaining a sample could be frustratingly long. From spring 1799, however, samples dispatched from England made possible trials of the practice in the Netherlands and Germany. A medical student in Leiden in 1798–9, John Walker, later resident inoculator of the RJS, brought cowpox to the attention of Dr Levie Davids of Rotterdam, obtained a sample of vaccine from Gloucestershire, and made a demonstration of the practice.[6] Curiously enough, however, the first successful vaccination in continental Europe took place in Vienna in late April 1799. The vaccine sent by Dr Marcet in London to his Genevan compatriot Dr Peschier had been taken from a patient in London as recently as 20 March. It is likely that it travelled by diplomatic courier.[7] In vaccinating two children of Dr Ferro, the government physician, Peschier was assisted by Dr Jean de Carro, another Genevan and an Edinburgh alumnus.[8] After inoculating his elder son with matter from one of Ferro's children on 11 May, De Carro wrote to Marcet, asking him to send a supply of cowpox and the latest publications on the new prophylaxis through the Foreign Office to the secretary of the British embassy.[9] On 20 May, amid some publicity, he inoculated his second son with lymph from his brother's arm. The arrival of a supply of vaccine from Marcet in autumn allowed him to resume his practice. Although the results were somewhat equivocal, he sent a sample to Dr Odier in Geneva, published an account of his experiments in the *Bibliothèque britannique*, and sent a positive report to Jenner, who, early in 1800, wrote to congratulate him on his achievement.[10] In Geneva, Odier and his colleagues failed to propagate the vaccine sent from Vienna, but finally succeeded with matter brought from London in June 1800.[11] Genevans were already playing a vital intermediary role in bringing vaccine to France. Early in 1800, J.-P. Colladon, a medical student, brought a sample from England that was used, unsuccessfully, in a trial in Paris at the Salpêtrière. A society established to promote the trial of the

---

[5] MS. 514, RSM; *Letters of Jean de Carro to Alexandre Marcet, 1794–1817*, ed. Henry E. Sigerist (Baltimore, MD, 1950).

[6] Epps, *Walker*, pp. 27–30, 106–7, 297; Willibrord Rutten, *'De vreselijkste aller harpijen'. Pokkenepidemieën en pokkenbestrijding in Nederland in de 18e en 19e eeuw* (t' Goy-Houten, Netherlands, 1997), p. 210.

[7] Jean de Carro, *Observations et expériences sur la vaccination* (Vienna, 1801), p. 67; Additional MS. 73,765, fos. 49r–56r, BL.

[8] De Carro acknowledged the value of his proficiency in English and connections in England: Jean de Carro, *Memoires du Chevalier Jean de Carro* (Carlsbad, 1855), pp. 10–11, 16–17.

[9] *Letters of de Carro*, ed. Sigerist, p. 30–1.

[10] BB, S&A, 13 (1799–1800), 112–16, 181–91, 315–16, 417–18.

[11] Gautier, *Médecine à Genève*, pp. 411–14.

practice in France funded another Genevan, Dr Aubert, to go to London to be instructed in the new prophylaxis and to obtain more vaccine.[12] After further failures, Aubert secured the assistance of Dr Woodville, who came to the French capital to introduce vaccination in the summer of 1800.[13]

The arrival of English cowpox in Paris ironically coincided with an escalation of the conflict between Britain and France. Deserting his army in Egypt, Napoleon returned to France to overthrow of the Directory and establish the Consulate through which he exercised increasing power. At the head of a new army, he crossed the Alps in winter 1799–1800 and reasserted control of Italy in a series of stunning victories. Fearing the collapse of the Second Coalition, the British government sought to counter French military dominance in Europe through its superior naval power, already demonstrated in Nelson's destruction of the French fleet in the Battle of the Nile. Britain planned to use its ascendancy in the Mediterranean in summer 1800 to dislodge the French from Malta and Egypt, secure the restoration of King Ferdinand and Queen Carolina to Naples and support Austrian attempts to recover its position in Italy.[14] Geo-political developments frame the early history of vaccination in the Mediterranean as well as in Austria. The couriers that carried cowpox from London to Vienna in spring 1799 also brought intelligence to Admiral Nelson, who was based at the Neapolitan court-in-exile in Palermo in the company of Emma Hamilton, the British ambassador's wife. Arthur Paget, who replaced Sir William Hamilton in spring 1800 and later showed himself to be a friend of vaccination, probably brought positive reports of the practice to Naples.[15] He may have been the impetus for the request for English cowpox. Full of ideas to reform and modernise the kingdom of the Two Sicilies, he believed nothing useful could be achieved except by the 'direct interference of foreigners'.[16] Given the build-up of Britain's armed forces in the Mediterranean theatre, the request for vaccine doubtless engaged the interest of government agencies as well as vaccination circles in London. If the mission to introduce vaccination to

---

[12] Darmon, *Longue traque*, p. 180.

[13] Elinor Meynell, 'Thomas Michael Nowell and his "matière de Boulogne": a neglected figure in the history of smallpox vacccination', *Journal of the Royal Society of Medicine*, 80 (1987), 232–8.

[14] J. W. Fortescue, *A history of the British army*, vol. 4, part 2, 1799–1801 (London, 1906), pp. 782–6.

[15] J. M. Rigg, 'Paget, Sir Arthur (1771–1840)', *Oxford Dictionary of National Biography*; Jean de Carro, *Histoire de la vaccination en Turquie, en Grèce, et aux Indes Orientales* (Vienna, 1804), pp. i, iii–iv.

[16] C. H. D. Giglioli, *Naples in 1799. An account of the revolution of 1799 and of the rise and fall of the Parthenonopean Republic* (London, 1903), pp. 383–5. For Paget's support of Marshall's work, see *Evidence*, ed. Jenner, p. 64; Ring, *Treatise*, 2, p. 677; Additional MS. 48,411, fos. 101r–102v, BL.

Naples was primarily private and philanthropic, it was facilitated by the royal navy and conducted under the sanction of the British government.

The Cowpox Odyssey

In July 1800 HMS *Endymion* set sail from Spithead, taking supplies, personnel and letters to Gibraltar, including instructions for Admiral Lord Keith and General Sir Ralph Abercromby. Among the passengers was Captain Philip Beaver, who was returning to service in the Mediterranean, and two physicians, Dr Joseph Head Marshall and Dr John Walker. Philanthropically inclined, Captain Beaver took an interest in the vaccine expedition and gave it material support in the following months. Dr Marshall had vaccinated on some scale in Gloucestershire in 1799 and his association with Jenner presumably gave him further credit among the men who organised the venture.[17] Dr Walker, whose wife was Marshall's cousin, volunteered to join him. He, too, had some experience with cowpox and had demonstrated the new prophylaxis in Rotterdam. The author of a popular textbook on geography, he relished the opportunity to extend his knowledge of the world and his narrative of his voyage, in the form of letters to his wife, is well observed and richly evocative.[18] A man of strong convictions, living as a Quaker, he undertook the mission of extending the blessings of cowpox somewhat in the spirit of a secular 'traveller under concern'. On his return, he was appointed as the Royal Jennerian Society's first resident vaccinator and dedicated his life, idealistically but not without controversy, to the cause of vaccination.[19]

Once at sea, Marshall and Walker looked for subjects for vaccination. Although they had samples of dried vaccine, they wished to increase the chances of the mission's success by propagating fresh lymph and maintaining it by serial vaccination. Beginning with a black sailor, they inoculated, a little over a week later, ten more sailors with lymph from his arm.[20] According to Walker, the sailors, 'so familiar with real dangers', shrunk from 'imaginary ones' and were hesitant about the procedure. He later admitted to qualms of conscience in winning their compliance by impugning their bravery and 'stirring up unworthy motives', but consoled himself with the thought that he had only done to them what he would have wished to have done to him. He and Captain Beaver experimentally inoculated themselves with cowpox. After

---

[17] Baron, *Life*, 1, pp. 324–6; Joseph Whitman Bailey, *The curious story of Dr Marshall, with a few side lights on Napoleon and other persons of consequence* (Cambridge, MA, 1930), pp. 10–13.

[18] John Walker, *Fragments of letters and other papers written in different parts of Europe, at sea, and on the Asiatic and African coasts or shores of the Mediterranean* (London, 1802).

[19] Epps, *Walker*, chs. 4–5, 12–13.   [20] Baron, *Life*, 1, p. 402.

a month at sea, on 9 August, the ship arrived in Gibraltar with a supply of fresh vaccine.[21] General Charles O'Hara, Governor of Gibraltar, authorised the offer of cowpox to members of the garrison and the infection followed the expected course: the symptoms were not exacerbated by the summer heat and the patients were able to continue 'their fatiguing duties' without special consideration.[22] Impressed by the new prophylaxis, the officers and medical men on Gibraltar established a vaccine institute, the first outside London, to support the practice. One practitioner professed an interest in making vaccine available in Spain and north Africa.[23]

Setting sail for Minorca three weeks later, the doctors again aimed to propagate fresh lymph by vaccinating a Spanish cabin boy. In Minorca, the British governor obtained permission from the local assembly for the vaccination of foundlings.[24] The examination of the first patients, however, raised doubts about the success of the procedure.[25] Marshall decided to return to Gibraltar to obtain a new supply of vaccine. Finding vaccination prospering there, he secured Admiral Keith's sanction to offer the procedure to the Fleet. On 19 October, Captain Beaver issued a memorandum encouraging soldiers and seaman who had not had smallpox to apply to Dr Marshall on the admiral's flagship, assuring them that the procedure was painless, required no preparation and excluded 'all possibility of the patient's ever being affected' with smallpox.[26] In the meantime, Walker pressed on to Malta, informing the authorities in Minorca of the uncertain results of the vaccinations and that his colleague was returning with fresh vaccine. He was anxious to forestall any claim that the British government had patronised 'a species of *charlatanerie* in place of a practice important to humanity'.[27] On his return to Minorca in November, Marshall conducted vaccinations that were entirely satisfactory and, in a public experiment, demonstrated the insusceptibility to smallpox of one of the patients by challenging him by variolation and exposure to a smallpox case. 'This trial so publicly made, and from which the little vaccinian came off triumphantly', he wrote, 'firmly established its character in Minorca' and 'everyone became anxious to participate in this most happy discovery, calling down blessings upon the head of its first promulger to the world'.[28]

On his arrival in Malta on 7 November, Walker found an earlier letter from Marshall, referring him to HMS *Regulus*, arriving from Gibraltar, on which there were men under vaccination. Going on board, Walker found,

[21] Captain's Journal, *HMS Endymion*, 1799–1801, ADM 15/1344, Part 8, TNA.
[22] Baron, *Life*, 1, p. 396.   [23] Walker, *Fragments*, p. 209.
[24] Walker, *Fragments*, pp. 251–2.   [25] *MPJ*, 12 (June–December 1804), 540–1.
[26] Baron, *Life*, 1, pp. 396–7.   [27] *MPJ*, 12 (June–December 1804), 540–1.
[28] Baron, *Life*, 1, p. 397.

'on the arm of a marine, the incipient vaccine pustule', from which he introduced 'the guardian affection among the Maltese'.[29] The formal inauguration of vaccination in Malta, however, took place after Marshall's arrival on 1 December. Captain Alexander Ball, Governor of Malta, was keen to ensure that the practice began auspiciously, and the first public vaccinations took place amid some ceremony. In 'going to the hospital we formed a small procession', Marshall wrote home, 'the Governor in his laced hat, the clergy in their canonicals, your friends Marshall and Walker, and the medical men bringing up their train'.[30] A week later Marshall demonstrated the insusceptibility to smallpox of the vaccinated children in the presence of the governor, the Tunisian ambassador, other notables and Malta's chief medical officers. Presenting the new prophylaxis as a blessing of British rule, Ball assigned Marshall and Walker a palatial residence, established a vaccination hospital under the name of the 'Jennerian Institution', funded a general vaccination and paid for the publication of a translation of Jenner's latest treatise.[31] With smallpox raging on Malta, hundreds of people accepted the new prophylaxis.

Back in Gibraltar, General Sir Ralph Abercromby received orders to sail eastwards, marshal British forces off the southern coast of Turkey, take on fresh provisions, and seek Turkish support to dislodge the French from Egypt.[32] Marshall and Walker saw the opportunity to expand their mission. It was decided that Marshall would complete the work in Malta and then proceed to Sicily and Naples, and that Walker would go east with the British expedition.[33] In a letter to Jenner in January 1801, Marshall reported on the progress of vaccination and the institute named in his honour in Valetta and informed him that he would be proceeding soon to Palermo and then Naples, 'at which places the introduction of the Jennerian inoculation is anxiously expected'.[34] For his part, Dr Walker had set sail, shortly before Christmas, with Captain Beaver on HMS *Foudroyant*, Nelson's old flagship, and soon found himself in the midst of the large British fleet assembling in Marmaris Bay. According to a report of Major-General Hutchinson, Walker oversaw a 'general vaccination of the army'.[35] Walker spent some time ashore, conducting some vaccinations in and around Marmaris. He later reminisced about 'his vaccinating mission up the Levant on the close of the past century'.[36]

---

[29] Walker, *Fragments*, pp. 170–1.   [30] *MPJ*, 5 (January–June 1801), 315–16.

[31] Paul Cassar, 'Edward Jenner and the introduction of vaccination in Malta', *MH*, 13 (1969), 68–70, plus figures.

[32] Fortescue, *British army*, 4, part 2, pp. 800–1.   [33] Walker, *Fragments*, p. 143.

[34] Baron, *Life*, 1, pp. 396–9, at 399.   [35] Walker, *Fragments*, p. 362.

[36] Epps, *Walker*, p. 112.

The New Prophylaxis in the Heart of Europe

For over a year De Carro's commitment to cowpox represented a triumph of hope over experience. In his experiments in Vienna, he was let down by the age and condition of the vaccine available to him and his own lack of expertise. He also found it hard to find patients willing to be inoculated with cowpox. By October 1799 he had completed only eleven vaccinations, most of which were probably unsuccessful.[37] He was then not able to vaccinate for some six months. Even after resuming the practice with new vaccine in April 1800, he met with only limited success. His first patient on 16 April was the son of a valet of the Princess of Monaco. His next ten patients, all in May, included the son of Count Mottet, the children of a banker, a Swiss entrepreneur and an English gentleman called Henry Smith.[38] He resumed the practice in September, this time with greater success. He added some seventy vaccinations to his tally by November. His eclectic clientele included the children of Countess Dembiska, a Polish noblewoman; the only son of Count de la Gardie, the Swedish ambassador; a French aristocrat about to return to France; Dr Moreschi from Venice; and the families of two Jewish merchants.[39] It was only shortly before Christmas, when he vaccinated some eightly children in the village of Brunn am Gebirge, south of Vienna, that De Carro extended his practice to a broader section of Austrian society. This opportunity was provided by a local clergyman, who promoted the new prophylaxis from the pulpit.[40] By March 1801, with a tally of 200 vaccinations, he could finally claim some mastery of the new prophylaxis.[41]

The faltering start in Vienna is hardly surprising. Even in England, the leading vaccinators only began to achieve a consistent level of success with the new prophylaxis during 1800. When Caroline Pichler, the celebrated Austrian poet, wished to immunise her baby in summer 1799, De Carro offered vaccination and lent her Jenner's treatise. Her physician was right to advise that the new practice was still experimental, and she had her daughter inoculated in the old mode.[42] The medical establishment in Vienna included some resolute conservatives. Dr Johann Stifft, the court physician, was struggling to hold the line against Brownism and other destabilising theories.[43] According to De Carro, Dr Ferro, who allowed his children to be inoculated with cowpox, sought to undermine him by preventing his

---

[37] De Carro, *Observations*, pp. 201–9.   [38] De Carro, *Observations*, pp. 209–15.
[39] De Carro, *Observations*, pp. 215–28.
[40] De Carro, *Observations*, pp. 231–5; *MPJ*, 5 (January–June 1801), p. 351.
[41] De Carro, *Observations*, pp. 235–42.
[42] Caroline Pichler, *Denkwürdigkeiten aus meinem Leben*, vol. 2, 1798 to 1813 (Vienna, 1844), pp. 8–9.
[43] Erna Lesky, *The Vienna Medical School of the nineteenth century* (Baltimore, 1976), pp. 4–12.

publicising the new prophylaxis. He likewise attributed the extension of the ban on smallpox inoculation in the city precincts to include cowpox inoculation to professional jealousy. Still, his representation of his colleagues was somewhat unfair. De Carro was an opportunist and self-publicist, making some effort to assure his own centrality in the new prophylaxis. He lamented the fact that, although the medical men of Vienna noted his experiments, none of them, apart from his colleague Dr Portenshlag, was prepared to take the practice up.[44] He resented being confused with Dr Luigi Careno, an Italian physician in Vienna, who prepared and published an influential Latin version of Jenner's *Inquiry* in September 1799.[45]

A major smallpox epidemic in Vienna in autumn 1800, in which 3,000 children died in three months, concentrated minds.[46] In October, De Carro informed Dr Pearson in London that the epidemic had brought 'a new lustre' to vaccination.[47] As he himself got into his stride with the new procedure, his anguish at the ban on cowpox inoculation, not lifted until early 1801, was real enough. De Carro recalled that one lady who brought three children from Hungary to avail herself of the new preventative was almost turned back at the city gates.[48] By spring 1801, vaccination began to win firm adherents among the medical fraternity. Dr Johann Peter Frank, professor of pathology at the University of Vienna and champion of social medicine, lent his support and Dr Ferro recommitted himself to the practice. De Carro wrote his own book on vaccination which was published both in French and in a German translation by his colleague Portenschlag.[49] In 1802 Dr Ferro, De Carro's old foe, likewise published a clear and succinct account of cowpox.[50] Reports of the success of vaccination in Britain and elsewhere strengthened its reputation locally. Colonel Meath, a British officer liaising with the Austrian army, brought early news of the Duke of York's vaccination of his regiments.[51] The Archduke Charles, the Austrian commander in chief, was keen to draft vaccine into service. In July 1801, he supported a clinical trial in which Dr Frank vaccinated patients in the General Hospital and, a month later, tested the procedure's effectiveness by challenging thirteen of them with smallpox. Advised of the success of the trial, the government commended the new prophylaxis and set in

---

[44] De Carro, *Memoires*, pp. 20–1.

[45] Edward Jenner, *Disquisitio de causis et effectibus variolarum vaccinarum*, transl. Aloysio Careno (Vienna, 1799).

[46] Pascal Joseph Ferro, *Über den Nutzen der Kuhpockeninfung* (Vienna, 1802), p. 6.

[47] *Philosophical Magazine*, 8 (July–December 1800), 305.

[48] *Letters of De Carro*, ed. Sigerist, p. 50. The lady may have been Madame de Dörry: De Carro, *Observations*, p. 238.

[49] De Carro, *Observations*; Joannes de Carro, *Beobachtungen und Erfahrungen über die Impfung der Kuhpocke*, transl. Joseph von Portenschlag (Vienna, 1802).

[50] Ferro, *Nutzen der Kuhpockeninfung*.   [51] *Letters of de Carro*, ed. Sigerist, p. 37.

train measures to generalise it in spring 1802.[52] With the massing of troops around Vienna, De Carro was asked to draft a plan for mass vaccination. In March 1803 copies of his book were issued to all army medical staff, and some 51,000 soldiers, half the number liable to infection, were vaccinated by September 1804.[53] The records reveal a remarkable drop in the annual number of smallpox deaths in Vienna from an average of 835 in the last decade of the eighteenth century to 164 in 1801, 61 in 1802, 27 in 1803 and, notwithstanding the military mobilisation, only 2 in 1804.[54]

De Carro could claim a larger achievement in the vaccination cause. In his letters, he reported his observations and experiments, commented on the latest literature, sought information about the new practice, passed on reports from his correspondents and generally promoted the cause. As his practice became more stable over the course of 1800, he played a considerable role in the extension of vaccination. He assisted Count Salm in introducing the new prophylaxis in Moravia and supplied information and vaccine to physicians in Bohemia and Hungary. After the government's endorsement in 1802, the new procedure gained support in most parts of the Austrian empire.[55] De Carro seeded the practice more widely in central Europe. Dr Friese of Breslau (Wrocław) used his vaccine to establish vaccination in Silesia. A Polish countess in exile in Vienna sent samples to Poland. De Carro's vaccination of the son of the Swedish ambassador and the daughter of Count Kaunitz, Austria's envoy to Denmark, raised the possibility that vaccine from Vienna would be the source for vaccination to Scandinavia.[56] Acknowledging his debt to De Carro, Dr Friese made Breslau a subsidiary node in the vaccination network and succeeded in sending viable vaccine to Moscow in autumn 1801. In addition to his role in central Europe, De Carro provided vaccine to the physicians who introduced the practice in Venice and the Adriatic and, most remarkably, supplied the vaccine first used in Istanbul in 1801 and in India in 1802.[57]

Despite its early attention to cowpox and receipt of samples from Vienna, Geneva was unable to obtain viable vaccine until June 1800. By this time, the groundwork for the new practice was well laid. After his summary translation of Jenner's *Inquiry*, Dr Louis Odier helped to make the *Bibliothèque britannique* a forum for reports of cowpox inoculation. In an early intervention, he declared his dissatisfaction with the term *la petite vérole des vâches*

---

[52] Heinz Flamm and Christian Vutuc, 'Geschichte der Pocken-Bekämpfung in Österreich', *Wiener klinische Wochenschrift*, 122 (2010), 265–75, at 267–8.

[53] 'Biographical account of Jean de Carro, MD', *Annals of Philosophy*, 10 (July–December 1817), 2; *The Times*, 6 September 1804.

[54] *Philosophical Magazine*, 23 (October 1805–January 1806), 371.

[55] Flamm and Vutuc, 'Pocken-Bekämpfung in Österreich', 267.

[56] De Carro, *Observations*, pp. 226, 242.   [57] See Chapter 10.

(smallpox of cows) and established the use of the term vaccine in the French-speaking world.[58] His experiments with the vaccine sent from Vienna, which turned out to be spurious cowpox (*faux vaccine*), introduced him to the challenges of the new prophylaxis, especially identifying a genuine vaccine response. Over summer, he oversaw the vaccination of 250 people and then confirmed their insusceptibility to smallpox by variolation.[59] Geneva rapidly became a major centre of vaccination and a trusted source of vaccine and advice in Switzerland, southeast France and northern Italy. Prior to approving the practice in France, the Minister of the Interior sought advice from Dr Odier. By their management and promotion of the practice, the Genevans impressed Jenner and his friends in England, who praised the role of the Genevan clergy in commending the procedure to parents presenting children for baptism.[60]

Italian Fronts

War and politics provided a volatile setting for the first arrival of vaccination in Italy. The French invasion of 1796 redrew the political map of the peninsula, with the establishment of the Cisalpine Republic centred on Milan, the defeat of an army raised in the south by Ferdinand, the Bourbon king of Naples and Sicily (the 'Two Sicilies'), led to the withdrawal of the royal to Sicily and revolution in Naples. Both the first Cisalpine Republic and the Parthenopean Republic in Naples proved short-lived. In April 1799, the Second Coalition restored Austrian rule in Milan and King Ferdinand, assisted by the British navy under Admiral Nelson, recovered Naples in May 1800. At this very time, however, Napoleon was restoring the Cisalpine Republic and consolidated French influence in the north in June 1800 by defeating the Allies at Marengo. No part of the Italian peninsula could resist the growing French hegemony. The smaller principalities and city-states found their constitutions remodelled and their identities occluded in an ever more explicitly imperial system. In 1802, the Cisalpine Republic became the core of an enlarged Italian Republic, under Napoleon's presidency, that was in turn transformed into the Napoleonic kingdom of Italy in 1805. The Republic of Venice saw its territory divided between French and Austrian spheres of influence and was then, in 1806, absorbed into the new kingdom. The Papal States, under French tutelage, were formally annexed in 1808. French expansion along the Adriatic coast made the Illyrian Provinces directly subject to metropolitan rule. After its conquest, the kingdom of Naples was set aside as an apanage for a Bonaparte prince or

---

[58] Gautier, *Médecine à Genève*, pp. 407–10.   [59] Gautier, *Médecine à Genève*, pp. 413–14.
[60] Gautier, *Médecine à Genève*, pp. 660–2.

general. Only Sicily remained outside the French empire, protected by the Strait of Messina and the British navy.

Physicians in Italy first heard about cowpox in the last quarter of 1798. After reading Jenner's treatise in Genoa, Dr Batt lent it to Dr Francesco Chiarenti in Florence.[61] In the second half of 1799, reports from Britain built interest in the new prophylaxis and the brief return of Austrian rule in northern Italy facilitated the circulation of Careno's Latin translation of the *Inquiry*. The British-backed restoration of the Bourbon regime in Naples raised the prospect that vaccine might first arrive in Italy in British ships. The progress of vaccination in Vienna and its establishment in Geneva in summer 1800 meant that it would be only a matter of a time before the new practice would commence with vaccine from the north. Professor Onofrio Scassi in Genoa is often accorded the honour of performing the first vaccination in Italy with vaccine from Geneva in April 1800.[62] This vaccine was spurious, however, and Scassi was not able to propagate it. The honour of the first successful vaccination can be assigned more confidently to Dr Alessandro Moreschi in Venice. Though he had had smallpox in his youth, he sought vaccination from De Carro in Vienna to gain experience of the procedure.[63] After being provided with some training and samples of vaccine, Moreschi inaugurated the practice in Venice, beginning 'with the children of people of the first rank' in the hope that their example would be emulated.[64] In December 1800, he vaccinated the fifteen-month-old son of Count and Countess Albrizzi in the presence of Dr Agliotti and many local notables.[65] A notable writer and saloniste, Isabella Teotochi, Countess Albrizzi, proved influential in her advocacy of the practice.[66] Early in 1801, her *nobile putello* was the source of vaccine for two other children and, over the course of January, many other children underwent the procedure.[67] In February, Moreschi published advice to the public on smallpox prevention and a translation of the plan of the Cowpox Institute in London.[68] The success of the new prophylaxis in Venice was widely noted. The authorities in Padua commissioned a report from Dr Fanzago, who recommended the adoption of the

---

[61] Batt, *Giustificazione dell'innesto della vaccina*, p. 6.

[62] Batt, *Giustificazione dell'innesto della vaccina*, p. 6; Vito Vitale, *Onofrio Scassi et la vita Genovese del suo tempo (1768–1836)* (Genoa, 1932), pp. 115–21; Bercé, *Chaudron et lancette*, p. 23.

[63] De Carro, *Observations*, p. 220.   [64] *MPJ*, 5 (January–June 1801), 352.

[65] Alessandro Moreschi, *Avviso al pubblico sull'antidoto, ossia preservativo del vajuolo* (Venice, 1801), p. 7.

[66] Adriano Favaro, *Isabella Teotochi Albrizzi: la sua vita, i suoi amori e i suoi viaggi* (Udine, 2003), p. 154; Susan Dalton, *Engendering the republic of letters: reconnecting public and private spheres in eighteenth-century Europe* (Montreal, 2004), p. 157.

[67] Franceso Fanzago, *Memoria storice e ragionata sopra l'innesto del vajuolo vaccino* (Padua, 1801), pp. 54–5.

[68] Moreschi, *Avviso*, pp. 56–69.

practice. Medical men in the Balkans likewise looked to Moreschi for vaccine, advice and inspiration.[69]

Napoleon's triumph at Marengo in 1800 added impetus to the extension of the new prophylaxis in Italy. Dr Michele Buniva, who had fled to France after the fall of the republican regime in Piedmont, took a close interest in vaccination during his exile, and on his return to Turin worked hard to make it available to his fellow-countrymen.[70] The most sensational development in vaccination in Italy, however, was the discovery of cowpox in Lombardy. Inspired by Careno's translation of Jenner's *Inquiry*, Dr Luigi Sacco began making enquiries about diseases among the cattle that grazed in the mountain valleys on the Swiss border.[71] On a visit to his hometown of Varese in autumn 1800, he found a cow in the market with a condition that matched Jenner's description. After monitoring the infection, he carefully took lymph from a ripe vesicle and, with some difficulty, found subjects willing to be inoculated with it in October.[72] It took him some time to convince himself that the procedure was a success.[73] The arrival of a sample of vaccine sourced from England subsequently gave him the chance to confirm that inoculation with English cowpox and the local cattle disease produced identical responses.[74] It was not until March 1801, however, that he had the chance to demonstrate the effectiveness of vaccination to the public at large. At the invitation of Luigi Lambertenghi, a former aristocrat with scientific interests, he used cowpox to suppress a smallpox outbreak in the district of Giussano, and then repeated the achievement, at the request of Citizen Zappa, in Sesto, not far from Milan.[75]

In Milan itself, Dr Sacco was beginning to attract attention. He was invited to vaccinate the children at the Foundling Hospital in December 1800.[76] His vaccination of the Visconti, Milan's most illustrious old regime family, was influential in some circles.[77] Seeking to promote vaccination as a public benefit, the government of the Cisalpine Republic provided critical support in its establishment. In April 1801 Sacco published *Osservazioni pratice sull'uso del vajuolo vaccine*, recording the names of colleagues already active

---

[69] Baron, *Life*, 1, p. 418.
[70] Dino Carpanetto, 'Buniva e il governo della sanità nel Piemonte Napoleonica', in Giuseppe Slaviero ed., *Michele Buniva introduttore della vaccinazione in Piemonte. Scienza e sanità tra rivoluzione e restaurazione* (Torino, 2002), pp. 27–72, at 35–6.
[71] Luigi Sacco, *Osservazioni pratiche sull'uso del vajuolo vaccino come preservativo del vajuolo humano* (Milan, 1801), pp. 20, 31–3, 60–4.
[72] Sacco, *Osservazioni*, pp. 60–4; Giuseppe Armocida and Ilaria Gorini, 'Nella Lombardia di Luigi Sacco', in *Il vaiolo e la vaccinazione in Italia*, ed. Antonio Tagarelli, Anna Piro and Walter Pasini, 4 vols. (Villa Verucchio, 2004), 2, pp. 673–97, at 683–5.
[73] Giuseppe Ferrario, *Vita ed opere del grande vaccinatore Italiano Dottore Luigi Sacco e sunto storico dello innesto del vajuolo umano del vaccino e della rivaccinazione* (Milan, 1858), pp. 16–17.
[74] Sacco, *Osservazioni*, pp 91–9.   [75] Sacco, *Osservazioni*, pp. 125–37.
[76] Armocida and Gorini, 'Nella Lombardia di Sacco', p. 685.   [77] Sacco, *Osservazioni*, p. 152.

in vaccination and outlining a plan for its generalisation in Lombardy.[78] In recognition of his leadership of the practice, the government appointed him director of vaccinations in the republic. In Piedmont, soon to be merged in the new Italian Republic, Michele Buniva was another strong champion of vaccination. After returning from Paris with a zeal for the new prophylaxis, he began vaccinating in Turin in November 1801 and proved very effective in establishing vaccination as a public health measure.[79] Still, Sacco retained his pre-eminence in Italy through his bold experimentation, his canny promotion of the new prophylaxis, his campaigns to introduce the practice in the countryside and his impressive personal tally of vaccinations. In a letter to Jenner in October 1801, informing him of his discovery of 'indigenous' virus, he claimed to have already vaccinated 8,000 people.[80] In July 1802, he told Dr Odier that, with 44,000 vaccinations, 14,000 of them by his own hand, 'vaccination in the Italian Republic cannot get any better'. He set great store on preparing for his campaigns, drafting proclamations to be issued by the government and enlisting local officials and priests to instruct people to attend his clinics. Reporting on the success of his recent mission in the department of Mella, centred on Brescia, he said that 'persuasion has spread like a firework show' and that 14,000 people had been vaccinated in just two months.[81]

In the meantime, a new front had opened in the war against smallpox in the Italian peninsula. After spending winter 1800–1 in Malta, Dr Marshall set sail in March for Palermo in Sicily. He was well prepared for the climax of his expedition, the introduction of vaccine in the Bourbon kingdom of the Two Sicilies. Like Dr Walker, who took lessons on the voyage out, Marshall probably gained some proficiency in Italian. He wrote, presumably with assistance, *Sul vaiuolo vaccinico* (On cowpox), and published it in Palermo in Sicily.[82] Welcomed by Arthur Paget, the British plenipotentiary, Marshall was presented to King Ferdinand, who established a hospital for vaccination and appointed Giovanni Vivencio, his chief physician, and Michele Troja, his surgeon, to assist Marshall and oversee the subsequent extension of the practice.[83] The first vaccinations on 14 March proved successful. A recent smallpox epidemic, in which 8,000 people died, inclined people to look favourably on the new prophylaxis.[84] 'It was not unusual', Marshall wrote,

[78] Sacco, *Osservazioni*, pp. 207–15.
[79] Carpanetto, 'Buniva e il governo della sanità', pp. 49–51.   [80] Baron, *Life*, 1, pp. 452–5.
[81] *BB, S&A*, 20 (May–August 1802), 398–405.
[82] John Chircop, '"Giusta la benefica intenzione del Re": the Bourbon vaccination campaign in Sicily', *Hygiea Internationalis. An Interdisciplinary Journal for the History of Public Health*, 9 (2010), 155–81, at 159, n. 11.
[83] Gaspare Rossi, *I manoscritti della Biblioteca comunale di Palermo* (Palermo, 1873), 384–5.
[84] *Evidence*, ed. Jenner, p. 66.

'to see in the mornings of the public inoculation at the Hospital a procession of men, women, and children, conducted through the streets by a priest carrying a cross, come to be inoculated'. He affirmed that 'the common people expressed themselves certain that it was a blessing sent from Heaven, though discovered by one heretic and practised by another'.[85] As well as vaccinating poor children at no charge, Marshall conducted experiments to test their subsequent insusceptibility to smallpox and provided instruction in the procedure to local medical men. Writing home in April, an English resident in Palermo attested the 'high reputation' of cowpox and noted its promotion from the pulpit. Interestingly, he also reported that Marshall took private patients, charging 'ten guineas in genteel families, and five in families of the middle class'.[86] Still in Palermo at the end of April, Marshall did not set out for Naples until King Ferdinand's own belated return in June 1800. He left the practice in Sicily in the capable hands of men like Dr Franceso Calcagni. Over the following three years, Calcagni was responsible for 2,754 of the 5,000 or so vaccinations, extending the new practice across the island by leading children vaccinated in one district to be put arm-to-arm with children in a neighbouring district. In 1804, he wrote a letter to the Marchioness of Spaccaforno, subsequently published, relating the history of cowpox inoculation and his own experience.[87]

The return of the Bourbon court to Naples in June 1801 lent drama to the arrival of vaccine in southern Italy. By no means popular with his war-weary subjects, King Ferdinand sought to project an image of regal beneficence. In an edict on 23 June, he declared that 'ever solicitous in all matters that could benefit his beloved subjects' he 'had interested himself in making available to the public the new method of smallpox inoculation discovered in England, with the greatest advantage to humanity'.[88] It was as if Ferdinand hoped that vaccination, made available by the 'King's charitable purpose', would inoculate his people against revolution. Dr Marshall began his work in Naples amid some ceremony. He may have been the source of the conceit, reported in England, associating Jennerian inoculation in Naples with the cult of San Gennaro, patron saint of Naples, on whose feast days a sacred vial containing his miracle-performing blood was displayed and assumed liquid form.[89] The medical faculty in Naples, however, comprised serious men of science.[90] Some

---

[85] Baron, *Life*, 1, p. 403.   [86] *MPJ*, 6 (July–December 1801), 95–6.

[87] Francesco Calcagni, *A letter on the inoculation of the vaccina, practised in Sicily* (Philadelphia, 1807), pp. 20, 28 and 35.

[88] Caterina Tisci, 'La vaccinazione antivaiolosa nel Regno di Napoli (1801–1809); il ruolo del clero', *Medicina e Storia*, 3 (2003), 89–117, at 91.

[89] Ring, *Treatise*, 2, pp. 809–10.

[90] Antonio Borrelli, 'Dall'innesto del vaiolo alla vaccinazione jenneriana: il dibattito scientifico napoletano', *Nuncius*, 12 (1997), 67–75.

took steps to assure themselves of the value of cowpox by conducting trials at the Foundling Hospital behind Marshall's back.[91] The extension of vaccination in the kingdom of Naples was entirely the work of local men and women. Michele Troja, who had observed Marshall's practice in Sicily, had the knowledge and experience to guide and reassure his colleagues. Dr Antonio Miglietta rapidly emerged as a powerhouse of the new prophylaxis. By the end of 1801, vaccination was firmly planted in the city of Naples and its hinterland. Five vaccine stations were established under the directorship of Troja and Miglietta in July 1802. To win over mothers to vaccination, midwives were given training and permitted to practice.[92]

Dr Marshall remained in Naples until the middle of November.[93] Appointed 'physician extraordinary' to King Ferdinand, and granted a gold medal on departure, he may have spent several months largely engaged in private practice. He later claimed that he had 'extended' the new inoculation to Rome, Leghorn [Livorno] and Geneva. Though there is no conclusive evidence, he may have demonstrated the practice in Rome or at least provided advice and vaccine to Cardinal Consalvi.[94] On his way home, he almost certainly called in at Livorno. A report that the vaccine used in the first trials in Siena was made available by a British admiral in Livorno may suggest that Marshall played some role there.[95] Marshall initially planned to travel home through Geneva. He was in Genoa with Dr Batt in mid-December, and in Turin at the end of the month, but severe weather prompted him to change his itinerary and entrust a packet that he intended to take to Geneva to a merchant.[96] Dr Marshall was in Paris on 26 January 1802, and back in London in late February, arriving in time to support Jenner's case for a parliamentary premium by appearing before the committee assessing his petition.[97] His subsequent life is shrouded in mystery. In May 1802, he took up residence in Paris. Though he established a medical practice there, he had other irons in the fire. During Napoleon's Hundred Days, he undertook clandestine missions between Naples, France and Britain.[98]

---

[91] *MPJ*, 8 (July–December 1802), 23.

[92] Tisci, 'La vaccinazione antivaiolosa', 92; Caterina Tisci, 'Le levatrici e la diffusione della vaccinazione antivaiolosa nel Regno di Napoli', *Revista Internacional de Culturas & Literaturas*, 3 (2005), 37–41.

[93] *BB, S&A*, 19 (January–April 1802), 73–4.

[94] *Evidence*, ed. Jenner, p. 67; Yves-Marie Bercé, 'Le clergé et la diffusion de la vaccination', *Revue d'histoire de l'Église de France*, 69 (1983), 87–106, at 89.

[95] G. Barsini and G. Bosco, 'La Vaccinazione Jenneriana in Siena agli inizi del secolo XIX', *Giornale Batteriologia Virologia Immunologia*, 69 (1976), 296–311, at 298.

[96] Add. MS. 48,411, fos. 101r–102v, BL; Add. MS. 8,099, fos. 136r–v, BL; *BB, S&A*, 19 (January–April 1802), 75.

[97] Baron, *Life*, 1, pp. 400–3; *Evidence*, ed. Jenner, p. 67.

[98] *MPJ*, 7 (January–June 1802), 480; Bailey, *Curious Story*, chs. 5 and 6.

Prophylaxis and Plunder in the Levant

News of cowpox found its way, early on, to the heart of the Ottoman world. The Earl of Elgin, with his pregnant wife, arrived in Istanbul as the new British Ambassador to the Sublime Porte in November 1799. The couple had sailed through the Mediterranean over autumn, calling in at Palermo where the Earl consulted Sir William Hamilton on the purchase of antiquities in Athens.[99] Since the Elgins were about to start a family, they may have taken note of the cowpox discovery prior to their departure. In April 1800, Lady Elgin gave birth to a son and heir in Istanbul.[100] From England, the Dowager Countess of Elgin, by this stage a convert to vaccination, sent a sample of cowpox for her grandson with Dr William Scott, but it almost certainly failed to survive the voyage.[101] By coincidence, Lady Elgin's parents, Mr and Mrs Nesbit, who were travelling overland to visit their new grandson, heard about cowpox inoculation at a dinner party, hosted by Lord Minto, in Vienna. Dr De Carro, another guest, reported his experiments and his enthusiasm for the new prophylaxis. In Istanbul in September, the Nesbits encouraged Elgin to write to Vienna for vaccine.[102] De Carro obliged by sending supplies of vaccine, first on threads and then on a piece of cloth. Frustrated in his first two attempts, Douglas Whyte, Elgin's surgeon, suggested applying a vesicatory to raise a blister, but his proposal was overruled by 'parental fondness'. Happily, he succeeded at a third attempt.[103] He made some of the vaccine that he propagated available to the captain of *George Washington*, an American frigate in port, who used it on members of his crew. On 23 December 1800, Elgin reported the happy turn of events to De Carro and thanked him for sending the means of introducing 'so salutary a procedure in this country'.[104]

Over winter 1800–1, Elgin's chief concern was to persuade the Grand Vizier to provide material support to the British expedition against the French in Egypt. Even as he wrote to announce the success of vaccine in Istanbul, the British fleet was assembling in Marmaris Bay and Dr Walker was offering vaccination ashore to subjects of the Ottoman empire. After more than a month at anchor, the British commanders gave up hope of Turkish assistance and headed south with limited provisions. Sighting Alexandria on 1 March, they launched an ambitious amphibian operation at Aboukir Bay a week later. After reaching the shore in the face of heavy fire, British soldiers won a major engagement among the Roman ruins at Canopus on 21 March, though General

---

[99] William St. Clair, *Lord Elgin and the Marbles* (London, 1967), ch. 3.
[100] St. Clair, *Elgin and the Marbles*, p. 46.
[101] Susan Nagel, *Mistress of the Elgin Marbles* (Chichester, 2004), p. 87.
[102] De Carro, *Histoire*, pp. 3–4.   [103] *MPJ*, 5 (January–June 1801), 243.
[104] De Carro, *Histoire*, pp. 5–6.

Abercromby was among the casualties.[105] Under the command of Major-General Hutchinson, the campaign continued with the occupation of Rosetta and the siege of the French position in Alexandria. With the assistance of local allies, the British army advanced on Cairo and secured the surrender of the larger part of the French army. Under the command of General Menou, Alexandria held out until July. Though giving the French garrison honourable terms, Hutchinson was prompted by a letter from Elgin to insist that Menou surrender the Rosetta Stone, the basalt slab whose inscriptions would provide the key to Egyptian hieroglyphs.[106] Although a pacifist, Walker played his part in the campaign, volunteering his services as a surgeon in Sir Sidney Smith's brigade.[107] He does not appear to have vaccinated in Egypt, probably for lack of viable vaccine. The main threat of contagion was in any case not smallpox but bubonic plague. In 1799, a French physician had conducted experiments in inoculating the plague prophylactically.[108] In 1802, Dr Whyte, an army medical officer, decided to inoculate himself with plague to prove his own theory that the plague was not contagious but took the disease fatally.[109] Indians serving in the British army may have heard reports of this episode. Two years later, there was concern in India about sepoys on leave from Egypt claiming that vaccination caused plague.[110] As the hostilities wound down, Walker borrowed money for a voyage to Jaffa, perhaps intending to visit the Holy Places.[111] Late in 1801, he returned to England by sea, re-joining his wife at his cousin's Gloucestershire home. In August 1802, he opened a 'vaccinium' in London in premises provided by Joseph Fox, a Quaker dentist and philanthropist. In 1803, he was appointed by the Royal Jennerian Society as its first resident vaccinator.[112]

In Istanbul, the Elgins maintained their interest in vaccination. Lady Elgin doubtless took some delight in introducing an improved version of the practice that Lady Montagu had brought from the Ottoman empire to Britain. The original stock of vaccine was lost early in 1801, but De Carro and Portenschlag sent new samples to an old friend, Dr Hesse, who succeeded in re-establishing the practice in late August.[113] It came in the nick of time for the second child

---

[105] Paul Fregosi, *Dreams of empire: Napoleon and the First World War, 1792–1815* (London, 1989), p. 193.

[106] Fregosi, *Dreams of empire*, p. 196.   [107] Walker, *Fragments*, p. 362.

[108] Richard Pearson, *A brief description of the plague: with observations on its prevention and cure* (London, 1813), p. 45.

[109] *MPJ*, 5 (January–June 1801), 245; William Wittman, *Travels in Turkey, Asia-Minor, Syria, and across the desert into Egypt during the Years 1799, 1800, and 1801, in company with the Turkish army and the British medical mission* (London, 1803), pp. 518–19; Pearson, *Brief description*, p. 46.

[110] John Shoolbred, *Report on the progress of vaccine inoculation in Bengal from the period of its introduction in November, 1802, to the end of the year 1803* (Calcutta, 1804), pp. 22–3.

[111] Walker, *Fragments*, p. 364.   [112] Epps, *Walker*, p. 73.   [113] De Carro, *Histoire*, pp. 7–8.

for the Elgins, who was born at the end of the month. Alarmed by reports that 'hundreds and hundreds of children' were dying each day in an epidemic in Smyrna, she arranged for daughter's vaccination a week after her birth. In a letter to her mother reporting her baby's vaccination, she observed that small-pox 'is so dreadfully fatal here, I think we shall compleatly establish the vaxine in this country'.[114] A month later, she announced her success in persuading the wife of Yousouf Aga, a court favourite, to have her child vaccinated. 'If so great a person as her, were to set the fashion amongst the Turks', she added, 'it would certainly take'.[115] In December, Dr Scott, Lady Elgin's physician, wrote to inform De Carro of the vaccination of Elgin's daughter and other embassy children, Dr Hesse's tally of vaccinations and Lord Elgin's distribution of packets of vaccine.[116]

In spring 1802, the Elgins set out on a tour of Greece. On the voyage to Athens, Dr Scott revaccinated their son, confirming the soundness of the original operation.[117] If Lord Elgin had other duties and interests, not least in acquiring antiquities, the party was also intent on introducing vaccination which, they discovered, was still little known in Greece. Dr Cassgitti, a leading physician in Athens, who had read about the practice, witnessed Scott's treatment of two children, one of whom provided lymph for Cassgitti to make the practice more broadly available in the city. 'It is astonishing how much the vaxine has taken here', Lady Elgin informed her mother, on 2 June, 'Doctor Scott is inoculating every day, with the best possible success; he has even inoculated a Turkish child. What an amazing thing it is to have introduced into a country where the smallpox is so fatal!' After reporting on the beginnings of vaccination in Greece, Lady Elgin told her about the Parthenon marbles. 'We yesterday got down the last thing we want from the Acropolis, so we may boldly bid defiance to our enemies. Captain Donnelly is to take all our remaining cases on board the *Narcissus*; how amazingly fortunate we have been'.[118] The Elgins could do little more than sow the seeds of vaccination. Dr Scott demonstrated the practice to surgeons from Argos, Corinth and other major towns.[119] The British Consul in Salonika (Thessaloniki), who came to meet Elgin on other business, was sufficiently impressed by what he learnt about vaccination to take a sample of vaccine to Dr Lafont, a French physician based in Salonika. After failing with the initial sample, three months old, Lafont solicited a sample from De Carro, playfully claiming it in recognition of Britain's debt to Salonika, the birthplace of the old woman who had

---

[114] *The letters of Mary Nisbet of Dirleton, Countess of Elgin*, ed. Nisbet Hamilton Grant (London, 1926), pp. 109–10.
[115] *Letters of Countess of Elgin*, p. 130.   [116] De Carro, *Histoire*, pp. 9–10.
[117] *Letters of Countess of Elgin*, pp. 176–7.   [118] *Letters of Countess of Elgin*, p. 199.
[119] De Carro, *Histoire*, pp. 9–10.

inoculated the son of Lady Montagu. In the first eight months, he vaccinated 1,130 people in the city.[120] The Elgins' enterprise in bringing vaccine to Greece complemented the endeavours of Dr Moreschi, who sent samples of vaccine on threads and glass from Venice to physicians along the Dalmatian coast, eventually reaching 'the famous Ithaca of Ulysses, and Patras in Peloponnese'.[121]

Although it circulated around the Mediterranean, vaccine made little progress in north Africa or the Levant. In January 1801, Dr Marshall reported that the Dey of Algiers was 'anxious for [cowpox] inoculation to be established among them'.[122] He also discussed with agents of Hammoudah Pacha, Bey of Tunis, the introduction of vaccine to Tunis, if the price was right.[123] When the British proconsul presented the Bey with a treatise on cowpox, probably Marshall's Italian pamphlet, and the Bey's physician explained what was involved, Hammoudah Pacha scoffed at the idea of inoculating a human being with matter from a cow infected with matter from a horse's heel and declared that the proconsul 'was always crazy and would die crazy'.[124] While Walker vaccinated some local people, probably Greeks, in and around Marmaris, he does not appear to have vaccinated in Egypt.[125] On his return to Istanbul in October 1802, Dr Scott found that the supply of vaccine had again failed, though it was soon re-established from Vienna. In 1803, Dr Auban, physician of the French embassy, estimated that over 5,000 people had been vaccinated since the beginnings of the practice, mainly Greeks and Armenians. Despite a few promising signs, the practice found little favour among the Turks.[126] Prior to returning home in 1803, though, Elgin supported moves to establish the practice in Aleppo and Basra, hoping to establish staging-posts for the transmission of vaccine to India.[127]

The Internationalisation of Vaccination

The dissemination of the new prophylaxis in continental Europe and the Mediterranean world between 1799 and the end of the Truce of Amiens in 1803 launched its international career. The early transmission of cowpox was almost literally diasporic, with cotton threads soaked in cowpox lymph

---

[120] De Carro, *Histoire*, pp. 13–15.   [121] De Carro, *Histoire*, pp. 16–17.
[122] *MPJ*, 5 (January–June 1801), 317.
[123] *Gazette nationale ou le moniteur universel*, 1801, 814.
[124] Salvatore Speziale, *Oltre la peste: sanità, popolazione e società in Tunisia e nel Maghreb (XVIII-XX secolo)* (Consenza, Italy, 1997), p. 101; Salvatore Speziale, 'Naissance de la santé publique en Tunisie au temps de Hammoudah Pacha (1782–1814)', in *Islam et révolutions médicales: le labyrinthe du corps*, ed. Anne Marie Moulin (Marseille, 2013), pp. 45–58, at 49–50.
[125] Walker, *Fragments*, p. 280; Ring, *Treatise*, 2, p. 798.   [126] De Carro, *Histoire*, pp. 79–82.
[127] AL40/6508, Herefordshire Record Office, Hereford; De Carro, *Histoire*, pp. 19–20.

dispatched in some profusion from England. To increase the chances of the virus surviving weeks rather than days, Jenner suggested rolling the threads tightly in paper and sealing the scroll with sealing wax. Dr Marshall perhaps used this method to send a sample of vaccine to Dr Walker in Rotterdam in 1799, as he did with samples sent to Göttingen early in 1800. In preparing for the mission to Naples, Marshall took the further precaution of varnishing packets of vaccine with a solution of wax and alcohol and storing them in vials.[128] Although the physicians in Vienna succeeded in propagating cowpox in May 1799, they were less fortunate with later samples. De Carro made a point of providing feedback on forms of packaging. In a letter to the *Bibliothèque britannique* in 1802, he reported that when he needed to keep vaccine for any length of time, or send it any distance, he used all the lymph from a ripe vesicle to soak a piece of English ribbon and placed the piece in a concave cavity between two pieces of glass. He observed, too, that storing vaccine in a small vacuum-sealed bottle worked well.[129] The low technology solution to the problem of transmitting vaccine from place to place was to move a child under vaccination. In the first years of cowpox inoculation in England and elsewhere, many doctors began their practice by taking a child, often their own, to be vaccinated in a town where the procedure was available and, on their return home, milking the child's vesicle to provide lymph to vaccinate locally. In vaccinating children of visitors to Vienna, De Carro likewise evidently soon saw that they might be the means of disseminating vaccine. The Hungarian lady who brought a child to De Carro for vaccination with the aim of introducing the practice in her homeland, however, may well have come to the idea independently.[130] Dr Marshall was the first to exploit the possibility of using successive vaccinations to transport vaccine over longer distances. His use of sailors to propagate vaccine on the voyage to Gibraltar and in the Mediterranean, and the deployment of children by Dr Calcagni, his disciple, to carry vaccine from village to village in Sicily, was purposeful and programmatic. Early in 1801, Jenner proposed to Lord Hobart a scheme of successive vaccinations to carry cowpox to India.[131] This method was subsequently used on a large scale, especially in Russia, British India and the Spanish empire, literally bringing the world arm-to-arm.

The extension of vaccination in Europe also involved the diffusion of technical expertise. The print media played a crucial role in underpinning the extension of the practice. Jenner's works and other publications, variously original and derivative, theoretical and practical, were noted and reviewed in newspapers and journals and circulated relatively easily among interested parties, at least until the abrupt end of the Truce of Amiens in 1803. When

---

[128] Ring, *Treatise*, 1, p. 61.   [129] *BB, S&A*, 20 (1802), 213–20, at 215–16.
[130] De Carro, *Observations*, p. 191.   [131] Baron, *Life*, 1, p. 409.

in June 1800 and June 1803, Dr Juncker and Dr De Carro sought the latest books on vaccination from London, they listed the publications they had read, revealing that they were less than a year behind their English colleagues.[132] Especially important in terms of the success of the practice were the plates illustrating the development of the cowpox vesicle that were widely consulted and copied in local publications. In 1801, De Carro eagerly awaited the new set of plates that he heard that Jenner was commissioning and that he rightly expected would provide a new standard for practitioners. Words and pictures, of course, were a poor substitute for direct observation. In addition to the Genevans, quite a few European doctors, including Gerhard Reumont of Aachen, Michele Buniva of Turin and Joseph Frank of Vienna, undertook fact-finding missions to Britain in the first years of vaccination.[133] Woodville's mission to Paris in summer 1800 and Marshall and Walker's vaccine odyssey in 1800–1 greatly accelerated the process by which local practitioners acquired competence and confidence with the new prophylaxis. If there had been peace in Europe, British medical men might have made a lucrative business out of vaccination on the continent. Alongside his charity work, Marshall charged ten guineas to vaccinate 'genteel' families in Sicily and may have done likewise in Naples and Paris.[134] More remarkable is the generosity and public-spiritedness shown in the diffusion of information about the new prophylaxis. Dr Batt sent his copy of Jenner's *Inquiry* to Florence and Marshall's copy of Jenner's latest work was translated for publication in Malta. Lady Elgin took her copy of De Carro's book to Greece, gave it to the British Resident in Salonika, and he in turn made it available to Lafont.[135] Dr Marshall, who sent vaccine to Istanbul, probably also sent his Italian book on vaccination to Dr Scott who, finding it 'to be well adapted for popular use', gave it to Dr Roiui, the Sultan's physician, to translate it into Turkish.[136]

The extension of the practice in new climatic and cultural zones helped to refine understandings of the new prophylaxis. In the light of discussion of possible differences in the nature and effects of cowpox in the English countryside and the metropolis, it was useful to discover that cowpox infection proceeded in the same manner and provoked no more severe response in Gibraltar in the height of summer than in an English winter. In reference to Marshall's reports from the Mediterranean, John Ring stressed that all his 'observations all terminate in one point, namely, the exact uniformity of the

---

[132] *MPJ*, 4 (July–December 1800), 141–5, at 144; *Letters of de Carro*, ed. Sigerist, pp. 48–53, at 48–9.

[133] *Deutsche Biographische Enzyklopädie*, VIII, p. 340; Carpanetto, 'Buniva e il governo della sanità', 36; *Letters of de Carro*, ed. Sigerist, p. 47.

[134] *MPJ*, 6 (July–December 1801), 95–6.   [135] De Carro, *Histoire*, p. 13.

[136] *Letters of Countess of Elgin*, p. 144; *MPJ*, 12 (July–December 1804), 450–1.

disease with its appearance in England'.[137] Dr Simmons of Manchester was quick to observe that cowpox would presumably also retain its mildness in Africa and the West Indies, where smallpox is 'dreadfully destructive', and the advantages of vaccinating slaves on the African coast, by which means 'their lives would be preserved, and their value enhanced by their security, when arrived at the place of destination'.[138] There appears to have been no doubt that cowpox would save people of all races from smallpox. Given the large number of men of African descent in London – including William Sancho, secretary of Pearson's Vaccine Institute – it is unlikely that the sailor on HMS *Endymion* was the first of them to be inoculated with cowpox. The assumption of a common humanity was qualified somewhat by recognition of possible differences in response to disease. Still, Marshall's selection of a black sailor as his first subject is instructive. Since he was seeking to begin a series of vaccinations, he must certainly have assumed that his racial background would not reduce the chances of a true vaccine response and that the transfer of lymph across racial lines would be biologically feasible and indeed culturally acceptable. He remembered the case well. Three years later, in response to an account of vaccination in Jamaica, he referred to his vaccination of the sailor, whose 'arm furnished the virus for our future inoculations', in support of the view that blacks were more susceptible to vaccine infection than Europeans. 'From my original memorandum, now before me', he observed, 'I find your observation upon the rapid progress of the disease in Negroes just; since the arm of this man yielded matter for inoculation on the third day'.[139]

The spread of vaccination in continental Europe from 1800 added significantly to the body of knowledge about the practice. Initially dependent on English expertise, European medical men were soon publishing their own experiments and observations, often adding new insights. The relative ease of communication, especially in 1802–3, created a vigorous transnational network of researchers engaged in what Randall Collins has termed 'rapid-discovery science': a community of scientists working 'on a fast-moving research front, making and discussing new discoveries for a few years before moving on to something else'.[140] De Carro's *Observations* and Sacco's *Osservazioni*, published in 1801, were reported in English medical journals as early as 1802.[141] Although all-important advances in virology and immunology were not possible for a century or more, the foundations were laid for international collaboration through shared understandings of smallpox and

---

[137] Ring, *Treatise*, 2, p. 748.   [138] *MPJ*, 5 (January–June 1801), 137.
[139] *MPJ*, 11 (January–June 1804), 39–40.
[140] Randall Collins, *The sociology of philosophies. A global theory of intellectual change* (Cambridge, MA, 1998), esp. 352–3.
[141] *MPJ*, 7 (January–June 1802), 169–88.

prophylaxis, the creation of a standard lexicon and protocols for clinical trial, and the formulation of new research questions.[142] Given the need to source cowpox, European medical men focused new attention on animal poxes, with Luigi Sacco's discovery of autochthonous cowpox in Italy generating great excitement. The effectiveness of the transnational network forged by vaccination is well illustrated by De Carro's speedy response to a report that Dr Loy of Whitby had successfully used horse grease. Obtaining a copy of Loy's work hot off the press, he published a French translation which he brought to the attention of his foreign correspondents. Originally sceptical of Jenner's horse-grease thesis, Dr Sacco found a horse with a similar affliction, probably horse-pox, demonstrated its prophylactic value experimentally and sent samples to Vienna and England. De Carro's translation was the inspiration, too, for Lafont to undertake experiments with equine matter in Salonika, which likewise produced positive results. A flurry of self-congratulatory correspondence flowed between Jenner, De Carro, Sacco and Lafont, who rather relished the idea that vaccination should, strictly speaking, be rebranded equination.[143]

The early vaccine diaspora likewise reveals the political, social and cultural factors in play in the reception of the new prophylaxis. In Britain, the level of government support for cowpox inoculation was negligible, largely limited to the sort of facilitation involved in the Mediterranean mission. In southern Italy, the Bourbon regime, notwithstanding its reactionary character, strongly supported the new prophylaxis. The Cisalpine and Italian Republics likewise welcomed vaccination and sought to embed it in broader public health agendas. It is quite startling to note the appointment of Luigi Sacco, probably within a year of the authorities first hearing about cowpox, as director of vaccinations, the first publicly funded position of this sort. The introduction of vaccination in European centres was generally associated with public demonstrations of its effectiveness, and the trials conducted in Vienna, Milan and elsewhere provided a firm base for government support, professional solidarity, and social acceptance that helped the practice to prosper. In Catholic Europe, the church played a surprisingly strong role in making the new prophylaxis culturally acceptable, with the clergy in Malta, Palermo and Naples involved in ceremonies to welcome the blessings of vaccine and in preparing their flocks for vaccination. In northern Italy, Luigi Sacco was able to enlist the clergy to support his work and was involved in the distribution of a

---

[142] Andrea Rusnock, 'Making sense of vaccination c. 1800', in Kenton Kroker, Pauline M. H. Mazumdar and Jennifer Keelan (eds.), *Crafting immunity: working histories of clinical immunology* (Aldershot, 2008), pp. 17–27.

[143] Baron, *Life*, 1, pp. 250–1; Edgar M. Crookshank, *History and pathology of vaccination*, 2 vols. (London, 1889), 1, pp. 387–8; *Letters of de Carro*, ed. Sigerist, pp. 50–1.

homily in favour of vaccination, purportedly issued by the Bishop of 'Goldstat' and allegedly translated from German to Italian.[144] In Geneva in December 1800, Dr Odier devised an address to parents on vaccination that ministers of the Calvinist church gave to parents bringing their children to be baptised that proved influential in northern Europe.[145]

The early success of cowpox in continental Europe assisted the cause in Britain. The vaccination of members of the armed services in the Mediterranean proved exemplary. Publishing Dr Marshall's letters from Malta, John Ring wrote, 'It is now, therefore, evident how little reason there was for the alarm excited with so much industry, that our brave tars were to be made the victim of experiment'.[146] The friends of vaccination contrasted the eager embrace of the practice in Vienna and Naples with the popular apathy at home. Testimonies to its success in Europe added to the impetus in the British parliament in 1802 to acknowledge Jenner's discovery by the award of a premium. The early vaccine diaspora saw the beginnings of a Europe-wide cult of Jenner. De Carro boasted his friendship with Jenner, named his third son in his honour and relished being dubbed 'the Jenner of the East'. In his first letter to Jenner, Luigi Sacco wrote, 'It is to the genius of medicine, to the favourite child of nature, that I have the honour to write'.[147] The idea of Jenner as a humanitarian hero was encapsulated in the appellation 'Immortal Jenner'. In Malta, Father Bellet called for a monument to Governor Ball for his efforts to establish vaccination and asked 'if Rome and Athens have raised statues to victorious generals for their destruction of human beings, what do we owe Jenner for having found the means to preserve life?'[148] In his poem *Vaccinatio*, Luko Stulli, who brought vaccine from Vienna to Dubrovnik in 1800, strikes a similar note, rebuking backward-looking classicists: 'Oh, let the one who remembers monuments to the old and does not glorify anything but what is under the soil, be ruined. What helps humanity and returns its happiness is what I want and admire with all my heart ...'.[149]

More generally, vaccination added to Britain's prestige. De Carro's enterprise prospered in the context of the close alliance between Britain and Austria. Liberated from French rule and anxious about the restoration of its old regime, Malta had an additional reason to embrace British protection. According to Dr Marshall, Governor Ball 'is the idol of the Maltese, [and] is establishing a botanic garden, interests himself in their hospitals and public regulations, and among other conciliating measures, boasts of the service England renders them

---

[144] Bercé, 'Clergé et vaccination', 91, 96–7.   [145] Gautier, *Médecine à Genève*, pp. 660–2.
[146] *MPJ*, 5 (January–June 1801), p. 354.   [147] Baron, *Life*, 1, pp. 452–5, at 452.
[148] Cassar, 'Vaccination in Malta', 69.
[149] A. Brovenčki and C. Pavlović, '200th anniversary (1804–2004) of the publication of the poem: *Vaccinatio; De Jenneriano invento optime merito; carmen elegiacum*; by Croatian scientist Luko Stulli', *Croatian Medical Journal*, 45 (2004), 655–73, at 673.

by the introduction of the cow-pox, and delights them by the offer of having the whole island inoculated'.[150] Many Sicilians, who welcomed increasing British influence as 'providing a potential escape from Bourbon misrule ... and a short cut to constitutional liberty', probably also regarded vaccination as part of the package.[151] Even in the Adriatic there was a positive assessment of Britain's role as a beneficent agent of progress. A long Latin poem in elegiac couplets, Stulli's *Vaccinatio* is a paeon to progress, with Britain's contribution to smallpox prophylaxis centre stage: 'Hail, England, great nourisher of heroes and virtues, dear home of charities and wisdom: our ancestors knew nothing bigger nor will the coming generation'.[152]

---

[150] *MPJ*, 5 (January–June 1801), p. 316.

[151] Robert Holland, *Blue-water empire. The British in the Mediterranean since 1800* (London, 2012), pp. 20–1.

[152] Brovenčki and Pavlović, '*Vaccinatio*', 667 [translation slightly reworded].

In June 1800, a small party crossed from London to Altona near Hamburg. The Danish-controlled port represented the only convenient point of access to the continent for British ships. Drs William Woodville, Antoine Aubert and Charles Nowell then boarded a neutral vessel for Boulogne. The French customs officers must have been bemused by the Quaker physician and his package of threads impregnated with cowpox. Britain and France were now in the eighth year of war. After consolidating his ascendancy as First Consul, Napoleon was preparing to escalate the conflict in Europe. In the increasingly tense atmosphere there was little reason to trust 'perfidious Albion'. The mission had been authorised, however, at the highest levels in both France and Britain. In Boulogne, Woodville vaccinated several local children, leaving them in Nowell's care. This proved a wise move as the vaccine from London proved inert on arrival in Paris. Happily, Woodville was able to send for fresh matter from the children vaccinated in Boulogne. The first successful vaccination in the French capital took place on 8 August. Ironically, Boulogne, where Napoleon later assembled forces for the invasion of England, served as the beach-head in cowpox's conquest of Napoleonic Europe.[1]

The French government and medical establishment were keenly interested in vaccination. Prior to 1789, there had been some acceptance of variolation in elite circles. The overthrow of the old medical regime, the abolition of corporative monopolies and controls and a new emphasis on public health created conditions even more favourable to smallpox prophylaxis. Though French newspapers carried notices of the cowpox discovery in autumn 1798 and the *Bibliothèque britannique* provided a summary of Jenner's treatise shortly afterwards, Paris had to wait almost two years before it could make a successful trial of *la petite vérole des vaches*. War-time restrictions compounded the challenges in delivering live vaccine matter and French medical men were unlucky with the samples that came their way. The delay in introducing cowpox, however, was not all loss. By summer 1800 France was

---

[1] Meynell, 'Nowell and "matière de Boulogne"', 232–8.

better prepared for vaccination – technically, organisationally and culturally – than even a year earlier. Interest in the new prophylaxis had led to the formation of a subscription society early in 1800 to fund initiatives to seek vaccine, assess its value and, if it lived up to its reputation, make it available in France. Coming to power at the end of 1799, the Consulate sought unity, order and 'regeneration' and was drawn to state-building initiatives. Vaccine had the potential to make the body politic immune to a deadly and costly disease and to promote national prosperity and welfare. The spread of the beneficent virus brought French people, literally, arm-to-arm, forging a new solidarity. Socially, the vaccination cause served the ends of *ralliement*, bringing together liberal aristocrats and former Jacobins. In the medical world, it helped to build a new professional identity based on scientific expertise and social responsibility. The arrival of cowpox in France opened a new chapter, too, in the global history of vaccination. Though the terms 'vaccine' and 'vaccination' were coming into use in England, the standardisation of nomenclature, and its subsequent generalisation in the age of Pasteur to cover other forms of prophylaxis, owed much to France. The French management of vaccination provided an especially influential model.

The Long Flirtation with Smallpox Inoculation

Smallpox inoculation had some profile in France but made only faltering progress. The Regent of France, Philippe of Orleans, was disposed to allow a trial of the practice, but his death in 1723 put experimentation on hold. The resistance to the practice was medical rather than theological.[2] The medical establishment in Paris, reluctant to endorse a procedure that involved significant risk, closed ranks against it. As reports from Britain in the 1730s indicated some loss of enthusiasm for inoculation, Parisian medical men congratulated themselves on their caution and good sense.[3] In the 1740s inoculation again became a serious proposition in Britain and a mounting body of evidence showed better outcomes from inoculation than from smallpox acquired casually. In a rousing address to the Royal Academy of Sciences in 1754, La Condamine declared that '*la nature nous décimoit; l'art nous millésime*' and made inoculation fashionable in aristocratic circles.[4] After organising his own inoculation, the Chevalier de Chastellux told Buffon: 'I am saved and my example will save many others'.[5] In a blaze of publicity in 1756, Louis

---

[2] John McManners, *Church and society in eighteenth-century France*, vol. 2 (Oxford, 1998), p. 306.
[3] La Mettrie, *Traité*, p. 9.   [4] La Condamine, *Mémoire*, 54.
[5] [G.-L. Leclerc Buffon], *Correspondance inédite de Buffon*, ed. Henri Nadault de Buffon, 2 vols. (Paris, 1860), 1, p. 343.

Philippe Duke of Orleans summoned Dr Tronchin to Paris to inoculate his children.[6] Another celebrity inoculator, the Italian Dr Gatti, built fashionable interest but made mistakes. In 1763, the Parlement of Paris banned the practice until it had been approved by both the Faculties of Medicine and Theology. The theologians deferred to the medical men who appointed a committee to seek information and advice from across France and Europe. Although most of the submissions were cautiously supportive of inoculation, the committee was divided on the issue. Deeply riven by the controversy, the Faculty held back from formally endorsing the practice, admitting it in 1768 to be merely 'admissible'.[7]

By the late 1760s, smallpox inoculation was gaining more support. Improvements in the practice were reducing the risk, stress and cost involved. In 1768 the Duke of Choiseul, the Foreign Minister, organised the inoculation of the cadets in the military academy at La Flèche. After Parlement's relaxation of the edict, British inoculators set up houses on the outskirts of Paris, including Simeon Worlock, Daniel Sutton's father-in-law, at the barrier of the Petit Charonne.[8] Louis XV's death from smallpox in 1774 set the scene for the acceptance of inoculation by Louis XVI and his siblings. In presenting Chastellux to the *Académie française* in 1775, Buffon declared that it was his 'great example' that had led to the still greater examples that provided reassurance regarding the lives of the adored princes.[9] In the 1780s, Marie Antoinette, Louis's queen, who had been inoculated in Vienna, made sure that their children were all inoculated. The well-publicised royal inoculations encouraged noble and bourgeois families to follow suit. While British inoculators remained active in Paris until 1789, French specialists also began to emerge. The physician Goetz and the surgeon Vaume built up a reputation in inoculation that would survive the Revolution. Still, only a small proportion of Parisians availed themselves of the procedure. Dr Desessartz, whose practice included 200 children in boarding houses in the Faubourg Saint-Antoine in the 1780s and 1790s, found that only 5 per cent had been inoculated.[10]

In the kingdom at large, inoculation was patchy. French aristocrats organised the inoculation of their families in their chateaux and often made the procedure available to their friends and dependents. In the ports and towns of Brittany and Provence, the practice was patronised by merchants, artisans and sailors. Learned medical men in the provinces made trials of inoculation. In 1777, Dr Calvet in Aix-en-Provence stated the procedure 'was one of the finest

[6] Catriona Seth, 'Esculape-Tronchin: le médecin à la mode' in Frédéric Charboneau ed., *La fabrique de la modernité scientifique. Discours et récits du progrès sous l'Ancien Régime* (Oxford, 2015), pp. 149–66, at 156–7.
[7] Hervé Bazin, *L'histoire des vaccinations* (Montrouge, 2008), p. 44.
[8] Bennett, 'Curing and inoculating smallpox', 29–33.
[9] *Correspondance de Buffon*, 1, p. 343.   [10] *Magasin encyclopédique*, 2 (1797), 20–1.

inventions of the human mind'.[11] Reform-minded ministers and officials, cognisant of the economic and social costs of smallpox, used their influence to promote prophylaxis. Minister Turgot patronised inoculation and several intendants followed his lead. Charles André de Lacorée, Intendant of Franche-Comté from 1761 to 1784, presided over a successful programme.[12] Jean-François-Xavier Girod, his chief physician, went to London to learn the technique and, on his return, inoculated several hundred people around Mignovillard in 1765. From the mid-1770s he oversaw the inoculation of thousands of villagers each year.[13] By the 1780s the French government was more active than the British state in encouraging the practice. In 1782 a substantial grant was given to set up an inoculation clinic at Caen.[14] In 1786 orders were issued for the inoculation of children in orphanages, establishing the practice in all regional centres. Dr Jauberthon, who had inoculated the royal family, toured the realm to supervise the initiative.[15] Bishops were called on to promote the practice from the pulpit. Aspiring to a new model of the *bon curé*, Dominique Chaix inoculated his flock in a remote parish in the Dauphiné in 1786.[16]

The outbreak of the French Revolution disrupted the advance of variolation. The aristocratic networks that had supported the practice were dispersed. Many of the revolutionary leaders supported inoculation but had other priorities. Maximilian Robespierre, scarred from smallpox as a child, declared his support for inoculation in his celebrated defence of the right of a town to erect a lightning conductor.[17] The Jacobins were alert to the class discrimination inherent in the old system. As Citizen Desessartz observed, the only beneficiaries of inoculation were people rich enough to 'buy from an inoculator the health, vigour and life of their children'.[18] The overthrow of the old medical regime and old prejudices, and the construction of a new professional identity based on clinical training and commitment to public health, created conditions favourable to the extension of the social base of the practice.[19] The establishment of the Directory brought a degree of stability that allowed professional

---

[11] L. W. B. Brockliss, *Calvet's web. Enlightenment and the Republic of letters in eighteenth-century France* (Oxford, 2002), p. 165.

[12] Darmon, *Longue traque*, pp. 127–32.

[13] Thérèse Ravard, *Histoire et médecins de Franche-Comté* (Yens sur Morges, 2002), pp. 44–5.

[14] Darmon, *Longue traque*, p. 137.

[15] Darmon, *Longue traque*, pp. 138–9; Laurence Brockliss and Colin Jones, *The medical world of early modern France* (Oxford, 1997), p. 743n.

[16] Timothy Tackett, *Priest and parish in eighteenth-century France. A social and political study of the curés in a diocese of Dauphiné 1750–1791* (Princeton, 1977), p. 162.

[17] Jessica Riskin, *Science in the age of sensibility: the sentimental empiricists of the French Enlightenment* (Chicago, 2002), p. 177.

[18] *Magasin encyclopédique*, 2 (1797), 19.

[19] Review of François Ignace Goëtz, *Traité complet de la petite vérole et de l'inoculation* (Paris, 1790) in *Journal de Paris*, 16 March 1791, no. 75, supplement no. 36, i.

and philanthropic networks to regroup. In 1797, Citizen Audin-Rouvière set forward a scheme for an inoculation hospital in Paris and a team of six inoculators to tour the surrounding *départements*. A government committee considering the scheme felt that the rural initiative was unworkable, as the peasants would not trust outsiders, but recommended the establishment of the hospital, and a plan for a hospital at Montrouge on the southern edge of Paris was drawn up.[20] A severe smallpox outbreak in Paris in summer 1798 underlined the urgency of the undertaking.

Vaccine en Voyage

The arrival of news of Jenner's cowpox in autumn 1798 provided fresh stimulus to medical interest in inoculation, old and new. In August 1799 Philippe Pinel, professor at the School of Medicine in Paris, obtained the Minister of the Interior's approval for experiments with smallpox and cowpox at La Salpêtrière, and soon afterwards made an unsuccessful trial of vaccine brought from London.[21] Around this time, too, there were trials of vaccine in Strasbourg that, although reportedly successful, did not establish the practice.[22] In January 1800, the National Institute and the Société de Médecine set up committees to investigate cowpox inoculation. In March, the former Count Larochefoucault-Liancourt and Dr Guillotin, an old friend, formed the 'Society for the Extinction of Smallpox in France through the Propagation of Vaccine' to support trials of cowpox and, if it proved a safe preventative of smallpox, to promote the new prophylaxis in France. In May, its medical committee sent Dr Aubert to London to observe the practice and return with vaccine for a trial in the Hôpital de la Pitié. Dr Pearson packed vaccine in a flask filled with hydrogen gas, sealed with mercury and stored in a bladder, but it failed when used in Paris.[23] Dr Woodville may have indicated his readiness, in the event of failure, to assist with the first vaccination. Dr Aubert was soon heading back to England with the necessary authorisation for Woodville's travel. Around the middle of July, the party crossed to Altona and then took another ship to Boulogne, where Dr Nowell had a medical practice. After pausing there to vaccinate several children, Dr Woodville arrived in Paris on 28 July.

The initiative to introduce vaccination evidently had high level support. Napoleon's seizure of power late in 1799 brought energy and direction to public affairs and ushered in a government that was more inclusive and

---

[20] *Magasin encyclopédique*, 2 (1797), 18–32; F/8/12, dossier 1-1, AN.

[21] William Woodville, *Rapport sur le cowpox ou la petite vérole des vaches*, transl. A. Aubert (Paris, An. 8), p. xxxii; Darmon, *Longue traque*, p. 142; [Robert John Thornton], *Preuves de l'efficacité de la vaccine*, transl. Joseph Duffour (Paris, 1808), p. xvi.

[22] Darmon, *Longue traque*, p. 177.   [23] Darmon, *Longue traque*, p. 180.

technocratic than its predecessors, which would serve the new prophylaxis well. Larochefoucault-Liancourt, a liberal aristocrat, had taken the opportunity of a pardon from the new regime to return to his homeland.[24] His leadership of the society for cowpox inoculation, a practice he had observed in exile, was in line with his earlier philanthropy and traditions of aristocratic *bienfaisance*. The participation of Lucien Bonaparte, Talleyrand, Fouché and Frochot, Prefect of the Seine and *ex officio* mayor of Paris signalled the collaboration of key members of the new regime. As Minister of the Interior, Lucien Bonaparte provided the crucial authorisations for the initiative and assured the co-operation of key officials. Foreign Minister Talleyrand provided a special passport for Dr Woodville to come to Paris. There was a new ethos abroad. At his installation as Prefect of the Seine in April, Frochot declared his readiness 'to welcome useful and beneficent ideas, projects of true public interest'.[25] On 14 July 1800, a fortnight before Woodville's arrival, Lucien Bonaparte made a speech to celebrate the national festival, recalling how at the storming of the Bastille 'the sacred fire burst forth and coursed through the arteries of the body politic; millions of arms rose up; the word "liberty" resounded on all sides'.[26] In looking to the potential of the new prophylaxis in France, he would have found it natural to imagine France in bodily terms, revitalised and united.

Dr Woodville arrived in Paris at the height of summer with vaccine already a month old. Dr François Colon had made his house at Vaugirard, southwest of the city, available for the trial. The hopes of the medical men turned to disappointment when it became evident, within a few days, that the vaccine was no longer fit for purpose. Fortunately, Woodville had taken the precaution of asking Nowell to send vaccine from the children vaccinated in Boulogne to Paris. By the time that the *'Matière de Boulogne'* arrived, Colon's senior colleagues had dispersed. In their absence, Colon took the opportunity to make a name for himself. On 8 August, Dr Woodville vaccinated Colon's only son, at eleven months old.[27] Over the following weeks, Colon succeeded in a series of vaccinations, entitling him to claim to have established vaccination in Paris. In a well-publicised move, he opened a clinic on the Rue de Faubourg Poissonière, stating that he could operate safely in the city because cowpox was not contagious. He offered to vaccinate the poor free of charge at 11am and promised private patients a refund in the event of failure. Declaring that it was not his intention to make his methods a secret, he invited other

---

[24] Henri Pigaillem, *Le docteur Guillotin* (Paris, 2004), pp. 173–4.

[25] Louis Paulin Passy, *Frochot, Préfet de la Seine* (Evreux, 1867), p. 227.

[26] *Choix de rapports, opinions et discours prononcés à la tribune nationale depuis 1789 jusqu'à ce jour*, vol. 17, 1799–1802, ed. G. N. Lallement (Paris, 1821), pp. 179–80.

[27] François Colon, *Essai sur l'inoculation de la vaccine, ou moyen de se préserver pour toujours et sans danger de la petite vérole* (Paris, 1800), p. 27n.

practitioners to witness them and offered to provide vaccine and advice to colleagues in the provinces.[28] Medical practitioners beat a path to his door to observe the practice and secure vaccine. Dr Antoine-Louis Blanche, who won notoriety for his experiments on prisoners during the Terror, came to Paris to consult him and obtain a sample for use in Rouen.[29]

Dr Colon was active in extending the new prophylaxis. In response to a request from Saint-Quentin, he set out with a recently vaccinated child to suppress smallpox in the town. He took steps to disseminate vaccine throughout France. An early triumph was the delivery of viable vaccine to Dr Roch Tarbès in Toulouse, an eight-day journey from Paris. Beginning the practice in late November, Tarbès in turn distributed vaccine through the Midi and even across the Pyrenees.[30] Colon enlisted the support of influential laymen in promoting the practice. He supplied the Minister of the Interior with over 500 copies of his pamphlet for distribution to prefects and mayors across France.[31] Citizen Corbigny, Prefect of Lois-et-Cher, sent a child, accompanied by a surgeon, to his clinic to be vaccinated and serve as the means of introducing the practice in Blois.[32] When his son caught smallpox in December, Prefect Frochot asked Colon to vaccinate his household in the Place de Vendôme. To inspire confidence in the procedure, Colon brought with him recently vaccinated children to be exposed to smallpox and a week later presented them at the house in good health.[33] Convinced by the demonstration, Frochot signed a memorial endorsing vaccination and made the *maison du Saint-Spirit*, near the Hotel de Ville, available as a clinic.[34]

In his clinical trials and moves to extend the practice, Colon stole a march on his colleagues on the medical committee. Dr M. A. Thouret, the president, was director of the *Ecole de Santé* and a busy man, but Professor Pinel made a trial of vaccine at La Salpêtrière. Dr Husson was more active, using vaccine from Colon to suppress smallpox in Reims and conducting experiments, including retro-vaccinating a cow.[35] The committee's approach was to move carefully and slowly before approving and extending the practice. In publishing his

---

[28] Colon, *Essai*, pp. 33–6.   [29] Pigaillem, *Guillotin*, p. 175.

[30] Roch Tarbès, *Mémoire historique et pratique sur la vaccine, contenant un procès-verbal de la contre-épreuve faite authentiquement* (Toulouse, 1801), p. 19; Roch Tarbès, *Rapport particulier sur la vaccine, prairial An 13* (Toulouse, 1805), p. 6. See Chapter 9.

[31] François Colon, *Mémoire présenté au Premier Consul, sur la nécessité et les moyens de répandre la vaccine en France* (Paris, 1803), p. 29.

[32] *MPJ*, 5 (January–June 1801), 556.

[33] Hugues Félix Ranque, *Théorie et pratique de l'inoculation de la vaccine* (Paris, 1801), pp. 118–23.

[34] *Rapport du Comité central de vaccine, établi à Paris par la Société des souscripteurs pour l'examen de cette découverte* (Paris, 1803), pp. 17–18.

[35] Henri Marie Husson, *Recherches historiques et médicales sur la vaccine, ou traité complet sur l'origine, l'histoire, les variétés, les avantages et la pratique de cette nouvelle inoculation*, 3rd ed. (Paris, 1803), p. 50.

Essai sur l'inoculation de la vaccine in autumn, which detailed his experiments, Colon broke ranks with the committee, making it clear that the views expressed were his own.[36] Thouret and his colleagues regarded him as a rash opportunist. In provisionally approving vaccination in November, they pointed to its success in Geneva and elsewhere but not to Colon's work.[37] Colon's bid for leadership in the establishment of the new prophylaxis misfired. It was Thouret's committee that secured the keys to the *maison du Saint-Spirit*, where the practice began under the supervision of Madame Dubois, a Sister of Charity. Colon found some support from the committee of the *Société de Médecine* which organised a public trial in August 1801, when the resistance of forty-eight vaccinated children to smallpox was tested in a 'solemn counter-proof'. In its report on vaccination, the committee acknowledged Colon as one of the practice's 'first and most fervent apostles'.[38] In his own history of the practice, Colon listed over 100 towns in France to which he had sent vaccine.[39] Professor Kluiskens of Ghent came to Paris to observe his practice and began vaccinating in Flanders with samples provided by him.[40] Marginalised by his former colleagues, however, Colon cut an increasingly sad figure struggling to maintain his standing. He attracted ridicule and censure for petitioning Napoleon for a place for his son at the elite school, the Prytanée. In his last publication, he pointed out that his son had claims on the French nation as the first child vaccinated in France and the source of much of the vaccine used to protect other children of *la patrie*.[41]

Fashion and Fear

In Paris and the provinces, most medical men embraced the new prophylaxis. In Lyon, France's second largest city, there was early interest in vaccination. The first French translation of Jenner was published there in 1800 and two local medical men, P. Brion and F. P. Bellay, publicised the new prophylaxis in their journal, *Le conservateur de la santé*.[42] They were unable to make a successful trial until March 1801, however, and, even then, failed to generate

---

[36] Colon, *Essai*, pp. 6–7.   [37] Ranque, *Théorie et pratique*, pp. 124–31.

[38] *Second Rapport de la Commission de Vaccine, à la Société de Médecine de Paris* (Paris, 1802), p. 61, 75; François Colon, *Observations critiques, sur le Rapport du Comité central de vaccine* (Paris, 1803), pp. 13, 29.

[39] François Colon, *Histoire de l'introduction et des progrès de la vaccine* (Paris, 1801), pp. 105–64.

[40] Colon, *Histoire*, pp. 116–17.   [41] Colon, *Mémoire*, p. 32.

[42] [Edward Jenner], *Recherches sur les causes et les effets de la variolæ vaccinæ, maladie découverte dans plusieurs comtés de l'ouest de l'Angleterre, notamment dans le comté de Gloucester, et connue aujourd'hui sous le nom de vérole de vache* [transl. Jacques-Joseph de

the demand necessary to make the practice self-sustaining. Acknowledging Lyon's suspicion of novelty, the doctors also noted the influence of some negative reports from Paris.[43] The main critics of vaccination were the specialist inoculators. In October 1800, Citizens Vaume and Goetz published letters raising doubts about vaccination.[44] After their struggle to win acceptance for the old mode of inoculation, they felt entitled to question the glib claims for the new system. Finding that the newspapers refused to print his letters, Vaume published them in a pamphlet, *Les dangers de vaccine*, in spring 1801.[45] By comparison with their English counterparts, the French anti-vaccinists were quite moderate, though their use of the term '*envachiner*', with its implication of bestialisation raised hackles in vaccination circles.[46] Older physicians, like Dr Calvet in Aix-en-Provence, were inclined to be cautious about a procedure whose long-term effects were unknown.[47] Overall, though, French medical men were united in their support of the new procedure. Dr Ranque was struck by the 'happy revolution in attitudes' that had led to such broad acceptance of 'this beneficent malady'.[48]

Many medical practitioners rose to the challenge of establishing the new prophylaxis. Quite a number followed Colon's example by beginning with vaccinating their own children. An *accoucheur* in Montreuil-sur-Mer began with his daughter, and Citizen Ducros, an *officier de santé* in Marseille, came to Paris to learn the technique, vaccinate his child and then return with the means to introduce vaccination in Provence.[49] Much early vaccination was *pro bono*. Colon and other pioneers vaccinated the poor at no cost and probably bore some expense in providing information and vaccine to colleagues. It was generally assumed that vaccination would become self-supporting, with doctors in private practice charging fees and doctors employed by towns and charitable institutions vaccinating as part of their salaried duties. Although it was possible for some medical men to make their name, advance their careers and win the gratitude of their patients, it soon became apparent that it was not a profitable specialism. There were gestures towards rewarding dedication to the cause. An anonymous citizen, later identified as Count Rouvroy, paid for the striking of a gold medal in 1804 to honour the most zealous vaccinator in the department of the Nord.[50] The French government

La Roque] (Lyon, 1800); *Le conservateur de la santé, journal d'hygiène et prophylactique*, 3 (February 1801–February 1802), 3–7, 9–15.

[43] P. Brion and F. Ph. Bellay, *Tableaux historiques de la vaccine, pratiquée à Lyon depuis le 13 Germinal, l'an IX, jusqu'au 31 Décembre de l'an 1809* (Lyon, 1810), p. 11.

[44] Colon, *Histoire*, pp. 38–46, 51–4.   [45] J. S. Vaume, *Les dangers de vaccine* (Paris, 1801).

[46] Colon, *Histoire*, pp. 41–54.   [47] Brockliss, *Calvet's web*, pp. 166–7.

[48] Ranque, *Théorie et pratique*, p. vii.   [49] Colon, *Histoire*, pp. 123, 158–9.

[50] Joseph Toussaint Lefebure, 'Exposé des travaux entrepris dans le département du Nord, pour l'extinction de la petite vérole et la propagation de la vaccine' in *Comité central de vaccine dans le département du Nord: traveaux des années 1840 et 1841* (Lille, 1842), pp. 13–43, at p. 23.

began to award medals annually for outstanding contributions to vaccination. Despite its strong commitment to the practice, however, it provided no more than token funding. Early enthusiasm in medical circles for committing time and energy to the new prophylaxis waned as it proved less straightforward and profitable than first assumed.

Awareness of high-level support for vaccination encouraged magistrates and public-spirited citizens to assist in establishing the practice. The mayor of Orleans sent two men to Paris with a child to be vaccinated to furnish lymph for the city's children.[51] Early in 1801, the Prefect of the Ourthe, acting on the advice of the local *bureau de bienfaisance*, set up a vaccination clinic in Liège.[52] In June 1801, the Prefect of Haute-Garonne took further steps to generalise and improve the practice introduced by Dr Tarbès in Toulouse by issuing forms to sub-prefects and mayors of communes on which the health officers were required to enter details and notes on observations in the appropriate columns.[53] The Prefect of the Gironde facilitated the establishment of a vaccination institute at Bordeaux.[54] In early summer the Prefect of the Rhône authorised the Society of Medicine in Marseille to test the immunity of vaccinated children at the Hospice of Humanity.[55] In Antwerp, the Prefect of Deux-Nèthes, the former Marquis of Herbouville, organised a vaccine committee in January 1802 and provided solid support for the practice in Brabant.[56] Many magistrates, like the mayor of Cherbourg, saw it as their duty to set an example by accepting vaccination in their families.[57] In response to Dr Blanche's request to be allowed to vaccinate foundlings in Rouen, Prefect Beugnot made six *enfans de la patrie* available on one condition, namely that his eighteen-month-old son be added to their number. A hundred or so parents followed Beugnot's example over the following weeks.[58]

The tentacular spread of vaccination from Paris into the countryside was assisted by the custom of sending children out to wet-nurses in the villages. Some of the publications on the practice were pitched to a lay audience, not least mothers.[59] Two broadsides in wide circulation combine, in text and image, basic information on vaccination by Dr François Chaussier and

---

[51] *Rapport du Comité central* (1803), pp. 39–40.
[52] Marcel Florkin, *Un prince, deux préfets. Le mouvement scientifique et médico-social au Pays de Liège sous le règne du despotisme éclairé (1771–1830)* (Liège, 1957), pp. 169–71.
[53] *Recueil de circulaires et de listes émanant de la préfecture de la Haute-Garonne, An 9-An 12, au sujet de la vaccine* (1804).
[54] *Rapport du Comité central* (1803), p. 35.   [55] *Rapport du Comité central* (1803), p. 141.
[56] G. Broekx, *Introduction de la vaccine à Malines* (Antwerp, 1856), pp. 21, 25.
[57] *Rapport du Comité central* (1803), p. 40.
[58] Yannick Marec, *Les hôpitaux de Rouen du moyen âge à nos jours: dix siècles de protection sociale* (Rouen, 2005), p. 42.
[59] E.g. Jean-Pierre Colladon, *Lettres a Madame de *** sur la Vaccine* (Paris, 1800).

well-executed images by Louis-Pierre Baltard of healthy cows and gracious mothers that represent the procedure as wholesome and benign.[60] More generally, citizens who embraced vaccination were presented as demonstrating their love of their children and heeding 'the paternal voice of the government'.[61] It was a patriotic duty. A trial of vaccination in Reims in 1801, in which twelve vaccinated children were inoculated with smallpox to demonstrate their insusceptibility, was aptly staged on the eve of the national festival of 14 July.[62] Citizen Desmousseaux, Prefect of the Marne, who had his children vaccinated to promote the practice in Liège, was moved to report an exemplary story concerning its spread in the Ardennes. A peasant from La Gleize, in the remote canton of Stavolet, heard talk about vaccine in summer 1802 and, prompted 'by love of his children', set off on a long walk to town in search of a health officer who could provide him with vaccine. On his return home, he attended to his own family, made his house 'a sort of centre for inoculation' and vaccinated over a hundred children in the district.[63]

In fashion-conscious Paris, the standing of vaccination was in some flux. A series of satirical prints published in May 1801 reflect some bemusement about the practice.[64] L'origine de la vaccine depicts an animated group of men inspecting the udders of a cow; La vaccine, ou l'inoculation à la mode presents an old woman inoculated with matter taken from an urchin; and La vaccine en voyage depicts vaccination as a bandwagon led by charlatans. Les malheurs de la vaccine hints at the self-interest of critics of the new prophylaxis: the proprietor of an inoculation house, clearly deserted, looks glumly at children vaccinating themselves in the playground. Admirable effet de la vaccine reflects anxieties about bestialisation. Unlike the English print with a similar title, the alarming consequence of the new prophylaxis is not that cowpox turns people into beasts, but that by using his house-calls as a cover for an adulterous liaison, the vaccinator is putting horns on the gullible citizen (see Figure 6.1). Fashion could be fickle and adverse outcomes seeded doubts. The uncertainties of the time found expression in an interlude presenting a dilemma over vaccination in disjointed snippets of conversation en famille.[65] His five-year-old daughter asks her father, as if she is asking for a treat, when she is going to be vaccinated; his wife reports that Citizen Lourdet has told her that vaccination is an English scam with no credit at the University of Louvain; his sister-in-law expresses her

[60] V0016508, Images, WLL.   [61] [Thornton], Preuves de l'efficacité, p. xxxix.

[62] Rapport du Comité central (1803), p. 140.

[63] Carl Havelange, Les figures de la guérison, XVIIIe-XIXe siècles: une histoire sociale et culturelle des professions médicales au pays de Liège (Paris, 1990), pp. 253–8, esp. 258.

[64] Marcel Roux, Un siècle d'histoire de France par l'estampe 1770–1871. Collection de Vinck. Tome IV. Napoléon and son temps (Directoire, Consulat, Empire) (Paris, 1929), pp. 625–30.

[65] Citizen D'Outant, Lettre aux citoyens composant le Comité de vaccine (c. 1801–2), attached to J. S. Vaume, Nouvelles preuves des dangers de la vaccine (Paris, 1801), separate pagination.

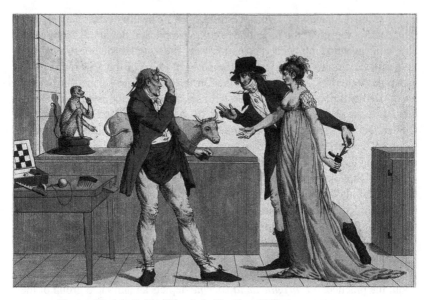

Figure 6.1 *Admirable Effet de la Vaccine*, 1801
(Wellcome Collections)

disapproval of her niece being 'envachinated'; and the chamber-maid hints at a
scheme to variolate the girl while her father is at work. The father seeks the
advice of four men: Lourdet and Mâdrénard, a notable inoculator, on one side,
and Prud-Homme, his own doctor, and Bonnez, an experienced vaccinator, on
the other. Once Prud-Homme and Bonnez explain the benefits of vaccination,
the mother and aunt begin to regard it more positively. As doubts remain, the
father decides to postpone his daughter's immunisation. Addressing his skit to
the *comité de vaccine*, he expresses the hope that it would eventually provide
clear guidance.

Fear of smallpox drove the practice. In observing that Parisians hesitated to
avail themselves of the boon of vaccine, the authors of a report to the *Société
de Médecine* declared, 'But smallpox, alas! too eloquent, has begun to cruelly
advise them of their interests'.[66] The epidemic that raged in Paris in summer
1802, in which vaccinated children were unscathed, helped to demonstrate the
value of the new prophylaxis.[67] Interestingly, there is little evidence of prejudice against vaccination as an English innovation. In D'Outant's skit, the
advocates of the old system point to the English provenance of cowpox and
stress the need to beware of Greeks bearing gifts. The supporters of the new

[66] *Second Rapport à la Société de Médecine*, p. 75.
[67] *Rapport du Comité central (1803)*, pp. 127–9.

practice, however, are given the better of the argument. They observe that variolation was learnt from England and, pointing out that, even in times of war, nationality is not a consideration in such matters, ask rhetorically, 'Are savants ever at war in the manner of peoples?'[68] The détente preceding the Truce of Amiens probably assisted the naturalisation of the practice in France. In 1801, the Prefect of Lot-et-Garonne congratulated the 'English *philosophes*, whose philanthropic and perceptive mind had by good deeds compensated for the bad outcomes of war'.[69] As diplomacy gained traction, vaccination was seen as a bond between the two nations. In October, the members of the jury of health of Amiens and the medical committee of the Somme made an address to the British Plenipotentiary Marquis Cornwallis, in which they reported how French doctors had repeated the experiments of the 'immortal Jenner' and confirmed his 'admirable invention'. 'England, my Lord, has the honour of this Discovery', they declared, 'we have received the Vaccine from your Physicians', adding the noble sentiment, 'The Friends of Science never interrupt their fraternal intercourse; and while their Governments wield the thunder of War to decide their political contests, men of Literature always remain in Peace'.[70]

Aux Armes, Citoyens

By the beginning of 1803 France and Britain were back on a collision course. Britain's declaration of war in May still came as a surprise. The lines of communication between the medical men on either side of the Channel were suddenly severed. The Napoleonic regime, whose military and naval manoeuvres had prompted Britain's pre-emptive action, was also mobilising in the war against smallpox. In March, the *Comité central de vaccine* published its long-awaited report with its unequivocal endorsement of the new prophylaxis.[71] In the third edition of his *Recherches historiques* in 1803, Husson provided more ammunition for the cause. After reporting on the many trials across France, including the *Comité*'s own 'grand and imposing experiment' on 102 previously vaccinated children in Paris in November 1801, he boldly claimed that it was 'to the glory of French medical men, that in three years they had done as much in this part of the science as the English had done in seven'.[72] Jean-Antoine Chaptal, the new Minister of the Interior, was a man of science and needed no urging to champion the practice. In a circular to the prefects in May 1803, he made vaccination a national cause. After recalling that, until recently, 'inoculation was the only resource that medicine could set

---

[68] D'Outant, *Lettre*, pp. 17–19.   [69] *Rapport du Comité central* (1803), p. 39.
[70] *MPJ*, 7 (January–June 1802), 200–3.   [71] *Rapport du Comité central* (1803), pp. 416–17.
[72] Husson, *Recherches historiques*, pp. 197–202.

against this formidable scourge', he instructed the prefects to promote the new prophylaxis in their *départements* by setting up clinics in the chief towns, introducing it into foundling houses and enlisting the cooperation of relevant societies, ministers of religion and public officials.[73] The official endorsement largely brought to an end debate about the new prophylaxis in the public sphere.[74] It was probably an open secret that Napoleon himself was an advocate of vaccination. In October 1803, he granted an interview to Dr Guillotin, who in presenting the committee's report on vaccination associated its progress with the wider achievements of the regime.[75]

From 1803, the vaccination cause in France gathered pace and purpose. The prefects who were already seeking to establish the new prophylaxis welcomed the support and recognition implicit in the minister's call to arms. The Prefect of the Ourthe expressed his frustration that, since its introduction in Liège in 1801, the city's health officers had promoted the practice but many citizens, more disposed to condemn than adopt the new discovery, had held back in *'sage defiance'*.[76] Conversely, the Prefect of Haute-Garonne was pleased to report in 1804 the issue of a revised set of forms to register vaccinations in which the column for deaths by vaccine, included in 1801, had been omitted as redundant.[77] In May 1804, Chaptal further strengthened the national framework. A new Society for the Extinction of Smallpox in France through the Propagation of Vaccine was established to replace its predecessors and its *Comité central de vaccine* in Paris became almost an arm of the state.[78] Acknowledging that many prefects 'were already impressed with a zeal worthy of the highest eulogies to fulfil in this respect the paternal views of government', Chaptal instructed all of them to establish local *comités de vaccine*, comprising medical men and other citizens 'distinguished by their rank, fortune and character', to be affiliated to the new Society. They were called on to make premises available in towns for vaccination, appoint health officers to introduce the practice in the countryside, to use children from orphanages to propagate vaccine, to collect and report data on smallpox and vaccination to the committee in Paris and generally to oversee, defend and promote the practice by a variety of means. In calling on 'a wise combination of efforts' and 'a union of measures which embrace every part of France', Chaptal adopted the tone of a Napoleonic

---

[73] *Circulaires du Ministère*, 1, pp. 277–9.
[74] Jean-Baptiste Fressoz, *L'apocalypse joyeuse. Une histoire du risque technologique* (Paris, 2012), pp. 100–1.
[75] Pigaillem, *Guillotin*, pp. 177–8.   [76] Florkin, *Un prince, deux préfets*, p. 176.
[77] *Recueil de circulaires*.
[78] Elinor Meynell, 'French reactions to Jenner's discovery of smallpox vaccination: the primary sources', *SCM*, 8 (1995), 285–303, at 297.

general: 'we must dispute every inch of ground with the enemy whom we wish to exterminate'.[79]

By 1805, France had a national system of vaccination, with activity in almost all *départements*. In May 1804, the Prefect of Pas-de-Calais issued a circular on vaccination, reporting that his infant son had been vaccinated, encouraging the adoption of the practice and commending the work of the vaccine committee established in the department.[80] In his zeal to suppress smallpox and promote the new prophylaxis, the Prefect of Saône et Loire banned the old style of inoculation in August, but Chaptal countermanded the order, insisting on the father's 'imprescriptible right' to choose for his children the method in which he had most confidence.[81] In the Basses-Pyrenees, in the far southwest of France, a vaccine committee was finally established in Pau in February 1805.[82] On a tour of the department in spring, the Prefect, the former Marquis of Chastelane, set up subcommittees in the four regional *arrondisements*. In Pau itself, vaccination was underway, with thirty-eight children immunised in the first month to build up a supply of vaccine.[83] In the first year, 5,000 children were vaccinated at public expense and probably the same number again privately. The committee acknowledged some problems. In Pau, mothers neglected to bring their children back for inspection and, once the threat of smallpox receded, became more negligent. Outside the town, however, interest remained strong and it was planned to secure the rural population by sending inoculators on tour, each spring and autumn, to immunise the new-born.[84]

The Minister of the Interior's circular gradually bore fruit in Lyon. D'Herbouville, the new Prefect of the Haute-Rhône, brought vigour to the promotion of vaccination. In parts of the countryside, the practice was already gaining traction. First used in the communes of Longes and Trèves, south of Lyon, around 1804, it was reported to be universal there four years later.[85] In Lyon and Haute-Rhône, the reappearance of smallpox in 1806–7 proved a great motivational force. By spring 1807, the city was totally infested, prompting over 1,600 vaccinations, not including those in private practice.[86] The mayor of Mornant published an address on vaccination, presenting it as the greatest discovery for humanity of the last century, and calling on parents 'in the name of the love that you have for your children' to heed the 'paternal recommendations of a wise and enlightened government' to embrace the practice as a means of eradicating smallpox. Concerned about female

[79] *Circulaires du Ministère*, 1, pp. 307–10, at 309.   [80] F/8/119/2 (Pas-de-Calais), AN.
[81] F/8/123/2 (Saône et Loire), AN.
[82] *Rapport général fait au Comité de vaccine du département des Basses-Pyrénées, dans sa séance du 15 janvier, au nom de sa commission de correspondance* (Pau, 1806), pp. 1–2.
[83] *Rapport des Basses-Pyrénées*, p. 3.   [84] *Rapport des Basses-Pyrénées*, pp. 12–15.
[85] *Bulletin de Lyon*, 15 March 1808.   [86] Brion and Bellay, *Tableaux historiques*, pp. 15–16.

practitioners who, though sensible and prudent, lacked the expertise to identify true vaccine, he urged people to use the services of the health officer who was willing to vaccinate the poor at no cost. In Larajasse a farmer successfully vaccinated his neighbours arm-to-arm: 'in a commune made up entirely of farmers', explained the mayor, 'a person of their own cloth inspires more confidence than all the doctors of the Empire'.[87] In the commune of Couzon, the practice was introduced and maintained in the most curious circumstances. After participating in a plot against Napoleon, Jean-Guillaume Hyde de Neuville, a liberal aristocrat, found refuge in the home of the mayor of Couzon in summer 1805. Under the assumed name of Dr Roland, Hyde sought to make himself useful by teaching himself to vaccinate and offering the procedure to the villagers. After making his escape from France, 'Dr Roland' came to the attention of the Prefect for his work and was nominated for a medal. In his memoir, Hyde relished the irony of Napoleon's spies hunting him as a traitor while other government agents were seeking to trace him to give him a medal.[88] An item in the *Bulletin de Lyon* in 1807, hailing Couzon as exemplary in vaccination, provides additional detail and reveals an intriguing discrepancy. It states that there had been no smallpox cases in the commune since the beginning of the practice in 1805 and that the annual tally of vaccinations had risen from 78 to 194. It gives the credit, however, to the mayor and his 'remarkable daughter', who applied herself to the practice 'with a zeal that honours her sex, her age and sensibility' and with a success that won her the blessing of mothers and the poor.[89] The conflicting reports can be readily reconciled. It is likely enough that 'Dr Roland' enlisted the assistance of his host's daughter and she had continued vaccinating after his departure.

In mobilising the nation, Minister Chaptal did not neglect the clergy. The Napoleonic regime expected the Catholic church, re-established in the concordat of 1802, to serve as a pillar of the state. Prior to this time, the clergy in the French heartland were not so well placed to assist even if they were inclined to do so. In September 1802, the Bishop of Versailles made a public statement that vaccination was lawful and could be regarded as an invaluable gift from Providence.[90] In the French countryside and the annexed territories and client states, the clergy had more influence, but were not necessarily well-disposed to smallpox prophylaxis. In the former principality of Liège, the Prefect of Ourthe believed that some priests were encouraging prejudice against vaccination and requested the bishop to direct them to reassure

[87] *Bulletin de Lyon*, 15 March 1808.
[88] *Mémoires et souvenirs du Baron Hyde de Neuville*, 2nd ed., 3 vols. (Paris, 1892), 1, p. 398.
[89] *Bulletin de Lyon*, 20 June 1807.
[90] Jean-Noël Biraben, 'La diffusion de vaccination en France au xixe siècle', *Annales de Bretagne et des pays de l'Ouest*, 86 (1979), 265–76, at 268.

parishioners as to its lawfulness.[91] In his circular to prefects in 1803, Chaptal instructed them to enlist churchmen in the cause. Claude Le Coz, Archbishop of Besançon, issued a pastoral letter promoting vaccination.[92] The vaccination lobby saw Pope Pius VII's visit to Paris in winter 1804–5 as a golden opportunity. After securing an appointment for an audience with the Pope, Dr Guillotin convened a meeting to which the prefects, bishops and savants in the capital were invited.[93] On the day of the meeting in March 1805, he released to the press a copy of the committee's address to the Pope that assured his Holiness that, if he deigned to give his protection to 'this sublime discovery', posterity would have additional reason to count him among the great benefactors of humanity.[94] Though the meeting was not minuted, the committee announced that the Pope had commended vaccination and invited the clergy to commend it.[95] In July, Chaptal called directly on the bishops 'to use the means of persuasion your ministry gives you to enlighten people on the happy results' of vaccination.[96] The Bishop of Mans assured the clergy of his diocese that the Pope, while in Paris, had given unambiguous signs of his approval and urged them to present it to their parishioners as 'God's precious gift'.[97] A number of clergymen turned their hands to vaccination, not least in the remote villages of the Jura.[98] The curé of Bessine near Niort responded to smallpox in June 1806 by vaccinating himself and then, after a sermon likening it to the plagues of Egypt, announced: 'My children, I carry with me today the remedy of the ills which will perhaps in a few days afflict your families; I have vaccinated myself; come to the presbytery; you will find there a man with no vested interests who will preserve you from this malady'.[99] In a well-meaning attempt to make vaccination more palatable to children, the curé of Saint-Roman (Côte d'Or) awarded the children a holiday on the day arranged for vaccination. Unfortunately, the children simply chose to remain at home.[100]

The expansion of vaccination took place in the context of national mobilisation on a massive scale. In May 1803, the regime conscripted 120,000 men for military service, with further levies of 60,000 men in December 1804 and September 1805.[101] Following the award of the imperial title to Napoleon in

---

[91] Florkin, *Un prince, deux préfets*, pp. 176–8.   [92] Bercé, *Chaudron et lancette*, p. 128.
[93] Pigaillem, *Guillotin*, pp. 178–80.
[94] *Voyage en France du Souverain Pontife Pie VII contenant des détails sur son départ de Rome, sa marche en Italie et sur le territoire français, son séjour à Paris* (Paris, 1807), pp. 177–84.
[95] Pigaillem, *Guillotin*, pp. 180–3.
[96] Robert B. Holtman, 'The Catholic Church in Napoleon's propaganda organization', *Catholic Historical Review*, 35 (1949), 1–18, at 7; Bercé, 'Clergé et vaccination', 91–2.
[97] 18 July 1805, F/8/123, 4 (Sarthe), AN.   [98] Bercé, *Chaudron et lancette*, p. 128.
[99] *Bulletin de Lyon*, 14 June 1806.   [100] Darmon, *Longue traque*, p. 206.
[101] Isser Woloch, *The new regime. Transformations of the French civic order, 1789–1820s* (New York, 1994), p. 394.

May 1804, over three and half million Frenchmen voted in the plebiscite to approve the new constitution.[102] Soldiers were probably offered vaccination on enlistment. It is something of a myth that Napoleon made the practice compulsory, but his high regard of it was probably well known.[103] As early as 1801, Brigadier General Noguès took up the offer of Dr Tarbès to vaccinate soldiers still susceptible to smallpox in the army based around Toulouse.[104] In spring 1806 Marshal Soult approved a scheme to vaccinate the 2,066 men in the Fourth Corps stationed in Germany. A clinic was set up in the military hospital at Passau and a supply of vaccine obtained. Two soldiers from each battalion went there to be vaccinated and on return their pustules were lanced to provide lymph for their comrades. Vaccination was still not obligatory, and less than half the men initially deemed at risk were vaccinated.[105] Although the increasing scale, intensity and cost of the war in Europe put a tremendous strain on France's resources and the good will of its citizens, the military mobilisation doubtless served to generalise the new prophylaxis among the populace. According to the returns to the central vaccine committee, some 425,812 people were vaccinated in 1806 and 1807.[106] Farmers reportedly showed their patriotism and humanity by taking part in campaigns to save their communes 'from invasion by smallpox'.[107]

Still, the response to Chaptal's call to arms was uneven. Although a vaccine committee was established in the department of the Manche in 1804, it made no reports to Paris for the first four years. In response to enquiries, though, Prefect Costaz advised that the practice was well accepted in the department. In 1808, he reported 4,329 vaccinations, noting that the tally was a minimum as some practitioners were not filling out forms.[108] The printing of a formal letter requesting returns from departments in 1808 suggests that the Manche was not the only laggard. Incomplete and unreliable practices mean that the reports do not fully represent the number of vaccinations, but the overall trend is clear enough. The secretary of the committee in the department of the Ain, who reported 1,516 vaccinations in 1806 and 2,711 in 1807, felt that enthusiasm was waning.[109] In the department of the Ourthe, vaccinations plateaued between 1806 and 1808.[110] In the department of the Nord, the annual tally,

[102] Louis Bergeron, *France under Napoleon*, transl. R. R. Palmer (Princeton, NJ, 1981), p. 88.
[103] Bercé, *Chaudron et lancette*, p. 70.   [104] Colon, *Histoire*, pp. 114–16.
[105] Bercé, *Chaudron et lancette*, pp. 70–1.
[106] Tableau des vaccinations pratiquées en France pendant 1806 et 1807, F8/97/III, AN.
[107] D.-M. Pacoud, *Notice historique sur la propagation de la vaccine dans le département de l'Ain, de 1808 à 1839* (Bourg, 1840), p. 7.
[108] F. de Lannoy, 'La propagation de la vaccine dans la Manche sous l'Empire', *Annales de Normandie*, 45 (1995), 431–8, at 434–5.
[109] Pacoud, *Notice historique de vaccine dans l'Ain*, pp. 4–5.
[110] Havelange, *Figures de la guérison*, p. 263.

which rose to over 13,000 in 1807, slumped to 5,000 in 1809.[111] The decline in numbers may overstate the decline in interest. The early vaccinees included adolescents and even adults as well as children. Parents were most keen to have their children vaccinated when smallpox threatened, so an epidemic one year would create a spike in vaccination that would be followed by a slump. Mishaps and failures provided excuses for procrastination. For the vaccine committee in Lille in 1812, it was as if the practice, after its initial happy success, had lost credit.[112] For some medical men, the business of vaccination may have seemed more trouble than it was worth. The lack or loss of vaccinators was a problem identified in parts of the department of the Ourthe in 1808.[113] All too often, the practice depended on individuals. Even in Dunkirk, a substantial port, the early practice of vaccination focused on one man, an American layman not a French medical man. Benjamin Hussey, a Quaker merchant, had moved his whaling and shipping business from Nantucket in the late 1780s. In his sixties, he vaccinated many thousands of Dunkirkers at no charge, including some 4,202 in 1807 alone.[114]

The Bonapartes and Vaccination

The Bonapartes had some acquaintance with smallpox inoculation, which was practised on Corsica prior to its acquisition by France in 1768. J.-S. Vaume, the Parisian inoculator, claimed that he learned his trade from Greek practitioners in Ajaccio and that the family, 'soon to become famous', that is the Bonapartes, 'added to the number of my inoculees'.[115] It is often said that an accident of history made Napoleon, born in 1769, a Frenchman. It also made him one of the first generation of Europeans to benefit from smallpox inoculation. It is not known when Napoleon recognised the potential of English cowpox. As he was childless in the first decade of vaccination, he had no compelling personal reason to enquire closely into it. Still, he presumably condoned, if he did not actively encourage the initiative to introduce cowpox inoculation, in which his brother, Lucien, was centrally involved in 1800. From this time, Napoleon was probably well briefed on the new practice. In his address to Napoleon in October 1803, Guillotin expressed an alluring vision of the role of the Napoleonic regime in the eradication of smallpox through the 'precious discovery' of vaccination. Was it not, he asked, the destiny of the Consulate to 'succeed in glories of all sorts, in all the advances

---

[111] *Annuaire statistique du département du Nord pour l'an 1812* (Lille, 1812), p. 134.
[112] *Annuaire statistique du département du Nord*, p. 134.
[113] Havelange, *Figures de la guérison*, p. 262n.   [114] Lefebure, 'Exposé des travaux', p. 25.
[115] J.-S. Vaume, *Traité de l'inoculation de la variole, méthode de faire cette opération avec facilité et avec un succès constant* (Paris, 1825), p. 7.

that can add to the distinction of France, and to bring happiness to the world.'[116] A medal struck in 1804 in honour of vaccination gave visual expression to the idea. On the obverse, it features the bust of Napoleon, newly acclaimed emperor, crowned with a laurel wreath. On the reverse, Æsculapius is presented shielding Venus, a bandage on her arm, flanked by images of a cow and a lancet.[117] Although the medal makes no reference to Jenner, there is no doubt that Napoleon held him in high regard. In June 1805, he responded to the English doctor's request to release two Englishmen interned in France with the exclamation, 'Jenner! Ah, we can refuse nothing to that man'.[118] Napoleon was intrigued by the concept of vaccination. Musing on the place of religion in 1806, he described it as 'a sort of inoculation or vaccine which, while satisfying our sense of the supernatural, guarantees us from the charlatans and the magicians'.[119]

The Napoleonic regime pushed vaccination in all the lands subject to its rule and influence. It is a matter of some debate how appropriate it is to talk about a French empire in Europe.[120] The championship of vaccination in France's annexed territories and client-states, the establishment of vaccine committees reporting back to the *comité central* and the emergence of new networks, centred in Paris, for the circulation of vaccine and information, made the new prophylaxis an 'imperial' project. Vaccination had an ideological dimension. A compound of natural remedy, empirical science and governmentality, it was emblematic of the enlightened, authoritarian state. In rural and remote districts, where ignorance and superstition held sway, the provision of vaccination was presented as an example of the empire's benevolence and civilising mission. Among the educated elite in northern Italy, the Rhineland and the Netherlands, it served the ends of *amalgam* and *ralliement*, with nobles and churchmen, liberals and former Jacobins, working with French commissars on *comités de vaccine*. It was axiomatic in 1811 that every effort should be made to establish vaccination in the Illyrian Provinces, ceded to France in 1809, as in other parts of the empire.[121] Napoleon's siblings proved great patrons of vaccination. Napoleon's sister Elisa began her rule as an enlightened despot in Piombino-Lucca in 1805 by prohibiting variolation and making vaccination compulsory. Her measures

---

[116] Pigaillem, *Guillotin*, pp. 177–8.
[117] Aubin Louis Millin and James V. Millingen, *Medallic history of Napoleon: a collection of all the medals, coins and jettons relating to his actions and reign* (London, 1819), p. 34–5.
[118] Baron, *Life*, 2, pp. 36–8.
[119] *The Corsican. The diary of Napoleon's life in his own words*, ed. R. M. Johnston (London, 1910), p. 227.
[120] Michael Broers, *The Napoleonic Empire in Italy, 1796–1814. Cultural imperialism in a European context?* (Basingstoke, 2005), esp. pp. 22–7.
[121] 5 October 1811, F/8/128, V (Provinces Illyriennes), AN.

to eradicate smallpox included the reporting of all cases, the use of soldiers to isolate them and the obligation of parents to have children vaccinated within their first months. In spring 1806, she had her own daughter vaccinated to show her confidence in the procedure and, in a letter to Count Ségur early in 1807, she claimed responsibility for 15,000 children being vaccinated in a month.[122] During the rule of Eugène de Beauharnais, Napoleon's stepson, as Viceroy of Italy, Dr Sacco's vaccination programme in Lombardy reached new heights. In his *Trattato di vaccinazione*, dedicated to the Viceroy in 1809, Sacco claimed that one and half million people had been vaccinated in the kingdom.[123] After his installation as the king of Holland in 1806, Louis Bonaparte greatly augmented the government's role in smallpox prophylaxis by introducing measures in 1808 that remained in force for over half a century. After the full integration of the Netherlands into the Napoleonic Empire in 1810, the appointment of a new set of prefects set the scene for creation of vaccination committees to entrench the practice.[124]

In France itself, Napoleon intervened to re-energise the vaccination cause. Though a fraction of the mortality a decade earlier, the 213 smallpox deaths in Paris in 1809 were presented as 'too considerable', because they were preventable. At its tenth anniversary meeting in May 1810, the central committee in Paris reported that the Emperor, as 'a signal mark of his paternal solicitude', had allocated an annual budget to support vaccination and announced new measures to streamline arrangements, generalise good local practice and provide new incentives to practitioners. A new network of vaccination committees and vaccine depots were established in twenty-four major centres across France and the empire. In addition to reporting on their vaccination activity to Paris, the local committees were again encouraged to recommend notable practitioners for medals and offer their own rewards. The new measures of 1810 included a prize scheme that aimed to reward outstanding performance across the empire. The first prize was 3,000 francs; there were two second prizes of 2,000 francs each; three third prizes of 1,000 francs each; and silver medals for a hundred runners up.[125] Napoleon's 'paternal solicitude' had a personal dimension. By summer 1810, his new wife, Marie Louise of Austria, was pregnant, presenting her husband with a son and heir, known as the king of Rome, in March 1811. Napoleon wasted no time in securing him from smallpox, specifying that the men drafted to his son's elite bodyguard have a

[122] Bercé, *Chaudron et lancette*, pp. 64–6.
[123] Luigi Sacco, *Trattato di vaccinazione con osservazioni sul giavardo e vajuolo pecorino* (Milan, 1809), p. 18.
[124] Rutten, *Pokkenbestrijding in Nederland*, pp. 226–34.
[125] *Edinburgh Medical and Surgical Journal*, 7 (1811), pp. 117–18.

certificate attesting their immune status.[126] The baby's vaccination took priority over his baptism. After selecting vaccine and testing it on other infants, Dr Husson vaccinated the royal infant at the Château de Saint-Cloud on 11 May. To make sure of the genuineness of the vaccine response, Husson took lymph from the baby to vaccinate three other children and then took lymph from them to vaccinate thirty-nine others.[127] News of the success of the vaccination of Napoleon's son was telegraphed to Brussels and Turin, prompting celebrations and praise of the father for setting an example to his people. As the Prefect of the Pô explained to the mayors of his department, the Emperor had

set the seal on the value of vaccination by subjecting to the procedure the object of his most tender affections, the hope of France, namely the King of Rome, feeling the need to inspire in you the desire to strive with all the means in your power for the propagation of a discovery which ought to be regarded as a gift of Heaven.[128]

The Advance and Retreat of Vaccination

The new impetus from Napoleon is reflected in an impressive scaling up of vaccination activity in the French empire between 1810 and 1812.[129] In Manche, the totals in 1811 and 1812 represented an increase of around 275 per cent on the tally in 1808.[130] In the department of the Nord, the number of vaccinations doubled in 1810 and then rose to over 17,000 in 1811 and 18,000 in 1812.[131] Though the prefects knew what the government wanted to hear, the ups and downs in the number of vaccinations and their attempts to explain them, would suggest that the totals are reasonably indicative.[132] The Prefect of Liamone (Corsica) was not afraid to report in 1812 that his department had lost its supply of vaccine and was unable to replenish it due to the war.[133] Elsewhere on the frontiers of the empire, there were solid results. In the department of the Roër, centred on Aachen (Aix-la-Chapelle), Baron Ladoucette built on successes in 1811 by instituting an annual scheme of general vaccination beginning in June 1812.[134] Baron Gandolfo, Prefect of Ombrone, centred on Siena, won praise for his paternal solicitude in supporting prophylaxis. Dr Barzelloti and his colleagues vaccinated 616 people in

---

[126] John Tyler Headley, *The imperial guard of Napoleon: from Marengo to Waterloo* (New York, 1851), p. 111.
[127] André Castelot, *King of Rome. A biography of Napoleon's tragic son* (New York, 1960), pp. 50–1.
[128] Bercé, *Chaudron et lancette*, p. 66.   [129] Darmon, *Longue traque*, pp. 207–10.
[130] de Lannoy, 'Vaccine dans la Manche', 436.   [131] Lefebure, 'Exposé des travaux', 26.
[132] Cf. Fressoz, *L'apocalypse joyeuse*, pp. 100–6.
[133] 20 December 1812, F/8/105, I (Corse), 2 (Liamone), AN.
[134] *Recueil des actes de la préfecture du département de la Roer: Sammlung der Praefectur Acten des Roer Departements. Jahr 1812* (Aachen, 1812), pp. 129–31.

1809, 3,021 in 1810, and 5,038 in 1811. The tally of 5,836 vaccinations in 1812 represented 77 per cent of the 7,909 births that year. In contrast, only six smallpox deaths were recorded, mainly in villages on the highway between Florence and Rome.[135] The publicity associated with the prizes may have helped to mobilise practitioners, amateur and professional, in the war against smallpox. In the French department of the Nord in 1810, they included sixteen physicians, nineteen surgeons, thirty health officers, eight midwives, one clergyman and ten others, including Benjamin Hussey at Dunkirk.[136] The most active vaccinator in 1811 was an anonymous lady who immunised 700 children in the canton of Bavay.[137] In the department of Ain, three farmers, who had first vaccinated in 1804, again took up the lancet, delivered vaccine to isolated communities, and 'saved for a second time the populations of their rich communes from invasion by smallpox'.[138]

In 1812, the war against smallpox might have appeared winnable. The number of vaccinations nationally rose by nearly 250 per cent between 1806 and 1810 and then doubled again between 1810 and 1812. In 1811 a total of 712,151 was recorded, and in 1812 a stunning 752,270.[139] The number of births is not recorded for these years, but the ratio of vaccinations to live births was probably over 80 per cent. The expansion of the practice in its first decade, though impressive, was by no means smooth. Large-scale vaccination activity, especially during epidemics, was often followed, especially when smallpox appeared to be in retreat, by periods of relative apathy and inertia. The reappearance of smallpox, flaring up in a city or town and then sweeping through the countryside, served again as a powerful inducement to seek prophylaxis. In the Italian town of Moldovi, for example, a major epidemic in 1812 prompted an increase in the percentage of vaccinations to live births from 3 per cent in 1811 to 105 per cent in 1812.[140] In official and medical circles under Napoleon, it was self-evident that vaccination had a vital role to play in protecting the nation's manpower. The number of smallpox deaths across France in 1810, that is 1,793, was substantially less than the number in Paris alone prior to the advent of vaccination.[141] The Napoleonic regime never sought to make vaccination compulsory, but a great deal of indirect pressure was applied. Over time, for example, it became requisite for children and adolescents entering elite schools and some occupational categories. Recruits to the army probably felt that they had no choice in the matter. On the Rhine

---

[135] Carteggio del comitato per la vaccinazione, 1809–13, Governo francese, 228, Archivio di stato, Siena.
[136] Annuaire statistique du département du Nord, p. 137.
[137] Lefebure, 'Exposé des travaux', p. 26.
[138] Pacoud, Notice historique de vaccine dans l'Ain, p. 7.   [139] Biraben, 'La diffusion', 269.
[140] Bercé, Chaudron et lancette, p. 319.   [141] Biraben, 'La diffusion', 269.

frontier in 1812, Baron Ladoucette felt justified in ordering the vaccination of all children susceptible to smallpox. In a letter to magistrates in Cologne, he stated that, if persuasion failed to induce parents to have children vaccinated, religion and humanity required them to use their authority and that, if 'unbelievers' objected, they were to tell them that the son of the Great Napoleon had been vaccinated.[142]

It is a moot point whether the expansion of vaccination could have been sustained. The ministerial drive from 1810 reaped dividends. Many prefects made a strong commitment to vaccination. Baron Ladoucette was proud to report that the districts in which general vaccinations had been instituted in 1811 resisted smallpox in 1812. Across France, the raising of more troops in that year and the return of the remnants of the *Grande Armée* were accompanied by epidemic smallpox that cost 9,019 lives.[143] Still, smallpox prophylaxis made a difference. Despite the adverse impact of the war on population and productivity, Count de Montalivet, Minister of the Interior, noted signs of demographic recovery in the French countryside in 1812 that he attributed to vaccination.[144] The basic problem was that the French government did not see it as its business to fund mass prophylaxis. Medals and prizes were all very well, but they did not provide vaccinators with an adequate income. The government rarely approved the allowances that some prefects felt necessary to support local vaccination campaigns. There was no clear advice as to whether public vaccinators who were contractually bound to vaccinate the poor were allowed to charge fees to parents who had the means to pay.[145] The expansion of vaccination between 1810 and 1812 drew heavily on the services of the lower echelons of the health profession, including *officiers de santé* and midwives, whose involvement may have had the further advantage of helping to build trust in the prophylaxis among poorly educated mothers. Some of the success can perhaps be attributed to the patriotic spirit and sense of purpose under Napoleon. The system came close to collapse, predictably enough, in the wake of defeat and invasion in 1814–15. During a smallpox epidemic in Normandy in autumn 1814, however, the practice itself proved resilient, albeit with reversion to older traditions with the Marquis d'Herbouville, who, as Prefect of Deux-Nèthes, promoted vaccination in Antwerp, presiding over the vaccination of seventy young children in his chateau.[146] In most parts of

---

[142] *Recueil des actes du département de la Roer*, p. 213.   [143] Biraben, 'La diffusion', 269.

[144] T. J. A. Le Goff and D. M. G. Sutherland, 'The revolution and the rural economy', in Alan I. Forrest and Peter Jones (eds.), *Reshaping France: town, country, and region during the French revolution* (Manchester, 1991), pp. 52–85, at p. 54.

[145] Darmon, *Longue traque*, pp. 263–75.

[146] *Rapport à monsieur le comte Stanislas de Girardin ... préfet du département de la Seine Inférieure, sur les vaccinations opérées dans plusieurs communes des environs de Rouen, ravages par la petite vérole en 1814* (Rouen, 1815), pp. 9–10.

France and the former empire there were foundations on which to rebuild. If its association with the Napoleonic regime may not have been a commendation in rural Italy, vaccination was probably more firmly rooted in the annexed territories in the Rhineland than in the French heartland. At his command post at Aix-la-Chapelle, Ladoucette may have felt he had more prospect of holding the line against smallpox than against the Russian host that dogged Napoleon's retreat from Moscow.

In July 1798, Henry Motz purchased Jenner's *Inquiry* in London. A Hessian serving in the commissariat of the British Army, he sent it as gift to his old school-friend, Dr B. C. Faust of Bückeburg, one of the authors of the plan for the eradication of smallpox addressed to the Congress of Rastatt.[1] Herr Scherer, a German visitor to London, brought a copy home to Weimar and made it available to Professor C. W. Hufeland in Jena.[2] In September, Charles Parry, the son of the dedicatee of the *Inquiry*, may have taken a copy to present to Professor J. F. Blumenbach at the University of Göttingen, where he was continuing his medical studies after a walking tour with S. T. Coleridge.[3] There were many close ties and connections between England and northern Europe. In addition to ruling Hanover, the British royal family were linked by marriage with many German princely families. Though religion was less important in international relations by this time, the common Protestant heritage made it more congenial for Britons and north Europeans to travel, pursue education and do business across the North Sea. Many Germans regarded Britain as a land of opportunity and a showcase of new ideas and technology. Britons found success in selling goods and services in northern Europe, not least practitioners of the 'new inoculation' from the late 1760s. Given the connections and cultural affinities, it is not surprising that doctors and laymen in northern Europe were intrigued by the cowpox discovery and, after the trials in London, disposed to give it some credit. The copies of the *Inquiry* that crossed the North Sea were not without impact. In the last quarter of 1798, Hufeland brought Jenner's cowpox to the attention of German medical men in his 'journal of practical medicine'. Dr Faust became a champion of vaccination and the founder of a children's festival on 14 May, the anniversary of Jenner's operation on James Phipps,

---

[1] Bernhard Christoph Faust, *An den Herrn Dr. Eduard Jenner, über einige Versuche zur weiteren Untersuchung der Wirkungen und zum Beweise der Unschädlichkeit der Kuhpocken-Materie* (Hannover, 1802), p. 24.

[2] *Hufelands Journal der practischen Heilkunde*, 6 (1798), 97–9.

[3] Saunders, *Cheltenham years*, p. 102.

174

that continues in Bückeburg to this day.[4] Interestingly, early German sceptics attributed the enthusiasm of their colleagues to 'Anglomania'.[5]

Around 1800, Germany and northern Europe were experiencing accelerating change. Demographic growth and economic development in the late eighteenth century created a more complex and dynamic society. An increase in literacy and the size of the reading public provided a broader foundation for the cultural and intellectual vitality associated with the Enlightenment. The absolutist regimes in Germany, Denmark and Sweden were powerful agents of economic and cultural modernisation. While population growth put pressure on resources, the economy was developing along with the ambitions of the new states. The French Revolution created new aspirations and anxieties and, after the outbreak of war between France and the Holy Roman Empire and Prussia in 1791, brought new challenges to an old order already in transformation. In the wake of French military success, the political map of the Holy Roman Empire of the German Nation was redrawn between 1797 and 1803, with the incorporation of many free cities and ecclesiastical states into the larger polities, setting the stage for the abolition of the Holy Roman Empire in 1806. In the titanic struggle between France on one side and Britain and a changing cast of allies on the other, the middle-sized northern powers found neither opportunism nor neutrality to be safe courses. After several French provocations, Prussia defied Napoleon in 1806, but then suffered humiliating defeat at Jena, an army of occupation through much of 1807, and territorial loss in the Treaty of Tilsit. For their part, Denmark and Sweden, key parties to the Armed Neutralities of the North, were subject to economic retaliation from Britain and bombardment from the British navy.

It has been observed that, while Britain had an industrial revolution and France had a political revolution, Germany had a 'reading revolution'.[6] The point simplifies and narrows the scope of the transformations taking place. It does, however, encapsulate distinctive features of northern Europe's path to modernity. The Dutch, Germans and Scandinavians were close observers of developments in Britain and France; they felt the impact of the momentous changes rapidly and uncomfortably directly; they sought to learn about them and discussed and debated their meaning and import; and found in them sources of inspiration or anxiety. The notion of a 'reading' revolution, moreover, indicates something more positive than merely experiencing life second hand. It points to an expansion in literacy, schooling, higher education and

---

[4] H. A. Gins, *Krankheit wider den Tod. Schicksal der Pockenschutzimpfung* (Stuttgart, 1963), p. 28.
[5] Sköld, *Two faces*, p. 374.
[6] David Blackbourn, *The long nineteenth century. The Fontana history of Germany 1780–1918* (London, 1997), pp. 40–3.

publishing – an expansion in the size of the 'public sphere' – that was well advanced in the Netherlands and more rapid in Germany than in Britain or France. Germany, after all, was the cradle of the print industry and the German Enlightenment had deep roots in strong traditions of craftsmanship, technology and natural philosophy. The Lutheran church provided the framework of public religion in most German and Scandinavian states and a set of values that proved accommodating of new imperatives and ideas. The Enlightenment in northern Europe proved eclectic in its blend of cosmopolitanism and localism and showed leadership and creativity in translating new ideas and aspirations into administrative measures and educational programmes. By the late eighteenth century there was growing interest elsewhere in Europe in German craftsmanship and art, its science, philosophy and literature, even its models of governance. Coleridge's walking tour in Germany reflects an engagement with Goethe and Romanticism and the enrolment of his walking companion, Charles Parry, at Göttingen indicates growing English regard for German scholarship. The reception of vaccination in northern Europe would by no means be passive.

Smallpox Prophylaxis in Northern Europe

The introduction of vaccination in the Netherlands, Germany and Scandinavia was facilitated by long and thoughtful engagement with smallpox inoculation. The dynastic link between Britain and Hanover gave it a foothold in Göttingen in the 1720s and the connections between German princely families facilitated its expansion. From the 1750s northern Europe learned to look to England as the fount of expertise. Dutch, German and Swedish physicians went to study inoculation in London and looked to Britain for developments in the field. Conversely, medical men from Britain made expertise in inoculation their calling card in northern Europe. Goethe recalled that in his youth the business in Frankfurt was in the hands of 'travelling Englishmen', while Madame Schopenhauer remembered being inoculated in Danzig (Gdansk) in the 1770s by an English doctor, 'one of a race of physicians who just then came into fashion' who 'set at defiance all the established rules of decorum and civility, and affected a simplicity of manners bordering on rudeness' and who, on this account, were 'especial favourites of fine ladies and princes'.[7] Inoculation was widely patronised by the elite in Germany and Scandinavia. It created and disclosed bonds of interest, intimacy and intrigue. After learning about the practice in Edinburgh and London, Dr J. A. H. Reimarus began inoculating in Hamburg in 1757, including the daughters of a Danish court official. Struck by

---

[7] Sarah Austin, *Germany, from 1760 to 1814; or, sketches of German life, from the decay of Empire to the expulsion of the French* (London, 1854), pp. 73–5.

the 'sharp and noble mind' of one of the girls, Sophie, he proposed to her and secured her hand. Dr Reimarus, his wife, nicknamed 'the doctor', and his sister Elise, known as 'the muse of Hamburg', were at the heart of Hamburg's scientific, literary and humanitarian endeavours, including support of inoculation, for several decades.[8] Inoculation brought another German physician a dangerous eminence in Denmark. As a court physician, J. M. Struensee undertook the inoculation of the Danish Crown Prince in 1770. His close attachment, personal and political, to the Prince's mother, Queen Caroline, was consummated by an affair during the Prince's passage through the disease. The adultery prompted a palace coup, the execution of Struensee for treason, and the confinement of Queen Caroline, sister of George III of England, in a remote castle.[9]

The politics of northern Europe generally proved hospitable to inoculation. Though politically and religiously divided, the states were at one in their desire to promote population growth in their lands. The Protestant states were served by men of similar ideological stamp – nobles who had been given a modern education as army officers or cameralist bureaucrats and clergy who saw themselves now as serving God through philanthropy and service to a beneficent state. Many princes regarded themselves as men of the Enlightenment who sought to use their power to make their states more prosperous and subjects happier. Frederick the Great of Prussia was an early champion of inoculation, though later in life he became more circumspect.[10] The Duke and Duchess of Saxe-Gotha, with his encouragement, made an early splash by espousing inoculation in 1759. Frederick V, king of Denmark, gave his people 'a convincing proof of his complete belief in the excellence and advantages of cure that he recommends to his subjects' by allowing the Crown Prince's inoculation in 1760.[11] After arranging their own inoculation in 1768, the Duke and Duchess of Anhalt-Dessau visited the celebrated Samuel August Tissot in Lausanne, prior to the inoculation of their children in the early 1770s.[12] To establish the practice among their subjects, the kings of Denmark and Sweden set up inoculation hospitals along English lines and Frederick of Prussia brought a British physician to Berlin in 1775 to run a workshop 'in the modern method' of inoculation, ordering the attendance of medical men from across

---

[8] *The account books of the Reimarus family of Hamburg, 1728–1780*, 2 vols., ed. Almut Spalding and Paul S. Spaldin (Leiden, 2015), 2, pp. 1174, 1235, 1321. Almut Spalding, *Elise Reimarus (1735–1805): The muse of Hamburg: a woman of the German enlightenment* (Würzburg, 2005), p. 157.

[9] F. C. Lascelles Wraxall, *Life and times of Her Majesty Caroline Matilda, queen of Demark and Norway*, 3 vols. (London, 1864), 1, pp. 223–4.

[10] *Correspondance de Frédéric le Grand Roi de Prusse*, vol. 11, ed. J.-D.-E. Preuss (Berlin, 1855), p. 663.

[11] Eriksen, 'Case of exemplarity', 356.   [12] Penschow, 'Wrestling *der Würgengel*', 67–8.

the kingdom 'so that the most distant of his subjects might partake of its benefits'.[13] The Lutheran pastors, who already served as government agents in their parishes, recording births and deaths, were enlisted to support the practice. Many of them, aspiring to a broader philanthropic vocation, became its champions and some took up the lancet themselves.

The medical men of northern Europe were generally well disposed to smallpox prophylaxis. As elsewhere in Europe, they were a diverse group, including university-educated physicians, guild-trained surgeons and apothecaries and a range of unlicensed operators. A distinctive element in the German scene, however, was the *Physicus*, a state-appointed physician whose responsibilities for public health gave them reason to take smallpox and prophylaxis seriously. In Brunswick (Braunschweig) in 1754, the medical college considered a plan for establishing an inoculation institute, and offered inoculation to the public during outbreaks in 1767–8, 1771 and 1787. The initiatives led to 350 inoculations, though doubtless more were done privately. As one layman observed, however, 'the life of one child', their child, 'weighs more heavily than the system' for most parents, and that he 'would really like to have more information from other places before we resolve that it is better to sacrifice every ninth child on the altar of science rather than every seventh child on the altar of nature'.[14] The medical faculties in German universities, more concerned than their English counterparts to prepare doctors for public service, ran informal workshops on variolation. Even so, medical men in Germany were more active in discussing inoculation than practising it and the influence of Pietism and later Kantian philosophy encouraged attention to the ethical issues.[15] Even as the practice became more common in the last quarter of the eighteenth century, moreover, new concerns were being raised about inoculation's role in spreading the infection. In 1791, a suspected outbreak of smallpox in Halle prompted an inoculation campaign that fuelled an epidemic in which there were 2,151 cases, of whom 430 died and 7 lost their sight.[16] After an enquiry into the tragedy, Dr Juncker formed a network of colleagues to gather data on smallpox outbreaks and inoculation activity in their districts and communicate them to an 'archive of doctors against smallpox'. He published

---

[13] Baylies, *Facts and observations*, pp. 130–1.

[14] Lindemann, *Health and healing*, pp. 331–2, 454.

[15] Andreas-Holger Maehle, 'Conflicting attitudes towards inoculation in Enlightenment Germany', in Roy Porter (ed.), *Medicine in the Enlightenment* (Amsterdam, 1995), pp. 198–222. Andreas-Holger Maehle, 'The ethics of prevention: German philosophers of the late Enlightenment on the morality of smallpox inoculation', in John Woodward and Robert Jütte (eds.), *Coping with sickness: perspectives on health care, past and present* (Sheffield, 1996), pp. 91–114.

[16] *MPJ*, 4 (July–December 1800), 141.

issues of the *Archiv* twice a year from 1796, dedicating the first issue to 'the father of our Fatherland', Frederick William II of Prussia.[17]

Inoculation also became increasingly well known in the Netherlands and Scandinavia. In the first decades of the practice in Britain some Dutch nobles sent their children to London for the operation. Théodore Tronchin offered inoculation in Amsterdam in the late 1740s and Charles Chais, pastor of the French Reformed church in The Hague, dispelled religious concerns about the practice and argued for its utility in 1754.[18] In the larger towns, however, there were concerns about the risk posed to the community and, in the countryside, there were pockets of Calvinist opposition. The improved mode of inoculation brought new interest in the late 1760s. Dr Sutherland and John Hewitt used The Hague as a base from which they offered their services to the princes of northern Europe.[19] Although they recognised the value of inoculation, Dutch medical men did not seem to have taken up the practice in any number. In 1774, the British ambassador expressed the hope that the 'sudden resolution' of the Prince and Princess of Orange to have their children inoculated would reverse 'the tide of prejudice' which 'runs strong against the practice in this country'.[20] Inoculation activity remained patchy. One true believer was Gadso Coopmans, rector of the University of Franekar who, despite the recent death of his daughter through variolation, wrote a Latin allegory about smallpox in 1783 that ended with the triumph of inoculation.[21] In the kingdoms of Denmark-Norway, royal and ministerial sponsorship gave inoculation an early boost. In 1754 Count Bernstorff recruited an English surgeon to inoculate his wife; a royal inoculation clinic was established in Copenhagen; the procedure was used during an epidemic in Trondheim; and the inoculation of the Crown Prince in 1760 was well publicised.[22] Still, the clinic and the practice languished for lack of patients. A decade later the Danish elite looked to German practitioners for prophylaxis. In 1797, the Medical Board still recommended inoculation, but was concerned about its potential to spread the disease.[23] In Sweden, the practice made slow but steady progress. In the 1790s, Dr Christopher Carlander conducted general inoculations in Gothenburg; a Lutheran pastor organised a general inoculation in his rural parish; and the owner of an ironworks inoculated his workforce.[24]

---

[17] *Archiv der Aerzte und Seelsorger wider die Pockennoth*, ed. J. C. W. Juncker, vols. 1 (Michaelmas, 1796), 2 (Easter, 1797), 3 (Michaelmas, 1797), 4 (New Year, 1798), 5 (Easter, 1798), 6 (Michaelmas, 1798), 7 (Michaelmas, 1799); Maehle, 'Attitudes towards inoculation', p. 213.

[18] Chais, *Essai apologétique.*   [19] MS. 7313/3, WLL.

[20] Amherst Manuscripts, U1350/C41/51–52, Centre for Kentish Studies, Maidstone.

[21] Sacré, 'Gadso Coopmans and his *Varis*', 520–38.   [22] Eriksen, 'Case of exemplarity', 356.

[23] Gerda Bonderup, *En kovending: koppevaccinationen og dens udfordring til det danske samfund omkring 1800* (Aarhus, 2001), pp. 27–8.

[24] Sköld, *Two faces*, pp. 333–5.

The idea of preventing smallpox remained a source of inspiration in northern Europe. Even in the 1760s, some German medical men envisioned the possibility of eradicating the disease.[25] There was certainly strong interest among princes and statesmen in the contribution that preventative measures could make to reduce high levels of child mortality and to the consequent increase in population and productivity. Though positive in principle about inoculation, and often using the procedure to secure their families, medical men and magistrates were increasingly less optimistic that smallpox inoculation could play a large role in suppressing the contagion. It was recognised that the inoculation of large numbers of people, especially cut-price inoculation in busy markets and towns, all too often served to spread the contagion. The sorts of 'general inoculations' that were practised in parts of England may have been feasible in more compact settlements east of the Elbe, but required a high degree of organisation and community acceptance. There was evidently little enthusiasm among the general populace. Given the risk and the cost in money and time, few people were willing to be inoculated except when smallpox was an immediate threat. Even then, it seemed easier to allow nature to take its course or to adopt the time-honoured practice of 'buying the smallpox', that is exposing children to less severe cases in the hope of a better outcome. For this reason, physicians like Dr Faust and Dr Juncker placed emphasis on measures to contain smallpox by isolating cases and looking to the establishment of special houses where people could be inoculated safely. Their scheme for eradication, of course, would be costly, albeit with corresponding economic benefits, and require strong political support, which meant, in Germany, the backing of some of the major states. Faust and Juncker cannot have had high hopes for the adoption of their plan at the Congress of Rastatt, preoccupied with more pressing political issues. The great hope that inoculation inspired in northern Europe and growing recognition of the pitfalls of the old practice nonetheless help to explain the highly positive response of most medical men and many laymen to the promise of cowpox. Faust had a copy of Jenner's treatise by autumn 1798 and in November cowpox was being discussed in medical networks that extended to Uppsala in Sweden.[26] In June 1800, Dr Juncker wrote a letter in Latin to Dr Pearson reporting on the *Archiv* on smallpox and the scheme for eradicating it, expressing an interest in the cowpox discovery and asking for a sample to be sent in a sealed glass container to inoculate some children in Halle.[27] Juncker died later in the year, perhaps before he could make a proper trial of the new virus. Dr Faust, however,

[25] Penschow, 'Wrestling der *Würgengel*', pp. 255–7.
[26] *Brevväxling mellan Christopher Carlander och Pehr Afzelius 1789–1822*, ed. Lars Öberg and Stig Cronberg (Tygelsjö, 1991), p. 66.
[27] *MPJ*, 4 (July–December 1800), 141–5; MS. 6914, WLL.

survived to see vaccination well-established in Germany and to lament the passing of Dr Jenner in 1823.

Cowpox (Kühpocken) to Guardian Pox (Schutzpocken)

From the spring of 1799 cowpox was dispatched across the North Sea. The vaccine sent to Vienna in May was the first to be successfully propagated outside England, but some successful trials took place in Hanover over the summer. Dr Ballhorn and Mr Stromeyer, who held positions at the Hanoverian court, saw themselves as the natural conduits for the English innovation and took on the task of translating Jenner's *Inquiry* into German. The connection between the British and Prussian royal houses assisted the introduction of vaccination in Germany. Early in 1799, Frederica, Duchess of York, was alert to the advantages of cowpox and a sample was sent to Louisa of Prussia, which was found to be inert on arrival. In November, Dr Sybil achieved the first successful vaccination in Brandenburg with vaccine supplied from Hanover.[28] Through the activities of De Carro, Vienna emerged as a major centre for the distribution of information and vaccine in the German *Reich*. Dr Friese of Breslau (Wrocław) established the practice in Silesia, with vaccine sent from the Austrian capital in December.[29] Despite the war and the disruption to communications, London continued to serve as a direct source of cowpox for medical men in western Germany, the Netherlands and Denmark. In 1800, Dr Gerhard Reumont, director of the Marienhospital in Aachen, ventured to London to learn about cowpox inoculation, bringing back vaccine to begin the practice in the Meuse-Rhine region.[30] Through the good offices of the Reverend Monod, pastor of the French Reformed church in Copenhagen, F. C. Winsløw received cowpox from Jenner to use in the first, albeit unsuccessful trials in Denmark in the summer of 1801.[31]

It took some patience to establish the practice in northern Europe. The inoculators in Germany had little time to explore the potential of cowpox before finding themselves in the thick of the confusion arising from early experimentation in England. The first samples sent by Dr Pearson came from patients inoculated at St Pancras and occasioned the generalised eruptions that suggested variolous infection. Jenner's advice about the need to distinguish between 'genuine' and 'spurious' cowpox was not always easy to follow. Still, German medical men rose to the challenge of mastering the literature, increasingly available in translation, on cowpox and its vagaries. In the spring of 1800, Strohmeyer contributed to the developing science by

---

[28] Gins, *Krankheit*, p. 15.   [29] *MPJ*, 9 (January–June 1803), 128–9.
[30] *Deutsche Biographische Enzyklopädie*, VIII, p. 340.
[31] Bonderup, *En kovending*, pp. 36–7.

providing feedback on the vaccines he received from London and Glouces-tershire.[32] With the early vaccinations often failing or producing ambiguous outcomes, it was a challenge to propagate good vaccine and maintain it over time. Medical men in northern Europe, as elsewhere, frequently began by inoculating their own children, both setting an example and securing a private supply of vaccine. In the cities and towns, patrician and professional families sometimes offered their children for vaccination to help begin the practice. The major towns, with orphanages and schools, offered the best chance of providing a stream of susceptible children to establish it properly. The large and cosmopolitan port of Hamburg emerged as an early centre of vaccination activity. It suffered mightily from smallpox: in 1798, 10 per cent of its inhabitants died from the disease and a further 5 per cent lost their health and beauty.[33] Dr Alexander MacDonald reportedly 'distinguish'd himself by introducing inoculation for the cow-pox' and overcoming the prejudices of his German colleagues.[34] His account of his experiments in Hamburg in 1800 concluded with 'a most animated address to fathers and mothers on the subject'.[35]

During 1800 supplies of cowpox became more broadly available. The war slowed communications between Britain and the Netherlands. Though he saw English cowpox in action in Rotterdam in 1799, Dr Levie Davids was unable to resume his experiments until after a visit to Paris in autumn 1800 enabled him to observe the beginnings of vaccination in France and return with the latest publications and a supply of vaccine. By the end of 1800 there were trials of the practice in The Hague, Haarlem and Amsterdam as well as Rotterdam and, over the course of the following year, the practice was being introduced, hesitantly in most places, in almost all the larger towns in the Netherlands.[36] In the meantime samples from London continued to find their way to Hanover and northern Germany. In summer 1800, Dr Heineke used a sample from Hanover to vaccinate some 200 people in Halberstadt. In autumn, Professor Christian Wiedemann and two colleagues obtained vaccine, probably from Halberstadt, to inaugurate the practice in Brunswick (Braunschweig) by vaccinating their own children. It took some time for Berlin to establish the practice. In February 1800, Dr Heim

[32] Ring, *Treatise*, 1, pp. 223–3.
[33] U. Frevert, *Krankheit als politisches Problem 1770–1880. Soziale Unterschichten in Prueßen zwischen medizinischer Polizei und staatlicher Sozialversicherung* (Göttingen, 1984), pp. 69–71; Richard J. Evans, *Death in Hamburg. Society and politics in the cholera years* (Oxford, 1987), pp. 218–19.
[34] [Thomas Rede Leman], *A sketch of Hambourg, its commerce, customs and manners* (Hamburg, 1801), pp. 81–2.
[35] Alexander Hermann MacDonald, *Abhandlung über die jetzt fast allgemein eingeführte Inoculation der Kuhpocken*, transl. J. P. F. Lochet (Hamburg, 1800).
[36] Rutten, *Pokkenbestrijding in Nederland*, pp. 209–18.

experimented with cowpox from London but proved unable to produce viable lymph. In October, Dr Johann Immanuel Bremer, physician at the royal orphanage, finally put the practice on a solid foundation by conducting trials, propagating a supply of vaccine, and dispatching samples to colleagues throughout Prussia.[37] During 1801, cowpox inoculation became available in all the main population centres. In January, Dr A. C. Reuß began vaccinating in Stuttgart with matter sent from Frankfurt.[38] In the east, Dr Friese made Breslau a centre of the new prophylaxis, distributing vaccine through Silesia and Prussian Poland and, indeed, as far as Moscow.[39] In Denmark, the first successful vaccinations also took place in 1801. From Sweden, Dr Eberhard Munch af Rosenschöld crossed the Sound twice to obtain samples from colleagues in Copenhagen. Finally, on 23 October 1801, in the port of Malmö, he inaugurated vaccination in Sweden.[40]

Cowpox attracted much publicity in the print media. The *Reichs-Anzeiger* kept the German reading-public up-to-date with the new practice. In a series of articles in the *Braunschweigisches Magazin* in autumn 1800, Dr Weidemann outlined its advantages and addressed points of concern.[41] Astonished by the number of German books on vaccination at the spring fair at Leipzig in 1801, an English reviewer wrote: 'The Easter-Catalogue swarms with treatises on this interesting subject, and with zealous calls to receive the new *Dea Salus*, whom the voice of Jenner has charmed forth from the cow-house'. The publications included a new edition of Dr Faust's *Catechism of health*, in which he commended cowpox and the first issue of a journal, the *Archiv für die Kuhpocken-Impfung*, dedicated to the new practice.[42] The focus on cowpox led to enquiries in Germany's dairy districts. It emerged that Peter Plett, a school-teacher in Holstein, had inoculated girls with cowpox in 1790, but the University of Kiel was unable to find any current cases.[43] In Scandinavia, news of vaccination arrived long before viable vaccine. Correspondence between Dr Carlander of Gothenburg and Dr Pehr Afzelius in Uppsala makes it possible to eavesdrop on two Swedish physicians reading about cowpox in autumn 1798, marvelling at its reception in Germany in 1800, relishing the debate

---

[37] Gins, *Krankheit*, p. 15.
[38] Eberhard Wolff, *Einschneidende Maßnahmen. Pockenschutzimpfung und traditionale Gesell-schaft im Württemberg des frühen 19. Jahrhunderts* (Stuttgart, 1998), pp. 110–11.
[39] *MPJ*, 9 (January–June 1803), 128–9.
[40] Dr Engelhardt successfully vaccinated in Lund around the same time: Sköld, *Two faces*, pp. 375–6.
[41] *Braunschweigisches Magazin,* 8 November, 15 November 1800; Lindemann, *Health and healing*, pp. 334, 454.
[42] *Monthly Magazine,* 12 (1801), 594.
[43] Peter C. Plett, 'Peter Plett und die übrigen Entdecker der Kuhpockenimpfung vor Edward Jenner', *Sudhoffs Archiv*, 90 (2006), 219–32, esp. 221–3. Cowpox and its prophylactic value were also reportedly known in Württemberg: Wolff, *Einschneidende Maßnahmen*, p. 135.

over bestialisation, reporting the beginnings of the practice in Sweden over winter 1801–2 and anticipating taking it up themselves in spring 1802.[44]

The idea of cowpox inoculation unsettled many people. An oblique and distasteful response to vaccination in Hamburg appears in a *Judensau* print. Ostensibly presenting cowpox inoculation as a Jewish fraud, it may be a satire on debate among Jews as to the merits of the old and new inoculation.[45] Early accounts of cowpox were followed by reports of failures, more sceptical assessments and savage denunciations. Following the anti-vaccinists in England, German critics denounced cowpox inoculation as '*Brutalimpfung*', bestial inoculation. In 1801 a controversy over the new practice erupted in Frankfurt am Main. After Dr Muller challenged the notion that cowpox could provide lasting protection against smallpox, Dr Ehrmann denounced the English 'cowpox swindle' and sharply criticised two local colleagues, Dr Sömmering and Dr Lehr, for subjecting children to *Brutalimpfung*.[46] The most strident antagonist was Dr Marcus Herz of Berlin, one of the first Jews to hold a medical degree and a favourite pupil of Immanuel Kant. After reading articles on cowpox inoculation in *Hufelands Journal*, he launched an attack on all aspects of it.[47] A basic concern was that it was unethical for a doctor to risk the life of a patient, even if it might benefit the population at large. More specifically, he thought that deliberately infecting human beings with a cattle disease was deeply repugnant. It has been well argued that his sense of identity, personal, professional and philosophical, required an absolute distinction between man and animals. He certainly attacked the new prophylaxis with some venom, referring to cowpox as '*eiterige Jauche eines kranken Rindviehs*' (suppurating muck from a diseased cow) and the procedure as '*viehlicher Impfung*' (beastly inoculation).[48] The supporters of vaccination took up their pens against the anti-vaccinists. Dr Jakob Aronsson, another Jewish physician in Berlin, published a cogent critique of Herz in July 1801.[49] Shocked by the

---

[44] *Brevväxling mellan Carlander och Afzelius*, pp. 66, 67, 70, 84–7.

[45] Isaiah Shachar, *The Judensau. A medieval anti-Jewish motif and its history* (London, 1974), plate 57b.

[46] Johann Valentin Müller, *Beweis, daß die Kuhpocken mit den natürlichen Kinderblattern in keiner Verbindung stehen, und also ihre Einimpfung kein untrügliches Verwahrungsmittel gegen die natürlichen Blattern seyn könne* (Frankfurt am Main, 1801); Johann Christian Ehrmann, *Über den Kuhpockenschwindel, bei Gelegenheit der abgenöthigten Vertheidigung des D. Ehrmann gegen die Brutalimpfmeistre den Hrn D. und Hofr. Sömmering und den Hrn. D. Lehr* (Frankfurt am Main, 1801).

[47] D. Marcus Herz and D. Dohmeyer, *Leibarzt des Prinzen August von England über die Brutalimpfung und deren Vergleichung mit den humanen* (Berlin, 1801).

[48] Martin L. Davies, *Identity or history? Marcus Herz and the end of Enlightenment* (Detroit, MI, 1995), pp. 134–44.

[49] Jakob Ezechiel Aronsson, *Rechtfertigung der Schutzblattern- oder Kuhpockenimpfung gegen die Einwendungen des Herrn Hofrath und Professors Marcus Herz und des Herrn Dr Joh. Valentin Müller* (Berlin, 1801).

intemperance of Herz's diatribe, Professor Remer of the University of Helmsted rebutted his arguments and presented the case for vaccination in the *Braunschweigisches Magazin*.[50]

Medical men in Germany and Scandinavia were evidently rallying to the cause of vaccination. It was a matter of some pride in Hanover that the first practitioners were associated with the Hanoverian court and that 'the learned men of Göttingen' helped to secure its reputation in the profession. Professor Arnemann and his students submitted 'the new practice to the most rigorous examination'.[51] In 1801, F. B. Osiander, a colleague at Göttingen, published one of the most thorough accounts of cowpox in any language. Presenting cowpox in the context of other livestock diseases, describing the experiments conducted in Göttingen and including coloured plates based on his own drawings 'from nature', he helped to 'naturalise' vaccination in Germany.[52] From the outset, however, the spread and promotion of vaccination was a national endeavour. Beginning in 1795, *Hufelands Journal*, edited from the University of Jena, provided a national forum for reports and discussion of vaccination, facilitating the emergence of a consensus as to its value. Following from a distance the German craze for cowpox and the rage over bestialisation, Swedish medical men were seemingly taken by surprise by the sudden triumph of vaccination: in March 1802, Dr Carlander conceded that he, too, would probably soon 'brutalise a bunch of kids' (*'brutalisera en hop ungar'*).[53] The solidarity among the German medical fraternity is the more remarkable in that it was divided socially and educationally as well as geographically, with a kaleidoscope of medical regimes reflecting Germany's fragmentation. An alumnus of the University of Marburg, Dr Sebastian Döring had to take further examinations to qualify to practice in Herborn, barely twenty miles away.[54] The imperatives of health could often override professional and political boundaries. The challenges of epidemic disease certainly required collaboration between not only physicians and other health workers, but also medical men in neighbouring states. In introducing vaccination in Herborn in 1801, Dr Döring looked to colleagues in other jurisdictions for advice and vaccine. Since most medical schools recruited students from

---

[50] *Braunschweigisches Magazin*, 26 September, 3 October, 10 October 1801.

[51] Michel-Ange-Bernard Mangourit, *Travels in Hanover, during the years 1803 and 1804: containing an account of the form of government, religion, agriculture, commerce, and natural history of the country* (London, 1806), pp. 49–50.

[52] Friedrich Benjamin Osiander, *Ausführliche Abhandlung über die Kuhpocken, ihre Ursachen, Zufälle, Einimpfung, Behandlung, Verhältnisse zu andern Hautausschlägen der Menschen und Thiere u. s w. nach eigenen und anderer Beobachtungen* (Göttingen, 1801); *MPJ*, 6 (July–December 1801), 253–4.

[53] *Brevväxling mellan Carlander och Afzelius*, pp. 66, 67, 70, 84–7.

[54] Dieter Wessinghage, *Die Hohe Schule zu Herborn und ihre Medizinische Fakultät, 1584–1817–1984* (Stuttgart, 1984), pp. 81–3.

outside their region, many physicians had access to networks that transcended territorial boundaries. A native of Saxony, Christoph Hufeland studied medicine at Göttingen and achieved celebrity in Berlin. The new medical newspapers and journals, especially *Hufelands Journal*, aimed for a 'national' audience.[55] In reading and writing about the new prophylaxis in books and articles, German medical men, inside and outside the Reich, found themselves engaged in a collective endeavour.

Over the course of 1801, the early debates about cowpox gave way to constructive appraisal. As in Britain and France, a new nomenclature emerged, as cowpox (*Kühpocken*) was rebadged. In a short account of the new practice for laymen, Dr Sternberg of Goslar offered '*Gesundheitblattern*' (health-pox) as an alternative.[56] '*Schutzblattern*' and then '*Schutzpocken*', however, won most favour. By analogy with '*Schutzengel*' (guardian-angel), '*Schutzpocken*' can be translated as 'guardian-pox' in English. Interestingly, Dr Döring of Herborn appears to have been one of the first to adopt the terms '*Schutzpocken*' and '*Schutzpockenimpfung*'.[57] In the first issue of *Hufelands Journal* for 1802, the inclusion of a section on vaccination under the heading '*Schutzpockenimpfung*' implicitly approved the new nomenclature. As 1801 drew to a close and with a truce in the war in prospect, there was more than a hint of triumph among the German friends of vaccination. In a handbook on the practice completed in October 1801, Professor Hecker of Erfurt hailed it as 'the greatest discovery of the eighteenth century'. When it was published early in 1802, the book bore the headline title 'Smallpox has been eradicated!'[58]

Princes and Public Health

In establishing and extending cowpox, medical practitioners in northern Europe generally found support and encouragement from government agencies. Although the princes who came to power in the shadow of the French Revolution were less inclined to authoritarian measures, enlightened or otherwise, than their predecessors, they were more conscious of the need to project a benevolent image of themselves as loving parents of their people. In Prussia and the Scandinavian kingdoms, they called on royal medical colleges to

---

[55] Thomas H. Broman, *The transformation of German academic medicine, 1750–1820* (Cambridge, 1996), pp. 85–6.

[56] J. H. Sternberg, *Kurze doch wahrhafte Nachricht von den Gesundheitblattern, auch Kuhpocken genannt. Zu Nutz und Frommen für Bürger und Landmann etc.* (Goslar, 1801).

[57] Sebastian J. L. Döring, *Kurzer Unterricht für die lieben Bürger und Landleute der Fürstlich Oranien-Nassauischen Lande über die Schutzpocken* (Herborn, 1801).

[58] August F. Hecker, *Die Pocken sind ausgerottet! Ein Handbuch für Ärzte und Nichtärzte, die die Geschichte der Kuhpocken in ihrem ganzen Umfange kennen lernen und die Impfung der Schutzblattern die grösste Entdeckung des achtzehnten Jahrhunderts, zweckmässig anwenden und befördern wollen* (Erfurt, 1802).

undertake trials of cowpox and present recommendations for introducing the practice. Nobles, patricians, landlords and businessmen likewise often combined a personal interest in the new prophylaxis, a recognition of its potential value to the state and the economy and a sense of responsibility to their dependents. The clergy, too, were increasingly feeling the need to demonstrate their social relevance by attending to the material as well as the spiritual needs of their parishioners.[59] School-teachers likewise often took it on themselves to promote schemes of improvement in the countryside. Although the promoters of vaccination in the public sphere were overwhelmingly men, women doubtless played a significant role in encouraging the practice in the private sphere.

The Prussian royal family led the patronage of vaccination in northern Europe. King Frederick William III was a conscientious ruler and family man.[60] From what is known of her character and influence, Queen Luise may have played a role in appraising and promoting the practice. In early 1799, when the first samples of cowpox arrived in Berlin, the royal couple already had three children under the age of four. Dr Brown, a royal physician, was responsible for the first successful vaccination and was the source of the vaccine that Dr Bremer used to establish the practice in Berlin.[61] The king took a close personal interest in Bremer's work, authorising the use of the royal orphanage for this purpose. In a handwritten letter to him in March 1801, he agreed to a salary increase, appointed him a state counsellor and exempted him from all fees 'as a sign of my special favour'.[62] In the controversy over cowpox in summer 1801, Dr Herz and Dr Aronsson both addressed their tracts directly to the king and, in October, Dr Hecker dedicated his *Die Pocken sind ausgerottet!* to him. In the meantime, the king issued guidelines for the investigation of cowpox and the regulation of cowpox inoculation.[63] In May 1802, he established the Royal Prussian Smallpox Vaccination Institute under the directorship of Dr Bremer.[64] Around this time, too, he arranged for his children's vaccination, the first European ruler to admit the practice into his immediate family.[65]

Almost all the princes of northern Europe played a role, direct or indirect, in the establishment of vaccination in their lands. In Denmark, the royal initiative in setting up a commission to investigate cowpox, presenting it as 'a discovery

---

[59] Robert Heller, '"Priest-doctors" as a rural health service in the age of Enlightenment', *MH*, 20 (1976), 361–83, at 364, 368.

[60] Christopher Clark, *Iron kingdom. The rise and downfall of Prussia, 1600–1917* (London, 2006), pp. 314–18.

[61] Gins, *Krankheit*, p. 225; Baron, *Life*, 1, pp. 456–7.   [62] Gins, *Krankheit*, p. 15.

[63] *Braunschweigisches Magazin,* 26 September 1801.

[64] Ragnhild Munch, 'Das Berliner Impfinstitut im 19. Jahrhundert', in Ragnhild Munch (ed.), *Pocken zwischen Alltag, Medizin und Politik. Begleitbuch zur Ausstellung* (Berlin, 1994), pp. 70–80.

[65] The date is inferred from a brief notice in the English press: *Ipswich Journal*, 12 June 1802.

of greatest importance', presumably reflects the interest of the future Frederick VI who exercised the regency for his mentally incapacitated father.[66] In Württemburg, however, the vaccination cause developed momentum in medical and ministerial circles. While the government provided strong infrastructural support, Duke Frederick himself remained cool about the procedure.[67] In Sweden, on the other hand, King Gustav IV Adolf demonstrably took a close personal interest in seeing vaccination established in the kingdom. As soon as vaccine became available in 1801, the Royal Medical College began a series of trials at the Masonic Orphanage in Stockholm. Early in 1802, the king wrote to the Count De la Gardie, his ambassador in Vienna, congratulating him on the vaccination of his son and expressing enthusiasm for the practice.[68] After receiving a positive report from the Royal College in October, he formally commended the new prophylaxis to his subjects and arranged the vaccination of Princess Sophia Wilhelmina.[69] Catholic rulers were moving in the lockstep with the Protestant princes. In August 1801, Maximilian I Joseph, Elector of Bavaria, broke with the conservatism of his predecessors by establishing a vaccine institute in Munich.[70] In June 1802, he arranged the vaccination of his twin daughters, just two months old, and shortly afterwards his eighteen-month-old son, Prince Max.[71] The Emperor Francis II followed this pattern, organising the vaccination of two daughters, Maria Clementina and Carolina, in September 1802 and then, in the following March, his only son, Archduke Francis.[72] In summer 1802, Frederick Augustus III, Elector of Saxony, the Catholic ruler of a predominantly Lutheran state, summoned Dr Magnus from Brunswick to Dresden to vaccinate two royal children.[73]

Vaccination was a sphere in which a prince could make a difference. In private correspondence in 1805, Dr De Carro regarded it as consequential that 'several crowned heads, among whom are the emperor of Austria and the king of Prussia, have submitted their own children to this beneficial operation'.[74] Royal acceptance of cowpox made it easier to counter popular repugnance of *Brutalimpfung*. In Bavaria, it was reported that Prince Max of Bavaria was vaccinated from the arm of a healthy peasant lad in Karlsruhe. In contrast to

[66] Bonderup, *En kovending*, p. 49.   [67] Wolff, *Einschneidende Maßnahmen*, p. 191.

[68] Sköld, *Two faces*, p. 388.   [69] Sköld, *Two faces*, pp. 388–9.

[70] H. Stickl, 'The development of vaccination, as demonstrated in the development of the Bavarian State Vaccination Institute in the 19th and 20th centuries', *Fortschritte der Medizin*, 95 (2) (1975), 76–8.

[71] Franz Seraph Giel, *Die Schutzpocken-Impfung in Bayern, vom Anbeginn ihrer Entstehung und gesetzlichen Einführung bis auf gegenwärtige Zeit, dann mit besonderer Beobachtung derselben in auswärtigen Staaten* (Munchen, 1830), p. 32.

[72] *Medicinisch-chirurgische Zeitung*, 30 September 1802. *Le Conservateur de la Santé. Journal d'Hygiène et de Prophylactique*, 5 (June 1803), 89.

[73] *Le Conservateur de la Santé. Journal d'Hygiène et de Prophylactique*, 4 (August 1802), 143.

[74] *Edinburgh Medical and Surgical Journal*, 2 (1806), 127.

the fanfare associated with some princely inoculations in the 1750s and 1760s or, indeed, with the vaccination of Napoleon's son in 1811, the vaccinations of European royal families were low-key affairs, reflecting a broader change in which the privacy of family life was increasingly valued by the elite. Although they were sometimes reported in the press, they were rarely given great publicity. In his first report as Director of the Royal Prussian Vaccination Institute in Berlin in June 1803, Dr Bremer drew attention to the example of the 'good king' in calling on all men of good will to promote the practice, but did not mention the vaccination of his children.[75] It was sufficient to affirm the paternal interest of rulers in commending vaccination to their subjects. In February 1805, in an edict to his 'his dear subjects' on the topic of *Schutz-pocken*, the Elector of Saxony explained how solicitude for their wellbeing moved him to promote its use as a preventative of smallpox.[76] In an address to the people of Prussia in 1805, King Frederick William presented vaccination as a gift of Providence, and declared that it was 'one of the first duties of fathers, mothers, guardians, educators, masters, and all authorities that are entrusted with the lives of children' to give them this blessing.[77]

German and Scandinavian regimes provided various forms of support for vaccination. In Denmark, a move to form a private society to promote the practice was rapidly superseded by an official vaccination commission.[78] Early in 1802, the Prince Regent approved the establishment of an institute that offered free vaccination to all who lacked the means to pay.[79] Royal patronage in Prussia led to the establishment in 1802 of the Royal Prussian Vaccination Institute. Housed in the Orphanage, it had responsibility for vaccination throughout Prussia, providing instruction, collecting data, conducting experiments, reviewing adverse reports, and disseminating vaccine throughout the kingdom. To ensure a continuous supply of fresh cowpox, Dr Bremer insisted that there should always be two boarders at the Institute undergoing vaccination. They were rewarded with choice food, comfortable beds and special care. He also offered cakes to children attending the clinic and awarded medals, depicting a child pointing to his vaccination scar and inscribed 'in remembrance of protection afforded', to children returning to have the success of the procedure confirmed and lymph taken from the vesicles on their arms.[80] After approving the new prophylaxis at the end of 1802, the Swedish government sought means to generalise it. In May 1803, the Medical Board approved a detailed plan, with the establishment of a Vaccination House in Stockholm

[75] Gins, *Krankheit*, pp. 24–5.
[76] *Handbuch der im Königreich Sachsen geltenden Medizinal-Polizeigesetze* (Lepizig, 1837), pp. 40–1.
[77] Munch, 'Berliner Impfinstitut', 70.   [78] Bonderup, *En kovending*, p. 38.
[79] Bonderup, *En kovending*, pp. 50–1.   [80] Gins, *Krankheit*, p. 225; Baron, *Life*, 1, pp. 456–7.

and regional vaccine depots at Uleåborg, Åbo, Karskrona, Lund and Gothenburg.[81] In 1804, all parishes were instructed to appoint vaccinators and submit reports to the capital.[82] Within a few years of the commencement of the practice, administrative systems for the support of vaccination were set in place in most German and Scandinavian states. The aim was to make vaccination available to all and the firm expectation was that everyone would avail themselves of its benefits.

Hearts and Minds

Cowpox was also winning hearts and minds. Early scepticism by some medical men was overwhelmed by the endorsement of their colleagues. Dr Ehrmann of Frankfurt am Main, whose French-inspired radicalism earned him the nickname 'the antivaccinarian Marat', was won over by its positive reception in France.[83] There were few theological misgivings about the vaccination. The Lutheran clergy, some of whom had reservations about the old form of smallpox prophylaxis, responded positively to the new. A new generation of Catholic priests, who were inspired by a new ethic of pastoral service, proved eager to preach the blessings of cowpox. Among the Jewish communities, leading rabbis approved vaccination and some actively promoted it.[84] Immanuel Kant's coolness regarding vaccination gave some of his disciples pause. On his deathbed in 1804, he reaffirmed his reservations, in relation both to the 'the absorption of a brutal miasma to the human blood' and the ability of cowpox to provide lifetime security against smallpox.[85] Few members of the German intelligentsia, with the notable exception of Dr Herz, were so negative in their assessments. What is remarkable is the exuberance with which many embraced vaccination, embedded it in cultural practices and invested it with meanings that reflected the ideals and sensibilities of the new age.

The bucolic provenance of cowpox had some resonance in the age of Romanticism. Germans were delighted to learn that there was some traditional knowledge of cowpox and its prophylactic power in their own land. A brief reference of the phenomenon in the *Allgemeinen Unterhaltungen* in 1769 was republished in *Der Deutsche Patriot* in 1802, and the story of Peter Plett, who reportedly used cowpox as a smallpox preventative in 1790, likewise

---

[81] Sköld, *Two faces*, p. 390.   [82] Sköld, *Two faces*, pp. 395–6.

[83] *MJP*, 17 (January–June 1807), 59.

[84] D. B. Ruderman, 'Some Jewish responses to smallpox prevention in the late eighteenth and early nineteenth centuries: a new perspective on the modernization of European Jewry', *Aleph: Historical Studies in Science and Judaism*, 2 (2002), 111–44, esp. 125–38.

[85] Thomas De Quincey, 'The last days of Immanuel Kant', in *Miscellanies: chiefly narrative* (Edinburgh, 1854), pp. 123–4.

achieved some circulation.[86] There was certainly a rapid cultural investment in the new prophylaxis in northern Europe. In a letter to Dr Faust in 1800, a friend in Oldenburg congratulated him on his cowpox experiments and enclosed a whimsical poem calling for a revival of the Egyptian cult of Apis, the bull-god, whose focus would be the cow now providing mankind with a remedy for smallpox. He proposed that Faust should organise a festival each year in which the children would dance, sing and scatter clover in honour of the animal that had saved the lives and beauty of thousands of people and had dispelled the mother's fear that she was suckling her baby to be given to the Minotaur.[87] On 14 May 1801, the fifth anniversary of Jenner's first vaccination, Faust invited the children of Bückeburg to a party, in which each vaccinated child was given a pretzel.[88] Dr Friese of Breslau also invested emotionally in the new practice. He and his colleagues held a celebration in 1802 to mark the anniversary of the first vaccination in Breslau. In a letter to England, he reported that a print of the 'immortal Jenner' was displayed, toasts were proposed and odes recited. After describing the scene, he added poignantly, 'Life affords but few occasions for joy and conviviality like this'.[89] Dr Faust's festival, the first *Krengelfest*, is still celebrated annually at Bückeburg, but there were similar festivals in Berlin, Brünn (Brno, Czech Republic) and doubtless elsewhere.[90] In the smaller towns and villages, vaccination assumed the character of a community event, with groups of children going through the procedure together. The sessions may have often been followed by a celebration, providing a treat for children with sore arms and an opportunity for parents to congratulate themselves that their children were now safe from the smallpox (Figure 7.1).

Clergymen and schoolteachers, Catholic and Protestant, played an important role in extending the new prophylaxis. Friedrich Lächelin, the Lutheran pastor who introduced vaccination in Botnang in Württemberg in 1801, boasted that his town was the first in Germany to be protected against smallpox.[91] Johan Georg Schmidt, pastor in Probsteier-Hagen and Schönberg (Schleswig-Holstein), had to wait until February 1802 to obtain vaccine to embark on 'the great beneficial work'. On the first day, 'a day I shall never forget', he penned a circular letter to schoolteachers in the district, providing information about the practice, outlining a plan for him and a medical friend to visit all the villages in turn and asking them to prepare lists of children who had not had smallpox. He stressed that there was a duty to seek protection from smallpox, just as there was to avoid other ills by taking medicine, fleeing from a burning

---

[86] Gins, *Krankheit*, pp. 5–7; *Edinburgh Medical and Physical Journal*, 3 (1807), 34–46.
[87] Faust, *Einige Versuche*, pp. 27–8. [88] Gins, *Krankheit*, p. 28.
[89] *MPJ*, 9 (January–June 1803), 130. [90] Baron, *Life*, 2, pp. 213–14, 378.
[91] Wolff, *Einschneidende Maßnahmen*, pp. 110, 116, 126.

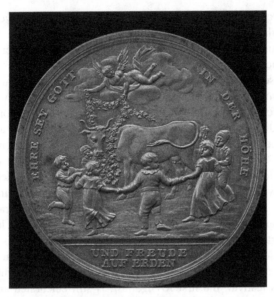

Figure 7.1 Medal celebrating vaccination (German, early nineteenth century), (reverse) children holding hands dancing around the cow, angel amid clouds above holding a garland of roses
(British Museum)

house and installing lightning rods.[92] In the Netherlands, Pastor Speckman, minister of the gospel at Elde, was sufficiently confident in commending vaccination to his congregation in 1806 that he offered ten ducats to anyone who subsequently caught smallpox. After reporting two years later on the practice's success at Groningen, where 5,000 had been vaccinated, and the lack of any claim in relation to his offer, he called on 'every true philanthropist' to promote the new prophylaxis, 'revealed as it were by Heaven for the benefit of the human species'.[93] In Prussia, Dr Bremer expected the cooperation of the clergy in organising vaccinations and Pastor Stumpf sent him a copy of his sermon commending vaccination for possible distribution.[94] In Sweden, the rural clergy were required, if there were no local practitioner, to perform the procedure themselves.

In Austria and southern Germany, the Catholic clergy were likewise enlisted in the enterprise by reformist and anticlerical regimes. In the diocese of Konstanz, a Habsburg enclave, the clergy were enjoined to portray vaccination

---

[92] Johan Georg Schmidt, 'Meinen lieben Schullehrern', *Neue Schleswig-Holsteinische Provinzial-berichte*, 5 (1) (1815), 84–8.
[93] *MPJ*, 20 (June–December 1808), 334–6.   [94] Gins, *Krankheit*, p. 21.

as a 'benefaction of Heaven', 'chase away silly fears' among their parishioners and assist medical men in their work.[95] In Austria, priests were instructed to preach two sermons a year on the importance of vaccination and to take every opportunity, as when a local child died of smallpox, to underline the point. In his sermons, Matthäus Priegl, an Austrian priest, combatted popular fatalism and superstition by deploying biblical and homely examples to show that it was right and sensible for them to make use of new discoveries to combat suffering and disease. To counter the notion that matters of life and death should be left in the hands of God, he observed that Joseph and Mary had wisely fled to Egypt to escape Herod's murderous plans, and presented smallpox in the role of 'a second cruel Herod'.[96] Johann Michael Sailer, a Jesuit at Ingolstadt, felt that the clergy should not be so involved. He expressed concern that 'some priests these days would rather talk about lightning rods, vaccination, clover, and the cultivation of trees' than about Christ. While he was not opposed to spreading information about such things at school, 'under the great linden tree on the common' or wherever, he believed that the 'Christian pulpit is dedicated to *the lesson of eternal life*'.[97] Still, Father Sailer's lament provides backhanded testimony to the enthusiasm of some priests for this aspect of their work. In presenting cowpox as a blessing, providing information and combatting prejudices and adding ritual and festive trappings to the procedure, the clergy helped to embed vaccination in the countryside. The association – temporal and metaphorical – between baptism and vaccination made it an important rite of passage for the child. The more secular-minded advocates of the practice sought to present vaccination as '*Aufnahme in die Gemeinschaft der Vernunftgläubigen*' (admission into the community of believers in reason).[98]

Consolidation and Compulsion

From the outset, there were elements of compulsion in vaccination. The overwhelming majority of people vaccinated in northern Europe, as elsewhere, were infants and children whose parents took the decision on their behalf. Foundlings and charity children lacked even the solace of tough love. Still, the governors of charitable institutions generally acted responsibly and circumspectly. They knew all too well the threat of smallpox to their charges and felt no qualms about making them available for trials of the practice and

[95] Wolff, *Einschneidende Maßnahmen*, p. 168.
[96] M. Pammer, 'Vom Bleichzettel zum Impfzeugnis. Beamte, Ärzte, Priester und die Einführung der Vaccination', *Österreich in Geschichte und Literatur*, 39 (1995), 11–29.
[97] Wolff, *Einschneidende Maßnahmen*, p. 171.
[98] Juliane Heinsdorff, 'Vakzination – Ein Geschenk Gottes', in Münch (ed.), *Pocken zwischen Alltag, Medizin und Politik*, p. 66.

propagation of vaccine. The line taken by princes, who presented themselves as fathers of their peoples, was likewise often hard to resist. There was strong pressure on soldiers not only to be vaccinated but also to make their children available for vaccination. Although it remained the duty of individuals to have themselves and their children vaccinated, it was the role of magistrates to make the line of duty clear. In an address to parents in 1804, the Austrian government left no room for doubt: since vaccination was a gift of God, it showed ingratitude for them not to make use of it; they would be conscience-stricken if one of their children, unprotected, caught smallpox and died; and they would be no less than the murderers of their children.[99] Since it was a basic duty of parents to have their children vaccinated, the Prussian Medical College insisted in 1805, they would feel great guilt if, through their negligence, their children died or were disfigured by smallpox.[100] Pastors and priests piled on the pressure. In 1808, the Austrian government instructed priests not only to promote vaccination in their sermons but also to participate in 'name and shame' exercises. The parents of children who died of smallpox were presented in local newspapers as 'people blinded by prejudice who would rather allow their dependents to die ... than keep them alive by so simple and safe a means as vaccination, offered to them by God and by the government'. Priests were required to press home the point in funeral services, which were held at night for smallpox victims, with the church bells kept silent 'as if they do not wish to make known the crime the parents have committed against their children'.[101]

The move towards compulsory vaccination in northern Europe was generally slow. Weary of his parishioners justifying their apathy by declaring that it was a matter of choice, J. P. Wallensteen, pastor of Kuddby, sought permission from the Swedish authorities to present vaccination as if it were compulsory. He would shout at his congregation from the pulpit, angrily banging his fist, that after all that he had told them about their duty to God and king to vaccinate their children he would no longer ask but order them to do so and if they did not comply he would call in the police to force their compliance. He then read out a list of the people who were required to attend the next vaccination session.[102] For the most part, governments restricted themselves to applying indirect pressure. Rules for the isolation of smallpox cases and the quarantining of infected households, which impinged most on the freedom of people

[99] Pammer, 'Vom Bleichzettel zum Impfzeugnis', 173–4.
[100] Munch, 'Berliner Impfinstitut', 70.
[101] Pammer, 'Vom Bleichzettel zum Impfzeugnis', 16 n.17, 19 n.51, 25 n.90.
[102] Peter Sköld, 'The key to success: the role of local government in the organization of smallpox vaccination in Sweden', MH, 45 (2000), 201–26, at 214.

who had not been vaccinated, were made more stringent.[103] Parents who did not acquiesce in vaccination were subject to further inconveniences and opportunity costs. In Austria, it was necessary to register children who had not been immunised.[104] Vaccination was often made a condition of admission to a school, apprenticeship or employment in public institutions. Vaccine institutes had initially issued printed certificates for record-keeping purposes. Increasingly, vaccination certificates became valuable passports for young people making their way in the world. One of the earliest extant vaccination certificates was issued in the principality of Liechtenstein in 1803.[105] From 1805, orphans and deserted children who were vaccinated in Denmark received certificates that served them well in later life.[106]

In 1805, two German states took 'the first steps in the medicalisation of the general public' by introducing compulsory vaccination.[107] In August, the newly constituted grand duchy of Hesse, a Napoleonic protectorate like Piombino-Lucca in Italy, led the way in Germany.[108] A few weeks later, Maximilian I Joseph, Elector of Bavaria, approved legislation, drawn up by his minister Montgelas, that required all children under three years old to be vaccinated before July 1808.[109] In the principality of Ansbach, where the Bavarian court was based at this time, 33,780 people were vaccinated in 1807.[110] In Denmark, too, there were early moves to mandate vaccination. Alarmed by an epidemic that spread through the country in the spring of 1808, the Danish government ordered the quarantining of smallpox cases and the vaccination of people at risk.[111] In the aftermath, legislation was devised that made vaccination very hard to avoid. In 1810, it became a requirement for marriage and apprenticeship and, in 1811, for admission to a school and confirmation in the church.[112] Most German states declined, at least for some time, to take coercive measures. The relatively liberal regime in Hamburg long resisted compulsory vaccination. The kingdom of Prussia likewise held back from making the practice mandatory. Its approach reflected the philosophical stance of the Prussian elite that stressed moral self-determination and held that 'the exaggerated solicitude of the state' would make people less active and sap

---

[103] Wolff, *Einschneidende Maßnahmen*, p. 197.

[104] Pammer, 'Vom Bleichzettel zum Impfzeugnis', 16, n.36.

[105] Rudolf Rheinberger, 'Zum 200. Geburtstag von Landesphysikus Gebhard Schaedler. Ein Liechtensteiner Arzt als Pionier der Pockenschutzimpfung', *Jahrbuch der Historischen Vereins für das Fürstentum Liechtenstein*, 76 (1976), 337–43.

[106] Bonderup, *En kovending*, p. 42.

[107] Claudia Huerkamp, 'The history of smallpox vaccination in Germany: a first step in the medicalization of the general public', *Journal of Contemporary History*, 20 (1985), 617–35.

[108] Peter Baldwin, *Contagion and the state, 1830–1930* (Cambridge, 1999), p. 260.

[109] Giel, *Schutzpocken-Impfung in Bayern*, pp. 96–107.

[110] Krauß, *Schutzpockenimpfung*, p. 53.   [111] Bonderup, *En kovending*, p. 81.

[112] Bonderup, *En kovending*, pp. 95–6.

their moral character.[113] There was nonetheless a strong expectation that parents would have their children vaccinated. Despite Dr Bremer's disappointment at the apathy of the poor in Berlin, the record of vaccination in the kingdom is very impressive, with the tally of vaccinations doubling each year from 1801 to 1804, and reaching 222,813 during 1805.[114]

Political fragmentation made for a range of measures for generalising vaccination in Germany and northern Europe. War, military occupation, political upheaval and changing boundaries disrupted initiatives and diverted energies after the significant progress in the first years of the nineteenth century. The kingdom of Prussia held itself aloof from the European conflict longer than the Rhineland, southern Germany and Austria. When the war came, however, it delivered Prussia a crushing blow, with defeat in the Battle of Jena (1806) and a period of French military occupation. The recovery of vaccination, with 160,329 people vaccinated between 1806 and 1810, showed the rootedness of the practice. In presenting the data in 1811, Professor Avelin of Berlin observed that, since not all vaccinations were reported, the overall total since 1801 would 'be at least 600,000 or even 800,000'. He was pleased to report, too, that 'the anniversary of the invention of the cow-pox inoculation, or the Jennerian Feast, was very solemnly celebrated' in Berlin on 14 May.[115] The drama of Napoleon's invasion of Russia and the German wars of liberation from 1813 to 1814 provided less than ideal conditions for vaccination in northern Germany. The disruption of the practice necessarily had an adverse impact on the supply and distribution of fresh vaccine, with consequential mishaps and failures. As the first decade of vaccination came to an end, there was growing concern, too, about cases of smallpox after vaccination and some doubts about the potency of the vaccine that was now many generations removed from the cow.[116] Overall, though, the reputation of vaccination in northern Europe was well maintained by government-supported institutes and the networks of concerned practitioners. Modest advances in the theory and practice of vaccination continued even in the most challenging circumstances. Napoleon's advance on Moscow in 1812, for example, provided the opportunity for a meeting between Dr Bremer and Adolphe Labouisse, surgeon-major in the French army, who had pioneered the use of cowpox scabs in vaccination.[117] Bremer had his own story to tell, which Labouisse communicated to the world. Visiting a patient on a farm outside Berlin, he paused to inspect a pustular lesion on a cow and after using the lymph in inoculation he announced, with Labouisse as a witness, the first

---

[113] Friedrich Meinecke, *The age of German liberation, 1789–1815* (Berkeley, CA, 1977), pp. 25–6.
[114] Baron, *Life*, 2, p. 378.   [115] Baron, *Life*, 2, p. 378.   [116] Gins, *Krankheit*, pp. 95–103.
[117] *Journal général de médecine, de chirurgie et de pharmacie*, 20 (1804), p. 224.

discovery of cowpox in Germany since the advent of vaccination. By coincidence, as Labouisse reported, the event took place on 14 May, the anniversary of Jenner's discovery.[118]

In the new European order after 1815, vaccination was better established in Germany and Scandinavia than in Britain, where it still lacked significant government support, and in France and its dependencies, where the Napoleonic regime that had so strongly supported it was being dismantled. The achievement in the small principality of Ansbach, now incorporated in the kingdom of Bavaria, was most impressive. In the year beginning in April 1812, 10,058 children were vaccinated, with only one case of smallpox, not mortal, reported. The numbers vaccinated rose at the end of the war to around 12,000 a year, with no smallpox cases reported.[119] Among the larger states, the kingdom of Sweden was making important advances. The requirement that the clergy should undertake vaccination, if necessary, made it available, in theory, through the entire country.[120] In 1812 the government required lists of people susceptible to smallpox and imposed penalties on the parents of unvaccinated children. In the spring of 1816, it became obligatory for parents to have their children vaccinated before their second birthday. Fines were imposed on negligent parents, with double the penalty for a second offence or recalcitrance during an epidemic.[121] The ratio of vaccinations to live births rose to 60 per cent which, given the high infant mortality rates, suggests that the overwhelming majority of school children were vaccinated. Smallpox mortality dropped significantly, from over 8 per cent of deaths 1802 to one in 5,000 deaths immediately prior to the introduction of compulsory vaccination.[122] Still, it was the principality of Ansbach that claimed the bragging honours in northern Europe. Only eight deaths were recorded in 1809, and over the following decade smallpox all but disappeared. In his book on the use of the 'guardian pox' in Ansbach, dedicated to the king of Prussia in 1820, Dr Krauß felt justified in announcing the local eradication of smallpox.[123]

---

[118] *Journal de Paris*, 3 September 1812; *Gaceta de Madrid*, 11 January 1813, pp. 43–4.
[119] Krauß, *Schutzpockenimpfung*, pp. 186, 213.
[120] Heller, '"Priest-doctors" as a rural health service', 381.   [121] Sköld, *Two faces*, pp. 445–9.
[122] Sköld, *Two faces*, p. 109.   [123] Krauß, *Schuzpockenimpfung*, pp. i–xvi.

8 Across the Pyrenees

Early Vaccination in Spain and Portugal

In the Catalan Pyrenees, the town of Puigcerdá was preparing to batten down for the winter. At the beginning of December 1800, Dr Francesc Piguillem i Verdacer, town physician, was becoming impatient. A native of Puigcerdá, he was probably hoping to make a name for himself by becoming the first physician to make a trial of cowpox in Spain. Perilously positioned close to the French border, Puigcerdá was briefly annexed by the French Republic in 1793, but with France and Spain again at peace there was now increasing traffic across the Pyrenees. The more alert Spanish physicians were following reports of the progress of cowpox in Paris. Piguillem himself wrote to a friend in the French capital for samples, hoping to receive them before the snow came to the high valleys. On 3 December, he took delivery of the vital package and an unnamed lady who had heard about the advantages of vaccination allowed her children to be the first subjects. Eleven days later, her children provided the lymph for the vaccination of six other children in the presence of the provincial governor and other notables. After vaccinating more people in the district, Piguillem set out with a supply of vaccine to establish the practice in Barcelona.[1] The physician from Puigcerdá had introduced a new disease into old Spain and, along with it, ideas and practices that were still novel and unsettling even in revolutionary France.

For eighteen months, cowpox lapped around the edges of the Iberian Peninsula. The British sent samples to Portugal in the summer of 1799, and Marshall and Walker brought cowpox to Gibraltar and Minorca in the winter of 1800–1. It might have been assumed that Spain would eschew the new prophylaxis. Conservative and Catholic Spain was as anxious to exclude contaminating ideas as it was to quarantine itself against infectious diseases. In the late eighteenth century, monarchs and ministers accepted the need to engage more positively with innovations that were delivering dividends in

---

[1] Francisco Piguillem, *[Transcipio de] La vacuna en España, os familiares sobre esta nueva inoculación, escritas a la señora* *** (1801) (Girona, 1979), pp. 8–12, 25–8; *Gaceta de Madrid*, 6 January 1800: Laura Martínez González, 'La medicina como noticia en España. La *Gaceta de Madrid* 1788–1808', Unpublished thesis, University of Valladolid, 2003, p. 550.

wealth and power elsewhere in Europe, but the reformist and progressive trends were somewhat arrested by the French Revolution. After taking up arms against the French Republic in 1793, King Carlos IV of Spain authorised his chief minister to seek terms with the regime that replaced the regicidal Jacobins. Awarded the title Prince of Peace, Godoy revived elements of the old centralising and reformist agenda and in his self-serving memoir he took pride in his public health measures, notably the patronage of vaccination.[2] Although Piguillem acted on his own initiative, it is likely that moves to introduce vaccine had the highest sanction. Another packet of vaccine from Paris was sent straight to the royal court at Aranjuez in the spring of 1801 and vaccine matter was soon made available for trials in Madrid. Progressive elements in elite circles evidently regarded the new prophylaxis as an innovation to be embraced. The traditionalists may have had forebodings about the arrival of the new disease from across the Pyrenees. The new prophylaxis would not provide immunity to the larger transformative forces emanating from France that would soon convulse the Peninsula.[3]

Smallpox in the Peninsula

Geography and history conspired to give smallpox a high profile in Spain and Portugal. Several centuries before it started to appear in epidemic form north of the Pyrenees, smallpox was well known in Moorish Spain. European physicians who owed their knowledge of classical medicine to Arabic intermediaries found in their commentaries the first accounts of smallpox and its treatment. Especially influential was Averroes (1126–98), a native of Córdoba, who was the first to record the observation that people only caught smallpox once.[4] At the street corner of expanding Europe, the Iberian Peninsula was especially exposed to viruses moving around the Mediterranean and along the Atlantic seaboard. The Portuguese empire linked the disease environments of the Guinea coast, Brazil and the Indian Ocean. By the late sixteenth century, Spain was a global superpower and Madrid was the hub of a political and military system that enmeshed much of Europe and the New World. It is probable that it was in the Iberian Peninsula that a new strain of smallpox made its European debut. The epidemic in Madrid in 1587, in which around 5,000 people died, marked the beginning of a new era.[5] In the eighteenth century,

---

[2] Manuel Godoy, *Memorias del Príncipe de la Paz,* 4 vols. (Madrid, 1836), 3, esp. p. 182; John Lynch, *Bourbon Spain 1700–1808* (Oxford, 1989), ch. 10.
[3] Richard Herr, *An historical essay on modern Spain* (Berkeley, CA, 1971), ch. 5.
[4] Hopkins, *Greatest killer*, pp. 297–8.
[5] Joaquín de Villalba, *Epidemiologia española; o, Historia cronologica de la pestes, contagios, epidemias y epizootias que han acaecido en España desde la venida de los cartagineses hasta el año 1801*, 2 vols. (Madrid, 1802–3), 1, p. 203.

smallpox was a great scourge in Spain and Portugal: 10,000 children reportedly died in an epidemic in Granada in 1726 and there were high levels of smallpox mortality in the Peninsula in the 1780s.[6] During his travels in Spain in the 1760s, Joseph Baretti witnessed the frantic grief of a Spanish woman who had just been told that her children had died from smallpox. In his journal, he expressed his sorrow that her children had not 'been inoculated like many in England', lamenting that 'in this part of the world, far from being introduced, inoculation has not yet been mentioned'.[7] During her travels in Spain in 1803, Lady Holland noted the large number of people bearing the marks of the disease, claiming that one out of ten were 'totally blind, or blinded in one eye, owing to the ravages of that fatal distemper'.[8]

In the Iberian Peninsula, there was folk knowledge of prophylaxis. From the 1730s, Feijóo's popular *Teatro crítico universal* offered the clergy and literate laity a balanced account of inoculation in Britain. Given its repudiation by the medical establishment in France, it is not surprising that there was little or no publicised inoculation activity in Spain in the first half of the eighteenth century. In 1754, La Condamine's championship of inoculation in the Academy of Sciences in Paris sparked some interest in Spain, but a proposal to publish a Spanish translation was not approved as it was held to be 'prejudicial to the public health'.[9] Exasperated by resistance to inoculation in France, La Condamine made a rhetorical point by declaring his gratitude to the Spaniards for ensuring that the French were not 'the last nation in Europe to adopt so salutary a practice'.[10] From the late 1760s, however, Iberian rulers and reforming ministers were showing interest in useful innovations like smallpox prophylaxis. Newspaper reports of the success of inoculation, especially in the Austrian imperial family in 1768, set the scene for more favourable assessments. In 1771, Dr José Luzuriaga inoculated the Count of Peñaflorida's son, presented a paper on the topic to the Real Societad Bascongada, and won support for a general inoculation campaign in 1772 involving over a thousand people.[11] In 1774, the Count of Campomanes, a reforming minister of King Carlos III, included inoculation among measures that he felt should be adopted to increase productivity and prosperity.[12] By the

---

[6] Villalba, *Epidemiologia española*, 2, pp. 179, 261–7; María Hermínia Vieria Barbosa and Anabela de Deus Godinho, *Crises de mortalidade em Portugal desde meados do século XVI até ao início do século XX* (Guimarães, 2001), pp. 22, 25–26.

[7] Giuseppe Marco Antonio Baretti, *A journey from London to Genoa, through England, Portugal, Spain, and France*, 4 vols. (London, 1770), 2, pp. 109–11.

[8] *The Spanish journal of Elizabeth Lady Holland*, ed. the Earl of Ilchester (London, 1910), p. 38.

[9] John Dowling, 'Smallpox and literature in eighteenth-century Spain', *Studies in Eighteenth-Century Culture*, 9 (1979), 59–77, at 61–2.

[10] La Condamine, *Journal of tour*, p. 110.

[11] Gratton, 'Smallpox prevention in Spain', pp. 127–33.

[12] Dowling, 'Smallpox and literature', 73.

1790s inoculation was endorsed by the Royal Academy of Medicine and taken up by some grandees.[13] The Irish-born Timoteo O'Scanlan established himself as Spain's first celebrity-inoculator. In 1798 Carlos IV had his three sons inoculated, issued a decree recommending the practice and ordered its use in royal orphanages.[14]

Foreign observers took a dim view of the medical profession in Spain. The university-educated physicians were highly conservative by European standards. They were few – around 4,300 in a population of ten million – and were concentrated in the cities. The surgeons were twice as numerous, but only a minority were formally educated and some were barely distinguishable in training from the blood-letters, barbers and healers on whose services many people depended.[15] Still, an English visitor's dismissal of the Spanish medical corps in 1780 as 'a distemper fatal to the country' is too severe. It fails to recognise the degree to which leading Spanish physicians and surgeons were keeping up with advances in medicine and the impulses that were beginning to change medical education, the structure of the profession and approaches to public health.[16] The professionalisation of the higher levels of surgical practice, associated with the foundation of three royal colleges of surgery in Cádiz, Barcelona and Madrid and the inclusion of some clinical training in the education of physicians, helped to build a constituency of interest in exploring the potential of smallpox prophylaxis. The government's centralising and modernising initiatives, though not always well accepted or successful, at least nourished the ambitions of practitioners who sought to advance their careers and contribute to the general welfare by keeping themselves well informed and embracing improvements.

The Circulation of the 'Precious Pus'

By the beginning of 1799 the Iberian Peninsula had news of Jenner's cowpox. In March, a brief report appeared Madrid in the *Semanario de Agricultura y Artes*.[17] Dr Pearson sent information and samples of vaccine to Portugal in the

---

[13] Luis S. Granjel, *Historia de la Real Academia Nacional de Medicina* (Madrid, 2006), p. 144.

[14] *Gaceta de Madrid*, 23 November 1798; Martínez González, 'La medicina como noticia', pp. 497–8.

[15] Antonio Domínguez Ortiz, 'Algunos datos sobre médicos rurales en la España del siglo XVIII', *Asclepio* 25 (1973), 317–21; Luis Blasco Martínez, 'Higiene y sanidad en España al final del Antiguo Régimen', PhD thesis, Centro de Estudios Historicos de CSIC, 1991, p. 22.

[16] Michael E. Burke, *The Royal College of San Carlos. Surgery and Spanish medical reform in the late eighteenth century* (Durham, NC, 1977), p. 23.

[17] *Semanario de Agricultura y Artes*, 5 (January–June 1799), 185–7; *Semanario de Agricultura y Artes*, 7 (January–June 1800), 380–4; José G. Rigau-Perez, 'La difusión en Hispanoamérica de las primeras publicaciones españolas sobre vacuna, 1799–1804', *Asclepio*, 44 (1992), 165–79, at 165, 174.

middle of the year.[18] There was early circulation of knowledge around the Mediterranean.[19] A small booklet entitled *Compendio de la vaccina ó vacuna* is dated 'Barcelona, 1799', though its section on vaccination cannot be so early.[20] In August 1800, Dr Luigi Careno, an Italian based in Vienna, sent King Carlos his Latin translation of Jenner's *Inquiry*. In response, the 'prime minister', perhaps Godoy, reported royal interest in introducing cowpox in his domains.[21] At the request of the Portuguese Prince Regent, Pearson sent further samples of vaccine to Lisbon in June 1800.[22] The propagation of vaccine in Paris over the summer provided a new source of vaccine, and closer diplomatic contact between France and Spain increased the opportunities for supply. For a brief interval, however, Piguillem's stock of vaccine held the field. Once vaccination had been established in Barcelona, Dr Salvá, doyen of Catalan physicians, sent samples for use in Madrid.[23] In the event, however, the Spanish court and capital received the first viable sample directly from Paris, where it had been obtained from the French National Institute by the Spanish embassy and dispatched by courier. On its arrival at the palace-town of Aranjuez, Dr Ignacio Jáuregui used it to vaccinate the children of Luis de Onís and another high-ranking official. A week or so later, Jáuregui sent newly-prepared dried vaccine to Madrid, where Dr Ignacio María Ruiz de Luzuriaga carried out the first vaccinations in May.[24]

By this time, vaccination was taking root in Catalunya. Dr Salvá and colleagues in the Medical Academy at Barcelona published progress reports in the *Diario de Barcelona*.[25] The Royal College of Surgery of Barcelona hosted a well-informed debate on the value of the new prophylaxis long before its counterparts in Madrid and Cádiz addressed themselves to the issue. By the spring of 1802, Piguillem himself had vaccinated more than 9,000 people.[26] If vaccine from Barcelona failed to reach Madrid, Jaime Nadal, physician of the royal hospital in Lleida (Lérida), was able to use a sample to vaccinate 300 children.[27] Piguillem supplied vaccine to Brigadier Juan Smith in Tarragona,

---

[18] *MPJ*, 2 (August–December 1799), 225.   [19] See Chapter 5.

[20] Anon, *Compendio de la vaccina ó vacuna* (Barcelona, 1799). Guillermo Olagüe de Ros and Mikel Astrain Gallart, 'Propaganda y filantropismo: los primeros textos sobre la vacunación jenneriana en España (1799–1801)', *Medicina & Historia*, 56 (1995), 1–16, at 4–5.

[21] Luigi Careno, *Sur la vaccine* (Vienna, 1801), p. 10.   [22] Pearson, *Examination*, p. 47.

[23] Guillermo Olagüe de Ros and Mikel Astrain Gallart, 'Una carta inédita de Ignacio María Ruiz de Luzuriaga (1763–1822) sobre la diffusion de la vacuna en España (1801)', *Dynamis*, 14 (1994), 305–37, at 319.

[24] Olagüe de Ros and Astrain Gallart, '*Carta*', 319–20.

[25] Olagüe de Ros and Astrain Gallart, '*Carta*', 318.

[26] Núria Pérez Pérez, 'Anatomia, química i física experimental al Reial Col-legi de Cirurgia de Barcelona (1760–1808)', Unpublished thesis, Autonomous University of Barcelona, 2007, pp. 119–39, at p. 129.

[27] *Gaceta de Madrid*, 16 February 1802.

who oversaw the vaccination of 1,900 men working on the reconstruction of the harbour.[28] By sending vaccine and copies of a small manual he published, Smith extended the practice through Valencia, including Alicante and the naval base of Cartagena, and seeded the practice in Zaragoza and elsewhere in Aragon.[29] In Alicante, an army physician vaccinated his two sons and eighty more children over the summer, reporting that the infection retained its mildness even in high temperatures.[30] Quite remarkably, vaccine sent from Barcelona seeded the practice at Navas del Madroño, close to the border with Portugal. Eager to propagate 'the wonderful discovery of the immortal Jenner', the town physician vaccinated himself to reassure his neighbours, then scores of local people, including the nephews of the Governor of Extremadura, and finally, desiring 'the good of mankind', all comers at his home.[31] By the end of 1801, too, medical men in Madrid were sending vaccine southwards and vaccination had begun in Córdoba and Seville.[32]

A range of initiatives brought vaccine to northwest Spain. In the autumn of 1801, Lope de Mazarredo, a Bilbao factory-owner, wrote to Jenner, presumably about cowpox.[33] After some early failures, Juan Antonio Ugalde of Bilbao succeeded in August with vaccine from Madrid.[34] On 15 September, Vicente Lubet began vaccinating in San Sebastián, near the Spanish border, with vaccine from Paris.[35] Establishing the practice remained a challenge. In Pamplona, the physician Vicente Martínez and his surgical colleague failed in early trials with vaccine from both Paris and Madrid. He solved the problem by securing permission to take two children from the orphanage to be vaccinated in San Sebastián and, on return, putting them 'arm-to-arm' with their playmates. By this 'costly but infallible' method, Martínez built up a supply of vaccine with which he immunised 16,000 people in over 200 townships.[36] In the mountainous Basque region of Navarra, a local mayor looked across the French border for vaccine. At his request, a French Basque physician from St Jean Pied de Port brought a recently vaccinated girl to go arm-to-arm with children in the Baztán valley.[37]

---

[28] [Juan Smith], *Progresos de la vacina in Tarragona ó instrucciones y reflexiones sobre la inoculacion de la vacina* (Tarragona, 1801), pp. 8–9.

[29] [Smith], *Progresos de la vacina*, pp. 14–15.

[30] *Gaceta de Madrid*, 25 August 1801; Martínez González, 'La medicina como noticia', pp. 566–7.

[31] *Gaceta de Madrid*, 18 December 1801.

[32] Olagüe de Ros and Astrain Gallart, '*Carta*', 326.   [33] MS. 3020, WLL.

[34] Blasco Martínez, 'Higiene y sanidad', p. 346.

[35] *Gaceta de Madrid*, 1 June 1802; Martínez González, 'La medicina como noticia', pp. 587–8.

[36] Vicente Martínez, *Tratado histórico-practico de la vacuna* (Madrid, 1802), pp. ix–xii, 22–3.

[37] J. J. Viñes, 'Las vacunaciones antivariólicas en Navarra (España) entre septiembre y noviembre de 1801', *Anales del Sistema Sanitario de Navarra*, 27 (2004), 359–71.

Embedding Vacunación in Spain

The geography of the Iberian Peninsula assisted the spread of vaccination around its maritime rim. Poor communications hindered the introduction and establishment of the practice in many places. Even in the Castilian heartland of Spain, where there were good highways radiating out from Madrid, the distances between towns could be considerable, slowing down the spread of new ideas and adding to the logistical difficulties of transmitting vaccine. Strong provincial and proto-national identities supported regional differences in the establishment of the practice. Early books on vaccination were published in provincial capitals. Barcelona led the way with Piguillem's translation of Dr Colon's *Essai sur l'inoculation de la vaccine* early in 1801 and his *La vacuna en España o cartas familiares sobre esta nueva inoculación* later that year.[38] In northwest Spain, Lope de Mazarredo published a translation of Dr Husson's instructions on vaccination in Bilbao late in 1801 and Dr Bances published his *Tratado de la vaccina* in Pamplona in 1802.[39] The pioneers of vaccination in Catalonia and northwest Spain likewise made their own moves to provide support for the practice. Late in 1801, Dr Piguillem set forward a scheme for a clinic in Barcelona to vaccinate the poor, accredit practitioners, keep records and monitor outcomes and publish the results. Although the Barcelona Medical Academy scotched the idea, the practice continued to find institutional support.[40] In Pamplona, Martínez and his colleagues had some success with their enterprise. In November 1802, they gained permission from the board of the Pamplona general hospital to vaccinate the '*hijos de la patria*' in the orphanage to provide a continuous supply of lymph. Plans were devised to extend the practice across Navarra. Since orphans and foundlings were sent into the countryside for fostering, they were to be vaccinated prior to departure so that they could be put arm-to-arm with local children on arrival. Posters advertising vaccination specified, for each parish around Pamplona, the day of the week that children could be presented. Surgeons in the *pueblos* were encouraged to bring children to the capital to be vaccinated, receive instruction in the practice and on their return to use lymph from them to immunise other children.[41]

---

[38] Anon., *Ensayos sobre la inoculación de la vacuna, ó metodo facil, y siguro de preservarse para siempre de las viruelas. Escritos en frances, y traducidos por el Dr.* *** (Barcelona, 1801); Piguillem, *La vacuna en España.*

[39] Olagüe de Ros and Astrain Gallart, '*Carta*', 325; Diego de Bances, *Tratado de la vaccina o viruela vacuna* (Pamplona, 1802).

[40] Guillermo Olagüe de Ros and Mikel Astrain Gallart, '¡Salvad a los ninos! Los primeros pasos de la vacunación antivariólica en España (1799–1805)' *Asclepio*, 56 (2004), 7–31, at 14–15.

[41] Jésus Ramos Martínez, *La salud pública y el Hospital General de la ciudad de Pamplona en el Antiguo Régimen (1700 a 1815)* (Pamplona, 1989), pp. 406, 409–10.

Madrid soon assumed national leadership in the new prophylaxis. As the capital, it was the centre for the dissemination of officially-approved news and useful information.[42] From the first mention of Jenner's discovery in the *Semanario* in 1799, it served as a clearing house and distribution centre for reports of vaccination. In June 1800, the *Diario de Madrid* advertised a book on the history of cowpox, 'discovered in England as a preservative against smallpox and preferable to inoculation'.[43] The *Gaceta de Madrid* published reports of the rapid progress of vaccination in Europe, including a notice of Piguillem's success at Puigcerdá. In the summer of 1801, the *Diario* reported the availability of a *'Breve instrucción sobre la vacuna'*, a translation of a French manual, and included, a fortnight later, an article on the advantages of cowpox inoculation as confirmed by the 'wisest and most experienced' physicians.[44] By this stage, of course, vaccination was well established in the national capital, presumably with the highest sanction. The headquarters of Spain's peak medical bodies, Madrid had the men and the institutions that could provide support for the new prophylaxis. Dr Ruiz de Luzuriaga, secretary of the Royal Academy of Medicine and son of the pioneer of inoculation in the Basque Provinces, was a key figure. After conducting trials in the hospital in Madrid, he and his colleagues began vaccinating on some scale. In August Dr Pedro Hernández, a Madrid colleague, published his influential *Origen y descubrimiento de la vaccina*, based largely on a French exemplar.[45] In the meantime, Ruiz de Luzuriaga made it his business to distribute vaccine across Spain and collect reports on the developing practice. In a letter to a friend in Paris in December 1801, he boasted that there was nowhere in Spain that vaccine had not penetrated by his means.[46]

In 1801, Spain moved to the forefront of vaccination in continental Europe. Its leading medical men eagerly participated in trials of the new prophylaxis and kept reasonably up-to-date with developments north of the Pyrenees. It is some recognition of Spanish mastery of vaccination that foreign residents in Madrid, including the ambassador of the king of Naples, the consul of the United States of America and Lucien Bonaparte, the French ambassador, were happy to have their children vaccinated locally.[47] In October, the Academy of Medicine formally requested King Carlos to establish a clinic to provide free vaccination to the poor, to allow surgeons to operate only on the advice of physicians and to ban unlicensed practitioners. Fiscal constraint and medical politics doomed an initiative that, though it reflected the Academy's ambition

---

[42] Antonio Calvo Maturana, '"Is it useful to deceive the people?" The debate on public information in Spain at the end of the Ancien Régime', *Journal of Modern History*, 86 (2014), 1–46.
[43] *Diario de Madrid*, 3 June 1800.   [44] *Diario de Madrid*, 22 August, 8 September 1801.
[45] Pedro Hernández, *Origen y descubrimiento de la vaccina* (Madrid, 1801).
[46] Olagüe de Ros and Astrain Gallart, '*Carta*', 327.
[47] Olagüe de Ros and Astrain Gallart, '*Carta*', 321–2, 331.

to extend its control over medical practice in the city, addressed real concerns about the stability and reputation of the practice. The Academy's publication of the *Primer informe sobre la inoculacion de la vacuna*, a translation of the report of the French Academy of Medicine on vaccination, was emblematic of its commitment to vaccination.[48] A notable feature of the Spanish version is the portrait of 'Eduardo Jenner' on the frontispiece, an engraving based on a mezzo-print portrait first available in Britain in June 1801. It describes Jenner as the man to whom 'the world owes the discovery of vaccine the prodigious and unique preservative'. Madrid was by no means behind the rest of Europe in promoting the cult of Jenner. Around the end of the year the Royal Economical Society of Madrid made Jenner an associate by merit, one of the first foreign honours for the English physician.[49] Ruiz de Luzuriaga had in mind an even greater honour. Feeling that the Spanish word '*vacuna*' (cow-like) was liable to misapprehension, he proposed a set of terms derived from Jenner's name, namely '*fluido yennerino*' for vaccine and '*yennerización*' for the procedure.[50] Even in authoritarian Spain, however, the new terminology was settled in the public sphere. First appearing in the *Gaceta de Madrid* in January 1801, '*vacuna*' became the popular usage and '*vacunación*' was in general use by the end of the year.[51]

Spain's search for self-sufficiency in vaccine in a time of war and shifting alliances in Europe was more than a matter of pride. After Dr Sacco's discovery of cowpox in northern Italy, there was a determined search for the infection among Spanish herds and reports of cases raised some hopes in 1801.[52] A member of the Royal College of San Carlos set out in 1803 to inspect cases of a cowpox-like disease in the Oro and Cadramón valleys in Orense.[53] Given Jenner's theory that cowpox was derived from an equine distemper, there was interest in the possible use of other animal poxes. In 1803, Juan José Heydeck, a German Jew, Catholic convert and professor of Hebrew in Madrid, informed Pedro Ceballos, Secretary of State, that he had discovered that goat-pox was a preventative of smallpox. Appointed to investigate the claim by the *Protomedicato*, Ruiz de Luzuriaga and Pedro Hernandez obtained a sample and bribed some parents in the *barrios* to permit their children to be inoculated with it. The surgeon, Nicolás Díaz Canedo, found that it had no prophylactic

---

[48] *Primer informe dirigida á la Sociedad de Medicina de Paris, por la Comision Médica establecida en aquella capital, en el Louvre, y encargada especialmente de hacer observaciones, y adquirir conocimientos, sobre la inoculacion de la vacuna* (Madrid, 1801).

[49] *Gaceta de Madrid*, 11 December 1801, p. 1246.

[50] Blasco Martínez, 'Higiene y sanidad', p. 343.

[51] Martínez González, 'La medicina como noticia', pp. 566, 567, 570, 572.

[52] Olagüe de Ros and Astrain Gallart, '*Carta*', 328.

[53] Guillermo Olagüe de Ros, 'La introducción de la vacunación jenneriana en España (1799–1805)', in Josep L. Barona, ed., *Malaltia i cultura* (València: 1995), pp. 251–73, at 266.

value, but there was no formal resolution of the issue. Shortly afterwards, Heydeck told his tale to an English physician in Madrid, giving him a translation of Díaz Canedo's report doctored to support his claim. The Englishman sent it to Richard Dunning who, with Jenner's encouragement, published it in the *Medical and Physical Journal*. The arrival of the relevant issue in Madrid, giving credit to Heydeck's claims, added to the confusion.[54] The discovery of a new animal pox, available in Spain, to add to the armoury against smallpox made a wonderful story. The irony is that Jenner and his colleagues in Britain briefly gave credit to a claim that the medical fraternity in Madrid had already investigated and found to be false.

Receptions and Rejections

Vaccination had a faltering start in Portugal in 1799. The early practice was largely dependent on foreign initiative. Dr Domeier, a German physician in the service of the Duke of Sussex, the asthmatic son of George III, who settled in Portugal for health reasons, vaccinated sixty-two individuals and published an account of the episode in Berlin. He hailed the Duchess of Cadavel, 'who, like an enlightened mother, spurned the prejudices of the vulgar against inoculation; thereby securing to her children life, health and beauty', but few seem to have followed her lead.[55] Early anti-vaccination sentiment in Britain may have hardened Portuguese scepticism: the Portuguese ambassador spread word in Madrid that the practice had been abandoned in England.[56] The death of his son from smallpox prompted the Prince Regent to lend his support to the practice. He commissioned a Portuguese translation of *Origen y descubrimiento*, published at the end of 1801, and the prologue shows his awareness of the success of vaccination in Spain.[57] Although he gave the practice his explicit endorsement in 1804–5, there was little progress before the French invasion of 1807 led to the flight of the Portuguese royal family to Brazil, political upheaval and full-scale war. By contrast, vaccination took root in Spain in the relatively favourable conditions of the Truce of Amiens in 1802–3. Though cautious, King Carlos and his wife were well disposed to the new prophylaxis. Godoy and other ministers gave it strong support. Luis de Onís y González, who helped to negotiate the alliance between France and

---

[54] *MPJ*, 10 (June–December 1803), 339–45. Guillermo Olagüe de Ros, 'De las falsificaciones en la historia: Juan José Heydeck (n. 1755) y su "portentoso" descubrimiento de una vacuna contra la viruela', *Asclepio*, 59 (2007), 275–284.
[55] Ring, *Treatise*, 2, pp. 892–3.   [56] Olagüe de Ros and Astrain Gallart, '*Carta*', 327.
[57] João Rui Pita, 'Manuel Joaquim Henriques de Paiva: um luso-brasileiro divulgador de ciência. O caso particular da vacinção contra a varíola', *Mneme. Revista de humanidades* 10, no. 26 (2009), 91–102, at 97–102.

Spain, used his influence to obtain vaccine from the National Institute in Paris. He was the first notable to allow his children to be inoculated with it on its arrival in Aranjuez. Zenón Alonso, Minister of Grace and Justice, demonstrated his confidence in the procedure by having himself vaccinated.[58]

Madrid gave the new prophylaxis a splendid reception in 1801. The approbation of the court and the government predisposed high society to adopt it in their own families. The Prince of Santo Mauro, the Marquises of Benavent and Villafranca, the Counts of Tilli and Polentinos were among the first to have their children vaccinated.[59] An early setback, when an infant's death was wrongly attributed to vaccination, prompted Godoy to restore confidence in the procedure by having his daughter and niece vaccinated. Aristocratic women embraced the new practice. The Dowager Marchioness of Villamejor submitted herself to the procedure and the Marchioness of Ariza had her only son, the Duke of Berwick, vaccinated.[60] From the outset, children of all ranks of society were vaccinated in the Spanish capital. Foundlings and other poor children were vaccinated in hospitals and other institutions. After arranging the vaccination of her sons, the Countess of Puebla del Maestre hired a surgeon to vaccinate the poor from the *barrio* at her house every ninth day.[61] Over the summer and autumn, Dr Ruiz de Luzuriaga and his surgeon vaccinated 1,126 people in Madrid and Aranjuez.[62] The enthusiasm carried vaccine into the provinces. The Duke of Osuna sent his surgeon to vaccinate on some of his estates and distributed copies of the *Primer informe* to medical men in neighbouring districts.[63] The pious Countess of Montijo promoted vaccination in Zaragoza and the kingdom of Aragon. Doña Xaviera de Mugartegui vaccinated her daughter herself to propagate vaccine in Guipúzcoa in the Basque country. The Duchess of Osuna invented a mechanism for wiping the lancet after use and applying lint to the incision.[64]

Elite support for vaccination is evident in the publication of Hernandez's *Origen y descubrimiento*, one of the most influential Spanish works on vaccination. Presented as a translation of a French work, it drew on the two broadsides, with text by Dr Chaussier and engravings by Baltard, that were published in Paris in May 1801. Despite the derivative nature of some of the text and illustrations, it is fair to see it as a distinctively Spanish production. The unnamed 'loving friend of humanity and the public good', who provided the original material and encouraged Hernández to translate it, probably

---

[58] Olagüe de Ros and Astrain Gallart, '*Carta*', 322.
[59] Olagüe de Ros and Astrain Gallart, '*Carta*', 320.
[60] Olagüe de Ros and Astrain Gallart, '*Carta*', 322.
[61] Olagüe de Ros and Astrain Gallart, '*Carta*', 322.
[62] Blasco Martínez, 'Higiene y sanidad', 346.
[63] Olagüe de Ros and Astrain Gallart, '*Carta*', 322–4; *Gaceta de Madrid*, 13 October 1801.
[64] Olagüe de Ros and Astrain Gallart, '*Carta*', 326, 328, 334.

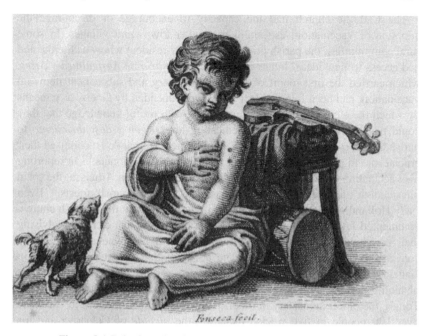

Figure 8.1 Baby boy showing vaccination scar, engraving by Jose de
Fonseca, adapting original by Louis-Pierre Baltard, 1801
(Hernández, Pedro, *Origen y descubrimiento de la vaccina* [Madrid, 1801])

selected it for its appropriateness for Spain. The short time between the
publication of the French prints in May and the completion of the Spanish
book in July suggest high level facilitation and sponsorship. Hernández was no
mere translator. In an original prologue, he dedicates the work not to the
medical fraternity but to the fathers of families and the parish clergy and
encourages women as well as men to take up the lancet. He was presumably
responsible for the dialogue at the end, a series of answers to frequently asked
questions about vaccination. The most arresting feature of the book, however,
are the four engravings by José de Fonseca. One is a basic depiction of the
progress of the vaccine pustule that was evidently designed to be of practical
use. The other three are images of a pair of cows at pasture, a woman at her
loom vaccinating a child with a needle and a bonny little boy showing his
vaccination marks (Figure 8.1). The first two are precise copies of Baltard's
engravings, but Fonseca credits himself with the design of the third, which
adapts Baltard's original but is arguably better composed. The three prints,
which associate the procedure with rural life, maternal diligence and love and a
safe and healthy child, give the work a certain élan.

The Catholic church had the capacity to encourage or discourage the adoption of vaccination, especially in smaller towns and villages. In some rural communities, the parish priest was the only resident who was literate and had access to new ideas. Interestingly, the *Semanario de Agricultura y Artes*, which carried the first report of Jenner's discovery and subsequent items on vaccination, had been founded in 1796 and commended by Godoy as a means by which the clergy could be kept up to date with useful knowledge that they could pass on to their flocks.[65] Dedicating his *Origen y descubrimiento* to parish priests (*párrocos*) as well as to family men, Hernández recognised their crucial role in promoting vaccination among their parishioners.[66] In reporting his vaccination of 200 people at Santa Cruz de Mudela in Amalgra, the town physician acknowledged the valuable assistance of two parish priests.[67] Even Lady Holland, who rarely had much positive to say about the Spanish church, commented favourably in 1803 on the role of the Spanish clergy in advising their parishioners to vaccinate their children.[68] Benedictine monks became converts to the new prophylaxis. The abbot of San Salvator, Celanova, in Galicia encouraged the house's monk-surgeon to take up the practice. After obtaining vaccine through the good offices of a monk at the abbey of Santo Tomás, the oldest monastery in Madrid, the monk-surgeon used it to vaccinate over 100 people in five weeks, including the *alcalde* of Celanova and his family.[69] While a friar in Madrid advised that vaccination was a mortal sin, a Franciscan in Palencia won praise from a surgeon for helping to persuade local people to accept the new prophylaxis, not least by volunteering his niece to be first to receive the beneficial procedure.[70]

Few of the initiatives to extend vaccination outside the major centres can have been sustained. Initially there was some hope that parents would be able to vaccinate their children by the simple expedient of dipping a needle in the vaccine fluid and inserting it under the skin on their children's arms. The success of the procedure, however, required rather more than a steady hand. The real challenges lay in securing a good supply of vaccine, using it in a timely fashion, and accurately assessing the success of the vaccination. Some laymen and laywomen, like Brigadier Smith, Lope de Mazarredo and Doña Xaviera de Mugartegui, had the intelligence and resources to play a role in extending and establishing the practice. In Vinaroz, in Valencia, a business-man showed initiative in securing vaccine from Madrid, performed the first vaccination himself and, with the assistance of a surgeon, vaccinated large

[65] Lynch, *Bourbon Spain*, p. 397.
[66] Hernández, *Origen y descubrimiento de la vaccina*, pp. 5, 16.
[67] *Gaceta de Madrid*, 30 July 1802, 751–2.   [68] *Spanish Journal of Lady Holland*, p. 39.
[69] *Gaceta de Madrid*, 6 August 1802, p. 781.
[70] Olagüe de Ros and Astrain Gallart, 'Carta', 327; *Gaceta de Madrid*, 7 September 1802, p. 900.

numbers of people in the district, including the sixty-two-year-old Governor of Valencia in Morella.[71] In the long-term, it made sense for specialists to acquire the technical facility and expertise to perform the procedure professionally, record it in a register, and take responsibility for maintaining a supply of vaccine. In the early stages of vaccination, many medical men sought to make a trial of a procedure that was well regarded by the aristocracy and leading physicians and surgeons. In Sacedon, in the Alcarria, the town physician obtained vaccine through the good offices of Josepha Xaviera de Sala, a local noblewoman, and won esteem by vaccinating his eldest son to propagate lymph for general use.[72] There were opportunities for medical men to make their name as friends of humanity and men of science by vaccinating the poor and conducting experiments. In May 1802, Dr Martínez and Mateo López, surgeon at the General Hospital in Pamplona, made a clinical trial in which they sought unsuccessfully to infect four foundlings vaccinated earlier in the year by challenging them with variolation and then exposing them to a soldier from the African regiment who had confluent smallpox.[73] For medical men who were not attached to institutions where vaccination was routinely practised, the business may have seemed too troublesome. From the outset, there were concerns that vaccination did not provide full or lasting protection. In 1802, the king and queen of Spain were troubled to hear that one of the first children vaccinated in Aranjuez had contracted smallpox and were relieved to learn, after the court surgeon had examined the case, that the child was suffering from measles.[74]

It remained a constant battle to generalise vaccination. Many people in Spain still saw smallpox as innate and inevitable and the failures encouraged scepticism about the claim that vaccination gave life-long protection. In Barcelona and in northwest Spain, where smallpox inoculation had made some headway from the 1770s, some people expressed a preference for the older mode of prophylaxis. More generally, though, the thirty-year polemic over the old inoculation in Spain, both in building arguments in favour of prophylactic intervention and in acknowledging the dangers of variolation, created a disposition to prefer vaccination. In his *elogio* to Jenner, Dr Salvá, inoculator-turned-vaccinator, made this point when he wrote that the long struggle on behalf of the 'older sister' (variolation) had removed the obstacles and smoothed the way for the 'younger sister' (vaccination).[75] It was crucial, too, that the royal family and the ruling class in Spain, which had only recently accepted smallpox inoculation, were so supportive of the new prophylaxis.

[71] *Gaceta de Madrid*, 14 February 1802, pp. 220–1.
[72] *Gaceta de Madrid*, 20 August 1802, 833.   [73] Ramos Martínez, *La salud pública*, p. 409.
[74] *Gaceta de Madrid*, 6 July 1802, 651–4.
[75] Jordi Nadal i Oller, *La población Española (Siglos XVI a XX)* (Barcelona, 1991), pp. 108–9.

The early champions of vaccination felt able to call on all who held positions of power and influence in Spain to promote the practice. Brigadier Smith made his pitch to office-holders, medical men and all 'who cared deeply for mankind' and Dr Hernández addressed himself to parish priests and loving parents. Between 1801 and 1803, the concerted efforts of the great and good achieved wonders in terms of the rapid extension of the practice across Spain. The great problem was to embed vaccination as a routine practice in the countryside. In 1801, Smith felt that most people in Spain would not trouble themselves to seek vaccination until a devastating epidemic dealt a vicious reminder of its benefits.[76] Smallpox outbreaks in Seville and elsewhere in 1802, however, also focused attention on some failures and encouraged recourse to variolation. The Spanish monarchy was far from countenancing the use of coercive measures to encourage vaccination.

During 1803, optimism that vaccination would become self-sustaining had largely evaporated. The collapse of the Peace of Amiens in May and the prospect that Spain would be drawn back into the maelstrom of war brought general gloom. Even in the Royal Foundling Hospital in Madrid, where 115 children were vaccinated prior to the autumn of 1803, the vaccination programme lapsed for a year and a half.[77] At the request of the Academy of Medicine, Dr Ruiz de Luzuriaga prepared a report on vaccination in December 1803 that pointed to the obstacles to its adoption: some residual preference for smallpox inoculation, the carelessness of practitioners in maintaining the supply of vaccine and the lack of interest by parents in making their children, after vaccination, available to pass on the lymph. He stressed again the necessity of institutional support, namely a central vaccination institute and a system of regional vaccine depots associated with hospitals and royal charities.[78] Inspired by the war effort, Dr Juan Peñalver, another member of the Academy, declared the need for the mobilisation of an army of determined partisans of *la vacuna* comprising parish priests, physicians, town and village surgeons, including *sangradores* (bloodletters), armed with an approved set of instructions.[79] The Spanish monarchy may have been prepared in principle to provide some of the support that the physicians saw as necessary. Bankrupt and at war with Britain, however, it had limited resources and pressing needs. In the spring of 1803, nonetheless, King Carlos and his ministers found some time to consider and some money to underwrite an expedition to carry vaccine to Spanish America and across the Pacific to the Philippines.

---

[76] [Smith], *Progresos de la vacina*, p. 48.

[77] *Gaceta de Madrid*, 27 August 1805; Martínez González, 'La medicina como noticia', pp. 712–13.

[78] Olagüe de Ros and Mikel Astrain Gallart, '¡Salvad a los niños!', 10–12.

[79] Olagüe de Ros, 'La introducción de la vacunación', 261.

Empire and Philanthropy

Even as the potential of vaccine was being acknowledged in the Iberian Peninsula, there was interest in making it available in the Portuguese and Spanish
empires. In 1800, the Portuguese government sent a positive report of the new
prophylaxis to the colonies, and British merchants in Lisbon attempted to send
vaccine to Madeira.[80] In late autumn 1800, Francisco Zéa, a Spanish American
botanist at the *Jardin des Plantes* in Paris, observed the beginnings of vaccination in the French capital and raised the possibility of sending seeds of the
disease to the New World.[81] At the end of 1801, Ruiz de Luzuriaga claimed that
he had already dispatched vaccine for use in Spanish America and China.[82]
A 'good hearted person' in Cádiz sent vaccine on a ship bound for the Philippines that was used unsuccessfully when the ship called at Callao in Peru in
1802.[83] On 1 October 1802 the Viscount of Anadia, the Portuguese Minister of
the Navy and Colonies, probably sent vaccine to Brazil along with a Portuguese
book on the practice.[84] By this stage it was well known that the shelf life of
vaccine was further reduced in hot and humid climates, adding significantly to
the challenge of transmitting viable vaccine through the tropics.

The need for smallpox prophylaxis in the New World was well recognised.
In Portugal and Spain, where smallpox was endemic or at least common, many
people acquired some resistance to smallpox. In Latin America, however, the
population, indigenous and creole, was subject to epidemics, perhaps a decade
apart, that hit children with cyclone force and high mortality rates. The severity
of the epidemic in the late 1770s led the authorities in New Spain to authorise
variolation and another major outbreak in the 1790s prompted the large-scale
introduction of variolation.[85] In 1802, the Council of the Indies received
harrowing reports from Santa Fé de Bogotá in New Granada of the impact
of an epidemic that was gathering force as it moved southwards to Peru. Aware
that private initiatives could not be depended on to introduce vaccine, still less
to establish the practice properly, the Council sought advice on a royal expedition to introduce vaccination. Dr José Flores, a native of Guatemala, who had
provided leadership in using variolation to suppress smallpox in his homeland
in 1780 and 1795, submitted a plan in February 1803, according to which two
ships would be sent across the Atlantic, one bound for Havana and New Spain

---

[80] *MPJ*, 9 (January–June 1803), 309.
[81] *Rapport du Comité central* (1803), pp. 47–8; Husson, *Recherches historiques*, p. 53.
[82] Olagüe de Ros and Astrain Gallart, '*Carta*', 327.
[83] [Alexander von] Humboldt, *Essai politique sur le Royaume de la Nouvelle-Espagne, Troisième partie*, 2 vols. (Paris, 1811), 1, p. 68.
[84] Carlos da Silva, *A vaca imortalizada a vacina antivariólica e as vacinas de Wright no Brasil* (Rio de Janeiro, 1972), pp. 71–2.
[85] See Chapter 12.

(Mexico) and the other for Cartagena and South America.[86] Each ship would carry cows infected with cowpox, children to be vaccinated during the voyage, a supply of lymph stored between glass plates, and a team of practitioners who would introduce the new prophylaxis in the colonies and work with local authorities and practitioners to embed it. Drawing on his experience in Guatemala, Flores stressed that the clergy needed to be involved in preparing their flocks for vaccination; keeping records of vaccinations; performing, if necessary, the procedure themselves; and presenting vaccine as a gift from God and the procedure as a sort of sacrament.

In the spring of 1803, the Council of the Indies forwarded the plan to the Minister for Benevolence and Justice, José Caballero, with the recommendation that Flores and a former army physician, Francisco Xavier de Balmis, be appointed as directors of the two arms of the expedition.[87] With a military background, ten years' residence in Mexico, experience in smallpox prophylaxis and credibility in vaccination circles through his translation of J. L. Moreau-Sarthe's *Traité historique et pratique de la vaccine*, Balmis threw himself into the task of transforming Flores's vision into a more practical plan.[88] In June, King Carlos appointed him the sole director on a salary of 2,000 pesos a year, made provision for three assistant directors, authorised the recruitment of boys from royal orphanage in Madrid and Santiago de Compostela to carry vaccine across the Atlantic and issued orders for the active co-operation of colonial officials, the clergy and all his subjects in the philanthropic enterprise.[89] In his turn, Balmis listed his requirements, including two thousand glass vials and a pneumatic machine to seal them. Conscious of the need to create a good impression in the colonies, he insisted on uniforms for his staff and for the children. More crucially, he set to work selecting a supply of good vaccine in Madrid to take in dried form. By this time, the idea of transporting cows to provide cowpox had been abandoned as infeasible and the focus was very much on the serial vaccination of children. From the British operations in the Mediterranean in 1800–1, this mode of delivering live vaccine must have been widely known. It may be, too, that a more immediate inspiration was the imperial vaccine expedition that set out from St Petersburg in the spring of 1802 to introduce vaccination through the Russian empire. Administered by a 'philanthropic' committee, it likewise involved the

---

[86] Susana María Ramírez Martín, *La salud del Imperio. La Real Expedición Filantrópico de la Vacuna* (Madrid, 2001), p. 41; Martha Few, *For all of humanity. Mesoamerican and colonial medicine in Enlightenment Guatemala* (Tucson, AZ, 2015), pp. 136–7, 144–5.

[87] Catherine Mark and José G. Rigau-Pérez, 'The world's first immunization campaign: the Spanish smallpox vaccine expedition, 1803–1813', *BHM*, 83 (2009), 63–94, at 67–8.

[88] Ramírez Martín, *La salud del Imperio*, pp. 89–94.

[89] Mark and Rigau-Pérez, 'World's first campaign', 68–9.

enlistment and collaboration of local authorities in setting up committees to maintain the practice.[90]

In September 1803, Balmis set out from Madrid for La Coruña. It was not until mid-October, however that he contracted with the captain of the *María Pita*, a 160-ton ship barely adequate for his needs. During this time, too, he selected his medical team, appointing José Salvany his deputy, recruited twenty-two boys, aged between three and nine years, and enlisted the services of Isabel Zendara y Gómez, rectoress of the La Coruña foundling hospital, to provide some maternal care.[91] On 30 November the Royal and Philanthropic Vaccine Expedition, as it became known, set out on the route familiar to Spanish sailors since the age of Columbus, heading southwards to the Canary Islands. Earlier in 1803, a group of notables in Tenerife had subscribed to a scheme to introduce vaccine and 395 children had been vaccinated before the supply was lost. The Marquis of Casa Cagigal, Commander General of the Canaries, who was instructed to prepare for the expedition, sent letters through the archipelago exhorting parents 'to run to present your innocent children to the arms of safety'.[92] There was a warm reception for the expeditioners, with the Marquis embracing the first of the La Coruña boys and other notables following suit until all had been welcomed individually.[93] There was clapping and cheering as Balmis and the children, accompanied by a military band, processed into town. On the first evening, ten children were vaccinated and they, around nine days later, provided vaccine for a second batch. It was Christmas season and the gift of cowpox was received by the children in festive spirit. On 27 December, Balmis led a procession to the main church and the preacher presented vaccination as a divine blessing bestowed by the king and his servants.

On the edge of the Old World, Tenerife was a trial run for the expedition. The omens were good. Vaccine was made available through the archipelago by escorting children vaccinated in Tenerife from one island to another. José Viera y Clavijo, one of Tenerife's luminaries, read a sonnet that apostrophised King Carlos as a beneficent ruler who 'extirpates the cruel empire of a tyrant' and teaches infants to revere *Vacuna*.[94] Balmis distributed so many copies of his book on vaccination that he had to write to his agent in Spain to dispatch 2,000 more to Havana.[95] The fact that vaccine had been earlier introduced and

---

[90] See Chapters 9 and 12.   [91] Mark and Rigau-Pérez, 'World's first campaign', 69.

[92] Víctor García Nieto and Justo Hernández, 'La Real Expedición Filantrópica de la Vacuna en Canarias (9 de diciembre de 1803–6 de enero de 1804)', *Asclepio*, 57 (2005), 151–68.

[93] *Gaceta de Madrid*, 20 January 1804. Martínez González, 'La medicina como noticia', 637.

[94] García Nieto and Hernández, 'La vacuna en Canarias', 157.

[95] Michael M. Smith, 'The "Real Expedición Marítima de la Vacuna" in New Spain and Guatemala', *Transactions of the American Philosophical Society*, new series 64 (1974), part 1, 1–74, at 20.

lost in the Canary Islands served as an object lesson of the need for a plan to embed the practice. The Marquis of Casa Cagigal obtained the lease of a private house in Tenerife to serve as a clinic and vaccine depot. In celebrating the expedition, there were opportunities for national self-congratulation. In presenting a child for vaccination, the French trade commissioner spoke of the expedition's noble aims and the glory that the king would gain for his philanthropy. In response, the Marquis highlighted Spain's commitment to science and humanity. 'While England and France', he declared, 'are prepared to spill blood and spread terror and war, this [nation] only tries to promote health and life!'[96] For Balmis and his colleagues, the month in Tenerife can only have heightened the sense of the significance and sacred character of the mission on which they were embarked. On Epiphany (6 January) 1804, the *María Pita* set sail for the New World with the precious vaccine inserted beneath the skin of the arms of two of the young boys.

War and Wreckage

In the Iberian Peninsula itself, there was less to celebrate. The renewal of war between Britain and France in 1803 brought a decline in trade, economic distress and political crises. Portugal, with its close links with Britain, and Spain, allied to France, both struggled to chart safe courses in an increasingly polarised Europe. With respect to vaccination, there was a perception of a loss of momentum and some attempt to arrest it. The Prince Regent of Portugal commissioned a translation of Jenner's *Inquiry* in 1803 and organised the vaccination of his surviving sons in 1804, but appears to have had little success in reviving the practice.[97] The king of Spain's philanthropic vaccine expedition in 1803 was a signal endorsement of vaccination and reports from Tenerife encouraged further activism. In 1804, King Carlos reminded his Spanish subjects of the value of vaccination and looked for further efforts from his officials to support its extension. In April 1805, he ordered the establishment of a *sala de vacunación* (vaccination hall) in each provincial capital to function as a clinic and vaccine depot.[98] Around this time, vaccination began again at the Foundling Hospital in Madrid and some 544 children were immunised.[99] In Barcelona, a *sala de vacunación* was set up in the

---

[96] García Nieto and Hernández, 'La vacuna en Canarias', 154, 158.

[97] Eduardo Jenner, *Indagaçaõ sobre as causas, e effeitos das bexigas da vacca, molestia descoberta em alguns dos condados occidentales de Inglaterra, particularmente na comarca de Gloucester, e conhecida pelo nome de vaccina* (Lisbon, 1803).

[98] Encarnación Santamaría, 'Las salas de vacunación en los hospitales peninsulares a principios del siglo XIX', *Dynamis*, 10 (1990), 303–11.

[99] *Gaceta de Madrid*, 27 August 1805; Martínez González, 'La medicina como noticia', pp. 712–13.

Hospital de Santa Cruz. The city of Alicante likewise appointed a vaccinator in response to the royal decrees.[100] Though a serious attempt to reinvigorate vaccination, the royal initiative achieved little in the longer term. In Seville, the plan to set up a clinic in the Hospital del Amor de Dios never got off the ground. The decision to establish clinics in hospitals, popularly associated with disease and death, may not have been wise. During this time, too, the escalation of the war with Britain was presenting new challenges for the crown. Even as there was growing recognition of the vital importance of government support for vaccination, the resources were wholly lacking. In October 1805, a British fleet destroyed Spain's navy at the Battle of Trafalgar.

Throughout Spain and Portugal there were many places where vaccination was still unknown. The introduction of vaccination often depended on a fortunate combination of circumstances. The people of Rota, north of Cadíz, had no experience of the new prophylaxis before 1804. When the Economic Society of Sanlúcar offered to make vaccine available, however, the town council seized the opportunity to make it available.[101] In Extremadura, on the Portuguese border, a smallpox epidemic in 1801 cost thousands of lives, including 2,000 in Badajoz, the provincial capital. In the winter of 1803–4 Juan Carrafa, Captain General of Extremadura, made vaccine available in Badajoz, oversaw 900 vaccinations and took steps to extend the practice elsewhere in the region.[102] In Portugal, the practice achieved little penetration of the countryside. In Avintes, in the north, Señora Doña María Izabel Van Zeller had her family vaccinated in 1805 and, from that time on, actively promoted the practice.[103] A physician in Portimão in the Algarve in 1806, however, depended on the Spanish garrison town of Alcántara, two hundred miles to the north, for a supply of vaccine.[104] In both Spain and Portugal, supporters of the new prophylaxis faced old prejudices. A physician charged with extending the practice in Asturias in 1806 reported to Madrid that the Asturians, like the Vizcayans, were too tradition-bound to accept it.[105] Dr Doglioni, a Portuguese physician active in the Algarve in 1806, found it hard to establish vaccination in the face of popular prejudice and the opposition

---

[100] Enrique Perdiguero Gil, Josep Bernabeu-Mestre and Mercedes Pascual Artiaga, 'Una practica inconstante: la vacunación contra la viruela en el Alicante del siglo XIX', *Asclepio*, 56 (2004), 111–43.

[101] 'Anales de la Villa de Rota, 1804': www.aytorota.es.

[102] *Gaceta de Madrid*, 1 May 1804; Martínez González, 'La medicina como noticia', pp. 661–2.

[103] 'Review of *Reflexoens, e observaçoens sobre a practica da innoculacaõ da vaccina, e suas funestas consequencias, feitas em Inglaterra pele Dr. Heleodoro Jacinto de Araujo Carneiro,' O Investigador portuguez em Inglaterra: ou, Jornal literário, político, &c,* 2 (1811–12), 173–89, 352–77, at 367–8.

[104] *Collecção de opusculos sobre a vaccina feitos pelos socios da Academia Real das Sciencias,* III–IV (Lisbon, 1813), pp. 122–3.

[105] Olagüe de Ros, 'La introducción de la vacunación', 261n.

of 'ignorant surgeons' who railed against it, insisting that it was too strange an idea to be accepted.[106] Even in places where vaccination was known, its reputation was by no means assured. It was a matter of some pride to Josef Martinez, a surgeon of Zaragoza, who began vaccinating in 1801, that he was able to vaccinate continuously from 1805 through to 1807.[107]

Securing good vaccine remained a problem. The use of old or poorly preserved vaccine increased the number of failures and misadventures. In a vicious circle, the reluctance of parents to have their children vaccinated, especially when smallpox was not an immediate threat, reduced the capacity to propagate fresh vaccine. The widow of the Viceroy of Navarra and her son-in-law the Count of Bureta, an Aragonese grandee, both felt the need to write to the Royal Jennerian Society for a supply of genuine cowpox.[108] In Hellín, in the province of Murcia, a smallpox epidemic in 1804 demonstrated the security of children vaccinated in 1801 but left no non-immune children to propagate lymph. Once some new vaccine was obtained, the town's medical practitioners undertook to keep fuller records and be more careful to maintain the local supply.[109] Medical men kept themselves informed of the latest developments in respect of the preservation of vaccine. The *Semanario* published an exchange of letters between Dr Jenner and a London physician about the best glass receptacles for the storage of vaccine lymph. The Minister of State, presumably Caballero, applied to London for the latest glassware but found it not entirely satisfactory. The French physician Dr Bretonneau championed the use of capillary tubes to store lymph, but they were fiddly to use.[110] Some Spanish practitioners looked for simpler solutions. Dr Josef María Daza, physician of San Vicente de Alcántara, was inspired by reports from Vienna to experiment with vaccine crusts. The Captain General of Extremadura called on others to follow his example.[111] In 1805, vaccine crusts were used in parts of Navarra and, perhaps experimentally, in the foundling hospital in La Coruña.[112] In the same year, a surgeon began vaccination in Dos Barrios in La Mancha using lymph from the son of a lawyer who had been immunised in Yepes. After vaccinating some sixty-five children, he preserved some scabs that he used successfully to vaccinate fifty-four children in the spring of 1806 and thirty-one more in the spring of 1807.[113]

[106] 'Review of *Reflexoens sobre innoculacaõ da vaccina*', 358–9.
[107] *Gaceta de Madrid*, 8 December 1807; Martínez González, 'La medicina como noticia', 780.
[108] *MPJ*, 12 (June–December 1804), 172.
[109] Martínez González, 'La medicina como noticia', 715–16.
[110] *Semanario de Agricultura y Artes*, 15 (1804), 237–9.
[111] *Gaceta de Madrid*, 1 May 1804; Martínez González, 'La medicina como noticia', 661–2.
[112] Martínez González, 'La medicina como noticia', 709, 221.
[113] Martínez González, 'La medicina como noticia', 218.

By this stage, the Bourbon regime in Spain was close to collapse. Though it sought to break out of the stranglehold of the French alliance, it was impossible to withstand Napoleon's demands for an allied invasion of Portugal in 1807 and a large French military presence in Spain. The Portuguese Prince Regent took ship for Brazil with the rest of the royal family, the government and the treasury. In Madrid, riots and a palace coup in March 1808 compelled King Carlos to dismiss Godoy and abdicate in favour of his son, Ferdinand VIII. There was little chance of political stability, still less a regime strong enough to resist the French military machine. Napoleon invited a group of Spanish notables to Bayonne in May and pressured them to repudiate their allegiance to the Bourbons and invite his brother, Joseph Bonaparte, to serve as their king. A popular rising in Madrid on 2 May 1808, though bloodily suppressed, set the scene for rebellions elsewhere in Spain. Napoleon himself crossed the Pyrenees and in the bloody conflict that followed there were battles, sieges, popular insurgency and atrocities. In the meantime, Britain sent an expeditionary force to defend Portugal and was soon poised to lend support to the Spanish Patriots. Under the leadership of Arthur Wellesley, the future Duke of Wellington, a large British army crossed the border in 1812, defeating the French at Salamanca and briefly liberating Madrid.

The Peninsular War, between 1807 and 1813, involved massive disruption and dislocation in Portugal and Spain. Even before the war, the new prophylaxis had made little headway in Portugal and, in the early stages of the conflict, old prejudices found reinforcement from anti-vaccination sentiment in Britain. Dr Heleodoro Jacinto de Araujo Carneiro, who went on a study tour in London, returned a convinced anti-vaccinist. In 1806, he began to list instances of failures and mishaps in Portugal to match the cases that he had heard about in London. The flight of the royal family, ministers and nobles to Brazil that followed the French invasion undermined the already narrow social base of vaccination. Back in London, Dr Carneiro wrote one of the most fluent and engaging, if tendentious, anti-vaccination tracts, publishing it in both English and Portuguese in 1809.[114] He reported the alleged death of the Duke of Miranda from 'cowpox fever' and a case in which a young girl from Azinhaga, near Santarém, 'vaccinated, as I have been informed, from the pus of a cow belonging to her uncle, had eight months afterwards her nipples covered with eruptions, which increased, together with the nipples, to such a size, that each breast was as large as her head.'[115] Applauding the 'good sense' of the Portuguese in not being swept up in the fashionable enthusiasm of cowpox

---

[114] Heleodoro Carneiro, *Reflections and observations on the practice of vaccine inoculation, and its melancholy consequences; with a true account of the late events which happened in Portugal and Brazil to the persons vaccinated* (London, 1809).

[115] Carneiro, *Reflections*, pp. 83, 86.

and making play on their reputation for superstition and resistance to change, he made ironic reference to other European countries, allegedly more civilised, in which cowpox was preached from the pulpit, celebrating the fact that in Portugal 'the sacred dogmas of religion' were not used to stifle debate.[116]

The Peninsular War may not have had a wholly negative impact on the cause of vaccination. The French generals and military surgeons had a high regard for the new prophylaxis and presumably encouraged local initiatives to maintain the practice. The Portuguese physician at Portimão began vaccinating with matter supplied by the French army. The arrival of the British army provided another source of expertise and interest. Marshal Beresford, the commander of the Portuguese Legion, was troubled about the susceptibility of his men and the lack of reliable vaccine. In April 1810, he sought from Britain 'a sufficient quantity' of vaccine for his troops, up to 12,000 men, around Coimbra.[117] A letter from a British officer suggests that all the soldiers were vaccinated.[118] The Portuguese supporters of vaccination began to assert themselves. Though acknowledging that vaccination had been neglected during the French occupation, Dr Bernadino Antonio Gomes wrote in 1811 that he had been vaccinating in Lisbon for eight years and that the value of the procedure had been amply demonstrated in the many smallpox outbreaks during this time.[119] Still, when British troops arrived at Alegrete they found the town full of smallpox, with victims dead or dying in almost every house and with the infection spreading among the Portuguese camp-followers.[120] In Spain, the grandees and ministers who collaborated with the French included men who had previously championed vaccination. Zenón Alonso, for example, was among the signatories to the new constitution agreed at Bayonne and subsequently held a ministry in the Bonapartist regime. Although he was briefly deported to France in 1809, the intercession of the Academy soon saw Ruiz de Luzuriaga back in Madrid. The Bonapartist regime certainly continued to promote vaccination. In May 1809, for example, the *Gaceta de Madrid* carried a long discourse, over several issues, in support of vaccination.[121] The author was probably José Miguel de Aléa, an enlightened cleric and director of the deaf-dumb institute, who translated into Spanish a French sermon on vaccination by G. K. Schaller, a Lutheran pastor in Strasbourg.[122] Acknowledging its debt to Schaller, the discourse sought to allay religious scruples against the practice and to stress the duty to

---

[116] Carneiro, *Reflections*, p. 83.   [117] New York Academy of Medicine, MS. 1184, New York.
[118] Gareth Glover, *Wellington's lieutenant, Napoleon's gaoler. The Peninsula and St Helena diaries and letters of Sir George Ridout Bingham, 1809–21* (Barnsley, 2005), p. 120.
[119] 'Review of *Reflexoens sobre innoculacaõ da vaccina*', 356–7.
[120] Glover, *Wellington's lieutenant*, p. 120.
[121] *Gaceta de Madrid*, 17, 18, 19, 21, 22, 28, 31 May, 3, 4 June 1809.
[122] *Gaceta de Madrid*, 17 May 1809.

embrace a God-given means of alleviating human suffering.[123] The complicated political context is evident in the favourable notice of King Joseph
alongside expressions of patriotic pride. In reference to the history of vaccination in Spain and the royal vaccine expedition, the author felt justified in
claiming that no nation had received vaccination more readily or had done as
much to spread it around the world.[124]

War, political crisis and social dislocation combined to set back the progress
of vaccination in the Peninsula. It may be that the fortunes of vaccination
recovered first, from a much lower base, in Portugal. A Portuguese-language
journal published in London in 1811 carried a lengthy and spirited two-part
refutation of Carneiro's anti-vaccination tract that included extracts of letters
from Portuguese practitioners who claimed that Carneiro's 'lies' had made
parents reluctant to have their children vaccinated.[125] The Royal Academy of
Medicine set up a vaccine institute in 1812 to collect information and promote
the practice.[126] In July 1813 the *Gazeta de Lisboa* published two government
decrees on vaccination, one addressed to the bishops and the other to the
provincial governors, both stressing the need to do everything possible to
achieve universal coverage.[127] In Spain, there was doubtless more vaccination
activity during the war years than has been recorded. Still, a great deal was lost
in terms of making vaccination available and normative. In Alicante, the home
town of the physician who carried vaccine round the world in 1803–6, there is
no record of public vaccination activity in the decade after 1805. The fact that
in 1815 the authorities were urged to require schoolchildren to have vaccination certificates, however, suggests that the practice had put down roots and
aspirations were rising.[128] In the wake of the divisions and humiliations of a
decade in which it had been occupied by foreign powers and its silver empire
began to disintegrate, Spain would find it hard to recover the sense of unity and
purpose that had assisted the early extension of vaccination. The glory of the
philanthropic vaccine expedition, largely unchronicled, already appeared to
belong to another age.

---

[123] *Gaceta de Madrid*, 18, 19, 21, 22, 28 May 1809.   [124] *Gaceta de Madrid*, 4 June 1809.
[125] 'Review of *Reflexoens sobre innoculacaõ da vaccina*', 173–89, 352–77, at 181.
[126] *Collecção de opusculos sobre a vaccina feitos pelos socios da Academia Real das Sciencias*
(Lisbon, 1812).
[127] *Gazeta de Lisboa*, 16 July 1813 [no page nos.] in vol. of collected issues (Lisbon, 1813).
[128] Perdiguero Gil, Bernabeu-Mestre and Pascual Artiaga, 'Una practica inconstante', 118.

9　Romanovs and Vaktsinovs

Vaccination in the Russian Empire

In autumn 1801, the holy city of Moscow prepared itself for the coronation of Emperor Alexander I. The Tsar, his wife, his mother, siblings and Romanov cousins and a host of courtiers, grandees and officials moved south from St Petersburg. Thousands of nobles and commoners from all corners of the vast Russian empire likewise converged on the old capital. The atmosphere was tense with anticipation and not a little apprehension. His father, the increasingly unstable Paul, had been assassinated in a coup d'état only six months previously. The twenty-three-year-old Alexander set out for the Kremlin with his father's murderers at his side and, as was wryly observed, with his grandfather's assassins and his own behind him.[1] From the outset the new regime cultivated an image of Alexander as a gentle, benign and angelic ruler who would govern by love and concern for the public good. During the ceremony itself, the sacral elements were played down to allow recognition of Alexander's personal qualities. In his sermon, Metropolitan Platon of Moscow presented an arresting image of mankind appearing before Alexander 'in all its primal and naked simplicity without distinctions of birth or origin', claiming to be his children and calling out 'for the rights of humanity'.[2] The imperial party remained in the city for four weeks, during which time the celebrations continued, with illuminations, balls and receptions and, finally, a great party for the people.

Shortly after the coronation, another auspicious event occurred in the Foundling House, a short distance along the river from the Kremlin. Since news of Jenner's discovery arrived in St Petersburg in 1799, there was considerable interest in making cowpox available in Russia. The Dowager Empress Maria Fedorovna, who six months earlier had felt obliged to have her youngest son variolated, was eager to see a trial of the new prophylaxis. When her physician obtained a sample of vaccine in St Petersburg in

---

[1]　C. Joyneville, *Life and times of Alexander I, emperor of all the Russias*, 3 vols. (London, 1875), 1, pp. 177–8.

[2]　Richard Wortman, *Scenarios of power: myth and ceremony in Russian monarchy from Peter the Great to the abdication of Nicholas II* (Princeton, NJ, 2006), pp. 100–2.

autumn 1800, she approved its use in the orphanage in the imperial capital and, when it proved inert, instructed her surgeons to make enquiries about the existence of cowpox in dairies on her estates.[3] The crisis in Anglo-Russian relations in 1800–1, in which Tsar Paul attempted to close the Baltic to British shipping, added a further delay to the delivery of English cowpox. By spring 1801, however, vaccination was well established in Vienna and spreading northwards towards the Baltic. Dr Friese of Breslau (Wrocław), active in seeding vaccination in northeast Europe, sent samples to colleagues in St Petersburg and then, after their departure with the court, to Moscow. After eighteen days on the road from Breslau to Moscow, the vaccine was used in a hastily arranged trial in the Foundling House under the Dowager Empress's patronage. Leading medical men from across Russia were on hand to witness the successful vaccination of Anton Petrov who, in commemoration of the event, was renamed Vaktsinov.[4] On leaving Moscow, the Dowager Empress took in her carriage a recently vaccinated girl who provided the lymph to vaccinate children in the orphanage in the imperial capital.

The first vaccinations in Russia coincided with the inauguration of a new reign, often regarded as a watershed in Russian history.[5] It is tempting to see some correspondence between the substitution of smallpox with cowpox and the replacement of the brutal Paul by the 'gentle, benign and enlightened' Alexander. Although his mother was the main sponsor of vaccination in its first years, the Emperor was involved in the initiative from the outset. He knew all too well the anxieties associated with smallpox inoculation: his severe illness following the procedure in 1781 may have been one of his earliest memories. During his time in Moscow, he visited and distributed gifts to the foundlings. By spring 1801, he was involved in measures to promote the new prophylaxis. Over the following decade, his government commissioned plans and sponsored expeditions to extend and embed the practice from the Baltic to the Black Sea and from Ukraine to Kamchatka. Imperial beneficence brought the new prophylaxis to millions of people, in their 'primal and naked simplicity without distinctions of birth or origin'. Although the Emperor's personal interest is not easy to distinguish from the rhetoric of his paternal care for his people, it is attested by his desire to meet Jenner in London in 1814 and his congratulating him on presenting his life-preserving discovery to the world.

---

[3] Anthony Cross, *By the banks of the Neva. Chapters from the lives and careers of the British in eighteenth-century Russia* (Cambridge, 1997), pp. 141–2, 420, n. 103.
[4] V. O. Gubert, *Ospa i ospoprivivanie [Smallpox and Inoculation]*, vol. 1 (St Petersburg, 1896), p. 492.
[5] David Saunders, *Russia in the age of reaction and reform 1801–1881* (London, 1992), p. 10.

Smallpox Inoculation under Catherine the Great

Russia was already well primed to accept vaccination. Along with bubonic plague, still a major killer in the 1770s, smallpox took a heavy toll across the empire. The Russian state saw the vital importance of population growth to colonise territory and exploit its vast resources, especially east of the Urals. The first smallpox hospital was established in 1763 at Tobol'sk in Siberia, where smallpox caused many deaths in a sparsely populated part of the empire.[6] Awareness of high mortality rates among neglected children led to the establishment of the foundling houses in St Petersburg and Moscow. When contagion spread, they were often death-traps. A smallpox outbreak in the Moscow foundling hospital in 1767 pushed the death-rate to 98 per cent.[7] Russia's sprawling and ethnically diverse empire had some experience with traditional techniques of smallpox prophylaxis. The Chinese practice of insufflation was practised, at least on a small-scale, on the frontier with Mongolia.[8] In the southern provinces of the Caucasus, too, there was long familiarity with the style of inoculation observed in Istanbul. The growing profile of smallpox inoculation in western Europe in the 1750s was matched in eastern Europe. In Dorpat in Livonia, Dr August Schulinus inoculated over 1,000 children, with only one fatality, in eight years.[9] Johann Georg Eisen, a Lutheran pastor, promoted the practice in the Livonian countryside in the 1760s.[10] In Russia itself, a journal article in the 1750s reported on its potential to increase population and productivity by reducing morbidity and mortality.[11] There was surreptitious experimentation in the St Petersburg area in 1758.[12] Still, the Russian authorities gave no countenance to smallpox inoculation until 1768, when Catherine the Great took the bold step of inviting an English inoculator to St Petersburg.

As a German princess, Catherine had a well-grounded fear of the disease. Shortly before her marriage in 1745, her fiancé, the future Peter III, caught smallpox and was horribly disfigured. In the following year, she had reason to suspect that hostile elements at court deliberately exposed her to the infection.[13] Early in 1768 she was shocked by Countess Anna Sheremetev's

---

[6] Alexander, *Bubonic plague*, p. 55.   [7] Alexander, *Bubonic plague*, pp. 93–4.

[8] Marta E. Hanson, 'On Manchu medical manuscripts and blockprints: an essay and bibliographic survey', *Saksaha. A Review of Manchu Studies*, 8 (2003), 1–32, at 3.

[9] William Tooke, *View of the Russian Empire: during the reign of Catharine, the Second, and to the close of the eighteenth century*, 3rd ed., 3 vols. (Dublin, 1801), 1, pp. 470–1.

[10] Donnert, *Johann Georg Eisen*, pp. 120–1.

[11] Philip H. Clendenning, 'Dimsdale in Russia', 115; George E. Munro, *The most intentional city: St. Petersburg in the reign of Catherine the Great* (Cranbury, NJ, 2008), p. 129.

[12] Tooke, *View*, 1, p. 471; Clendenning, 'Dimsdale in Russia', 115.

[13] *The memoirs of Catherine the Great*, ed. Dominique Maroger (London, 1955), p. 157.

smallpox death and alarmed that her son had been in her company.[14] She would have known, too, that European princely families were beginning to embrace inoculation, and that Empress Maria Theresa of Austria, after losing a daughter-in-law and a daughter to smallpox in 1767, was contemplating its use to protect her family. Through her ambassador in Britain, Catherine secured the services of Dr Thomas Dimsdale, whose book on the new method of inoculation was known to Baron Cherkasov, a key adviser in the affair.[15] The Quaker physician arrived in St Petersburg in autumn and began preparing the Empress for the operation. He made a trial on a young man of obscure parentage, taking smallpox matter from him to inoculate the Empress in October. Happily for the physician as well as his patient, the operation proved successful. Dimsdale then inoculated the Tsarevich and other members of the court. In addition to making Dimsdale a baron of the Russian empire and rewarding him extravagantly, Catherine granted the young man who supplied the smallpox lymph a patent of nobility with a crest depicting a bare flexed arm holding a red rose.[16]

The inoculation of the Empress was a public as well as a private act. It was widely reported in Europe and applauded in enlightened circles.[17] In Russia itself, the success of the procedure was the occasion of celebration and thanksgiving.[18] Many nobles and their ladies were inoculated, prompting Catherine to declare, 'See what setting an example can do! Three months ago, no one wanted to hear about it, and yet now they look on it as salvation'.[19] As part of the celebration, an allegorical ballet, entitled *Prejudice Overcome*, was performed by pupils from the dancing school at the Foundling Hospital, who themselves were among the earliest candidates for the new prophylaxis. The plot of the ballet was simple. Ruthenia (Russia) lives in fear of smallpox until Minerva (Catherine) issues forth from the Temple of Æsculapius and, as an example to the people, submits to inoculation. Ruthenia then seeks inoculation herself, and rejoices in driving out superstition and ignorance.[20] In 1772, a commemorative medal, in which the empress and her son are depicted as receiving 'Russia' and her children into a temple, on the steps of which a monster, representing smallpox, lay prostrate, proclaimed a similar message.[21] By this stage, Catherine had embedded the practice in the empire. Prior to his

---

[14] Virginia Rounding, *Catherine the Great* (London, 2006), pp. 205–6.
[15] Clendinning, 'Dimsdale in Russia', 117–19; Dixon, *Catherine*, pp. 188–9.
[16] Clendinning, 'Dimsdale in Russia', 120–3.
[17] Dixon, *Catherine*, p. 190; Lentin (ed.), *Voltaire and Catherine*, p. 56.
[18] Rounding, *Catherine*, pp. 212–16.   [19] Dixon, *Catherine*, pp. 190–1.
[20] Stephen Lessing Baehr, *The paradise myth in eighteenth-century Russia: Utopian patterns in early secular Russian literature and culture* (Stanford, CA, 1991), p. 60.
[21] Baehr, *Paradise myth*, pp. 219–20.

departure from Russia, Dimsdale oversaw the establishment of a smallpox and inoculation hospital in St Petersburg. Inoculation was made mandatory in the foundling houses in St Petersburg and Moscow, which served as showcases for the practice. The procedure was also made available in smallpox hospitals across the empire, notably in Irkutsk in 1772, where 15,580 people were treated in the first five years.[22] The intelligentsia was generally supportive of prophylaxis. The Free Economic Society organised the publication of articles on smallpox prevention.[23] Although the Medical College lacked the conviction and resources to take up the scheme proposed by Pastor Eisen for the extension of the practice in the countryside, some aristocratic families, like the Vorontsovs, saw the value of inoculating the peasants on their estates.[24] Though the leaders of the Orthodox Church accepted the imperial initiative, however, many rural priests shared the prejudices and strengthened the reservations of the peasantry.

In the last quarter of the eighteenth century imperial patronage and direction assured the progress of inoculation. By 1780, around 20,000 people had been inoculated in European Russia and more than that number east of the Urals.[25] In 1781, Dimsdale returned to Russia to inoculate the Empress's eldest grandsons, including the future Tsar Alexander. From 1783, the smallpox hospital offered accommodation, at the empress's expense, to children of the poor who were undergoing inoculation.[26] Between 1780 and 1790, some 1,570 children were inoculated in the institution, with only four fatalities.[27] The accession of Tsar Paul in 1796 involved no lessening of commitment to the practice. His wife Maria Fedorovna followed her mother-in-law in promoting variolation. During an epidemic on her estate at Pavlovsk in 1789, she arranged for her British physician Dr Halliday to inoculate her peasants, instructing her bailiff to 'persuade their parents to agree, making them to understand that we have two children who have not yet been inoculated and who will truly be in danger'.[28] Many aristocratic families adopted inoculation for their children and some sponsored it on their estates. In 1795 Madame de Krudener, later Tsar Alexander's spiritualist confidant, organised the inoculation of the serfs on her estates in Estonia.[29]

---

[22] Clendinning, 'Dimsdale in Russia', 120; Tooke, View, 1, pp. 472–3.

[23] Joan Klobe Pratt, 'The Free Economic Society and the battle against smallpox: a "public sphere" in action', The Russian Review, 61 (2002), 560–78, at 562.

[24] R. P. Bartlett, 'Russia in the eighteenth-century adoption of inoculation for smallpox', in R. P. Bartlett, A. G. Cross and K. Rasmussen (eds.), Russia and Europe and the world of the eighteenth century (Columbus, OH, 1988), pp. 193–213.

[25] Tooke, View, 1, pp. 472–3.   [26] Munro, Most intentional city, p. 75.

[27] Heinrich F. von Storch, Historisch-statistisches Gemälde von Russland am Ende des 18ten Jahrhunderts, vol. 1 (Riga, 1797), pp. 426–7.

[28] Cross, Banks of Neva, pp. 141–2.

[29] Clarence Ford, The life and letters of Madame De Krudener (London, 1893), p. 43.

In 1797 Heinrich Storch, a political economist, reported that inoculation was well accepted in St Petersburg and noted a slight decline, from one in thirty-one to one in thirty-eight, in smallpox's contribution to the death toll.[30]

By early 1800, the imperial family was aware of cowpox and its advantages. Trade and diplomatic networks facilitated communications between London to St Petersburg, at least during the months when the Baltic was not ice-bound. British medical men resident in the Russian capital kept themselves up-to-date with developments back home. Britain's conflict with the Baltic powers from 1799 and the breakdown of relations with Russia in the second half of 1800, however, served to somewhat delay the arrival of vaccine. In March 1800, the Tsarina Maria Fedorovna had her youngest son, Archduke Michael, inoculated in the old fashion. In autumn, she authorised Dr Halliday, who had acquired vaccine 'by chance', to conduct a trial of it in one of the charitable institutions under her patronage. When it proved inert, she instructed her surgeons in the countryside to examine cows in the hope that a local source of the virus might be found.[31] At the end of the year, vaccine became available in the Baltic provinces, making possible successful trials by Dr Otto Huhn in Riga (Latvia) and Dr G. A. F. Schutz in Harju (Estonia).[32] Impatient to obtain vaccine, two Russian physicians wrote to request samples from Paris.[33] In spring, British naval action in breaking the Sound and bombarding Copenhagen and the assassination of Tsar Paul reopened lines of communication between Britain and Russia.[34] The new British ambassador, Lord St Helens, arrived in St Petersburg at the end of May and it is likely that some vaccine came with him. Dr Buttats, a Russian-born graduate of the University of Göttingen, who had observed vaccination in London, arrived at this time eager to assist in introducing the new prophylaxis.[35] During spring and summer, samples of vaccine probably arrived from many sources, including a sample from Dr Friese in Breslau (Wrocław) to his friend, a surgeon in the imperial household, but none of them were successfully propagated.

---

[30] von Storch *Historisch-statistisches Gemälde*, 1, p. 359.

[31] Cross, *Banks of Neva*, pp. 141–2, 420 n.103.

[32] A. V. Dirbe, 'The Riga surgeon Otto Huhn – a popularizer of vaccination in Russia', in V. I. Valeskeln and Ia. P. Stradyn' (eds.), *Nauchnye sviazi Pribaltiki v XVIII–XX vekakh: Materialy VII Pribaltiiskoi konferentsii po istorii nauki* (Riga, 1968), pp. 183–85; Isidorus Brennsohn, *Die Aerzte Estlands vom Beginn der historischen Zeit bis zur Gegenwart. Ein Biographisches Lexikon* (Riga, 1922), pp 328–9.

[33] *Rapport du comité central* (1803), p. 46.

[34] Janet M. Hartley, *Alexander I* (London, 1994), pp. 58–62.

[35] N. Kul'bin, 'Buttats, Frants', *Russkii Biograficheskii Slovar'*, ed. Polovtsov, IV, pp. 26–7; Ring, *Treatise*, 2, p. 749.

Vaccination by *Ukase*

In the event, vaccination in Russia began not in St Petersburg, its new capital and 'window on the West', but in Moscow, the old capital of Holy Russia. From his friend in the imperial household, Dr Friese knew that the Dowager Empress Maria was keen to see the introduction of vaccination and that the Emperor and his court were travelling to Moscow for the coronation. A few weeks before the event, he sent samples of vaccine from Breslau to Moscow, a journey of almost 1,000 miles. On 1 October Dr Efrem Muktin, professor of medicine at the University of Moscow, one of whose assistants had recently defended a thesis on cowpox, presided over the vaccination of Anton Petrov, a boy from the Foundling House.[36] The governors of the hospital board, leading physicians from St Petersburg and Moscow, and many notables in the city for the coronation witnessed the procedure. After demonstrating his insuscepti-bility to smallpox, the surgeon took lymph from the vesicle on the boy's arm to vaccinate more children. The boy himself was renamed Anton Vaktsinov in honour of the event. After the return of the imperial court to St Petersburg, Mukhin assumed responsibility for bedding down the practice in Moscow. As president of the Slavonic-Greco-Roman Academy, he was at the hub of a network of Russian savants who were open to new ideas and interested in promoting the new prophylaxis. From late 1801, the Foundling House served as an institutional focus for vaccination. The medical men generated a supply of vaccine by vaccinating the foundlings and offering free vaccination to the children of the poor. Since there was constant movement of children back and forth between the Foundling House and the families in the countryside who variously nursed, fostered and apprenticed them there was a ready means of distributing live vaccine through the province. From Moscow, samples of dried vaccine were likewise sent out on request to doctors in more distant towns and regions. Under Mukhin's leadership, the vaccination programme was refined and systematised over time: children were vaccinated at a young age but in batches so that fresh matter was always available; the few children who did not respond to vaccination were sent into the country for greater safety; and, in 1807, the vaccination of foundlings was made mandatory. The Foundling House likewise provided facilities for medical men from all parts of Russia to gain instruction in the practice.[37]

In St Petersburg, the Dowager Empress arranged for the girl she had brought under vaccination from Moscow to go arm-to-arm with the first set of children in the St Petersburg Foundling House.[38] By the end of the year, 161 orphans had been vaccinated in groups and, in the new year, the effectiveness of the

---

[36] Gubert, *Ospa i ospoprivivanie*, 1, pp. 496–7.   [37] Gubert, *Ospa i ospoprivivanie*, 1, p. 496.
[38] Gubert, *Ospa i ospoprivivanie*, 1, p. 492; Baron, *Life*, 1, pp. 459–60.

procedure was demonstrated by the resistance of a sample of them to smallpox inoculation. In her patronage of vaccination in Russia, the German-born Maria Fedorovna emulated the achievement of her redoubtable mother-in-law in respect of the old prophylaxis. In late 1801, Dr Buttats dedicated to her his book on vaccination, the first original work in the Russian language. 'Many thousands saved from an early death by this divine method, and the countless multitudes of their future descendants', he declared, 'will all owe their lives to your care, Great Sovereign!' Unbiased posterity will ever gratefully recall your deathless name and charitable institutions. For only that which tends to the good of all mankind and to the solace of the suffering has import, in your lofty thoughts'.[39] In August 1802, the Dowager Empress sent diamond rings to both Jenner and Friese as expressions of gratitude. In thanking her for the gift, Jenner declared that her sanction of the practice would help to extinguish prejudice and 'hasten the universal adoption of vaccine inoculation'.[40] Like its counterpart in Moscow, the Foundling House at St Petersburg served as an important centre for the practice. Maria Fedorovna continued to involve herself personally in the cause, requiring both houses to provide monthly reports on vaccination activity. She was still reading the reports and following up with questions in 1805.[41]

As the imperial capital, St Petersburg was the centre for state-sanctioned schemes to generalise the practice in the empire. Several imperial agencies supported the work and the arrival of vaccine and information from Britain and elsewhere established the practice on firm foundations. The College of Medicine was centrally involved. In 1801, it published *Observations on Inoculation with Cowpox*, a Russian translation of a German work, and, in the following year, prepared a report on the new prophylaxis for the government. On receipt of the College's advice in 1802, Tsar Alexander issued a *ukase* authorising and endorsing vaccination. The Foundling House remained a hub of activity in the capital. The total number of vaccinations rose to 1,523 in 1802, and then incrementally to over 2,000 in 1806.[42] The figures include the children who were billeted in the countryside and who were often the means of extending the practice to local children. They do not include the vaccination of children outside the system, including poor children vaccinated charitably in the capital. In addition, many families in the upper and middle ranks were having their children and servants vaccinated privately. Early in 1802, there may not have been complete confidence in the vaccine in Russia. Count Markov, the Russian ambassador to France, arranged for his daughter to

---

[39] Franz Buttats, *Nastavlenie o Privivanii korov'ei Ospy [Instructions on Inoculation with Cowpox]* (St Petersburg, 1801), cited in Gubert, *Ospa i ospoprivivanie*, 1, p. 493.
[40] Baron, *Life*, 1, pp. 462–4. [41] Gubert, *Ospa i ospoprivivanie*, 1, p. 493.
[42] Gubert, *Ospa i ospoprivivanie*, 1, p. 499.

be brought to Paris for vaccination by Dr Colon. She was accompanied by the family physician, Dr Hakenszmit, who obtained training in the procedure and returned with his own supply of vaccine.[43]

From its beachheads in Riga and elsewhere late in 1800, vaccination was making progress in Russia's Baltic provinces. Dr Huhn distributed vaccine throughout Latvia and sought to enlist Lutheran pastors in the new practice. He organised the translation, publication and distribution of a booklet written by a French army surgeon. Acting as a one-man institute, he collated reports and passed them on to the Minister of Internal Affairs and the College of Medicine, recommending the adoption of his system in other parts of the Russian empire.[44] In Estonia in 1803, Dr Harder and Dr Bornwasser consolidated the practice in Tallin and Torma by organising trials in which vaccinated children were challenged with smallpox.[45] In April 1802 the Dowager Empress sought to establish the practice in the grand duchy of Lithuania, recently incorporated in the Russian empire. She sent vaccine to Professors Johann Lobenvien and Augustas Bekiu, both of whom took up the practice with alacrity and effect.[46] An English traveller in eastern Europe at this time wrote to Jenner about Lobenvein's 'indefatigable exertions' in the cause and was probably the source of a report that 2,760 people had been vaccinated in Lithuania in 1803.[47] Augustas Bekiu, who had lost eight out of nine of his siblings to smallpox, wrote a treatise on vaccination in Polish, the language of the educated elite in Lithuania.[48] The appointment of Dr Johann Peter Frank, the doyen of social medicine, to a chair at the University of Vilnius and the arrival of his son Dr Joseph Frank, who had studied vaccination in Britain, lent further weight to their endeavours.[49] All in all, Vilnius was putting itself on the map of global vaccination. In May 1804, the medical fraternity held a special festival on Jenner's birthday in honour of his discovery and, in December, the University

---

[43] *Journal politique de Mannheim*, 20 January 1802.   [44] Dirbe, 'Otto Huhn', pp. 183–85.

[45] Kh. Gustavson, 'The beginning of vaccination in Estonia, up to the establishment of vaccination committees in 1811', in V. I. Valeskeln and Ia. P. Stradyn' (eds.), *Nauchnye sviazi Pribaltiki v XVIII-XX vekakh: Materialy VII Pribaltiiskoi konferentsii po istorii nauki* (Riga, 1968), pp. 186–89.

[46] Michael J. Bennett, 'The beginnings of vaccination in Lithuania', *Lithuanian Papers: Annual Journal of the Lithuanian Studies Society at the University of Tasmania*, 24 (2010), 23–8; *Russkii biograficheskii slovar'*, ed. A. A. Polovtsov, 25 vols. (St Petersburg, 1896–1918), II, p. 677, X, p. 566.

[47] Baron, *Life*, 2, p. 52; *The Times*, 18 August 1804.

[48] *MPJ*, 14 (June–December 1805), p. 149. A copy of *O wakcynie czili tak zwanei ospie krowiey [On the effect of so-called vaccination against smallpox]* survives in the library of the University of Vilnius.

[49] G. Bagenskii, *Znachenia Imperatorskago Vilenskago Meditsinskago Obshchestva v dele rasprostranenii ospoprivivaniia [The significance of the Vil'na Medical Society in the matter of disseminating vaccination]* (Vilnius, 1896).

elected Jenner as an associate member.[50] Early in 1805, Dr Bekiu went to Britain to present the certificate to Jenner and acquire the latest information on vaccination.[51]

In spring 1802, Tsar Alexander, wishing to make the new prophylaxis available throughout the empire, gave his support to a plan set forward by Dr Franz Buttats, who would have heard in London about the methods used to deliver live vaccine to the Mediterranean. The aim was for Buttats and two colleagues to take cowpox from province to province in 'European' Russia and then to the 'Asiatic peoples' of the empire. The plan required the collaboration of multiple agencies and high-level support. The College of Medicine was to prepare the ground by sending instructions, copies of Buttats' manual and English steel lancets to the provincial capitals. Once the practice had been introduced in each centre, local medical officers were to continue vaccination, submit monthly reports on the number and outcomes of vaccinations and co-operate with officers in neighbouring districts in maintaining the supply of vaccine. Small hospitals were to be established in each province, 'each capable of holding 50 beds, for the purpose of inoculating with cowpox – at certain fixed hours – anyone who appears and desires it'. The governors of the provinces were to play a critical role in facilitating the enterprise, especially in setting up the medical councils and making available groups of children, some for immediate vaccination, some to be vaccinated subsequently to maintain the supply of vaccine, and some to be taken under vaccination to go arm-to-arm with children in the next district. Funds were to be made available to cover the expenses of relatives accompanying the latter group of children. The itinerary was to include Novgorod, Moscow, Kiev, Astrakhan, Kazan', Irkutsk and Kiakhta. The plan was costly but, according to Buttats, it was 'the only way of effecting the beneficent intentions of so great and mighty a monarch, who will ever be reckoned the most magnanimous and benevolent of rulers, and whose name will be praised by the people from generation to generation'.[52]

The Tsar issued a *ukase* for the vaccine expedition in April. It was part of a broadly reformist and humanitarian agenda. He was considering a plan for the new Ministry of Internal Affairs whose remit was 'to look after the well-being of the people everywhere' and to 'endeavour by all means to avert shortages of food and all other life necessities'.[53] It was reported overseas, including in Spain, that he was amalgamating the Councils of Beneficence and Utility into a

[50] Baron, *Life*, 2, pp. 52–3.   [51] *MPJ*, 13 (January–June 1805), 427–9.
[52] Gubert, *Ospa i ospoprivivanie*, 1, pp. 503–5.
[53] Daniel T. Orlovksy, *The limits of reform: the Ministry of Internal Affairs, 1802–1881* (Cambridge, MA, 1981), pp. 5, 17–19.

single 'Philanthropic' Council.[54] In June 1802, Buttats and his colleagues left St Petersburg and began their work by vaccinating forty-seven children at Novgorod. The expedition moved more slowly than expected and, in addition to administrative problems, it was found not to be easy to persuade parents to have their children vaccinated, let alone have them used to deliver vaccine to a distant town. In 1802–3, however, he made his way through seven provinces and completed 6,000 vaccinations.[55] By this stage, it was felt to be more practicable to send dried vaccine to the capitals of the *gubernias* along with instructions as the management of the practice. Supported by the Ministry of Internal Affairs and a Philanthropic Medical Committee in St Petersburg, however, the new prophylaxis was steadily extended through 'European' Russia. In 1804, over 64,000 people were vaccinated in nineteen provinces, including fifty-four in Perm' on the border of 'Asian' Russia. During 1805, the practice was introduced in almost all the *gubernias* of the empire. In the far north, 296 people were vaccinated in Archangel'sk.[56] In May, viable vaccine arrived in Irkutsk, over 2,700 miles from St Petersburg.[57]

Trans-Siberian Vaccine

Tsar Alexander's dispatch of a diplomatic mission to China in 1805–6 provided a further opportunity to consolidate and further extend vaccination east of the Urals. Headed by Count Golovkin and including luminaries like Count Jan Potoki and the Orientalist scholar J. H. von Klaproth, the mission had a strong scientific dimension. Three months before the mission's departure, Dr Joseph Rehmann, the mission's physician, submitted a plan to the College of Medicine to include a vaccine expedition. In addition to stressing the need for the co-operation of agencies on route to maintain the supply of vaccine, he requested a second physician to concentrate on establishing the practice in Siberia while he continued with the embassy to China.[58] Although a second physician could not be funded, Rehmann achieved a great deal, with the assistance of a competent surgeon, in extending and strengthening vaccination. As the embassy moved southwards and then eastwards, he reported that the practice was established at Kazan', including among some of the Tartars in the district, and commented favourably on the situation at Perm'. At Ekaterinburg,

---

[54] *Gaceta de Madrid*, 12 April 1803.
[55] *Russkii Biograficheskii Slovar'*, ed. Polovtsov, IV, pp. 26–7.
[56] *Moskovskoe Otdelenie Obschego Arkhiva Glavnogo Shtaba, raport ... ob ospoprivianii [Moscow Division, Head of Staff, report regarding vaccination]* (Moscow, 1911), p. 513.
[57] *BB, S&A*, 34 (1807), 284–6.
[58] Joseph Rehmann and Alexander A. Thesleff, *Mongoleireise zur spaeten Goethezeit: Berichte und Bilder des J. Rehmann und A. Thesleff von der russischen Gesandtschaftsreise 1805–06*, ed. Walther Heissig (Wiesbaden, 1971), pp. 9–10, 147–51.

he found that the health department had set up a small vaccine institute and commissioned the glassworks to make special glassware for storing lymph. At Tomsk, he was less impressed with the state of affairs and could do no more than vaccinate five children rounded up by the garrison commander. The embassy's need to make progress prevented his following up the results of his vaccinations at Tomsk or the outcome of his vaccination of two Cossack children at Krasnoyarsk.[59] On arrival in Irkutsk in September, he reported that vaccine had arrived four months earlier and had been successfully maintained. Over the following weeks, he worked hard to expand the practice in and around Irkutsk and to build up a supply of vaccine to take to China. He also prepared an address to the Chinese nation, translated into Manchu and Chinese by Klaproth, outlining the history of cowpox inoculation and its successes.[60]

The Russian embassy halted at the border of the Celestial Empire. Count Golovkin was accorded an imperial banquet in Urga (Ulaanbaater) on 20 December but his refusal to prostrate himself before burning candles, proxies for the emperor, was reported back to Beijing and early in the new year the embassy was summarily dismissed.[61] Rehmann, who had been left behind at Troizkasafsk, passed his time usefully, exploring the countryside, collecting specimens and learning about the Mongol peoples. He was delighted by the Buryats and found them disposed to accept vaccination. Along with Surgeon Petrov, who spoke their language, he was invited to their settlements, given milk, spirits and a special tea at the lodgings of the lamas and led to their holy places. Vaccination took on the character of a festival. Nomads, young and old, arrived on horseback from miles around. In a month or so, 744 Buryats were vaccinated. In a rare depiction of vaccination, Rehmann painted his colleague vaccinating one of the Buryats inside a yurt (Figure 9.1).[62] On his return to Irkutsk, he was disappointed to find that only 200 people had come forward for vaccination. On a more positive note, he met Mr Schilling, who had served as director of the smallpox hospital at Irkutsk for over thirty years, variolating 18,272 people, with only 237 deaths. After the hospital's closure, he became district physician at Verkhneudinsk, where he took up the new prophylaxis with a zeal that belied his age. To assist his work, he trained a lama and other Buryats who spread the practice among their people on the Chilok River and in the districts of Verkhneudinsk and Barguzin.[63] Several

[59] *BB, S&A*, 34 (1807), 283–5.   [60] *BB, S&A*, 34 (1807), 285–7.

[61] Alain Peyrefitte, *The collision of two civilisations. The British expedition to China 1792–4* (London, 1993), pp. 500–3.

[62] Joseph Rehmann, 'Bericht über die Einplanzung und Ausbreitung der Schutzpocken in Siberien in den Jahren 1805 und 1806, an den Minister des Innern, geschrieben in Irkutsk am Ende des Jahres 1806', in Joseph Rehmann (ed.), *Sammlung auserlesener Abhandlungen und merkwürdiger Nachrichten Russischer Ärste und Naturforscher* (St Petersburg, 1812), pp. 212–25.

[63] Rehmann, 'Schutzpocken in Siberien', pp. 215–17.

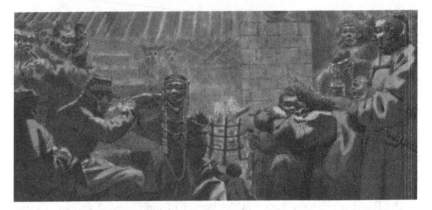

Figure 9.1 Vaccinating among the Buryats, 1805–6, watercolour by
Dr Joseph Rehmann
(Württembergische Landesbibliothek, Stuttgart)

other Russian practitioners were energetic in the cause. Assistant surgeon
Miron Stepanitch Britakov vaccinated some 2,129 Buryats around Tunka, a
tally rivalled only by Petrov in Troizkasafsk.[64]

In his report to the Minister of Internal Affairs in 1806, Rehmann advised
that greater pressure should be applied to establish vaccination in Siberia. After
all, he observed, the government enlisted the sons of peasants into the army
without seeking their consent. He expressed his belief that if Count Golovkin
were to appoint two medical practitioners to travel around Siberia, accompanied by police officers, tasked with treating venereal disease and vaccinating,
the province would be well populated within thirty years. It was a false
principle of philanthropy, he reasoned, to give people freedom to ignore a
measure so vital for the population.[65] More positively, he reported the recent
progress of vaccination northwards and eastwards from Irkutsk. From
Yakutsk, where vaccine had arrived late in 1805, Dr Roslein had established
the practice among the Yakuts and supplied vaccine to Ivan Redovski, who
had left Golovkin's embassy to explore and botanise in Kamchatka and the
Kuril Islands. He expressed concern that a repetition of the lethal smallpox
epidemic that ravaged Kamchatka thirty years earlier would devastate the
indigenous peoples and threaten the survival of the Russian settlements. Given
that it was difficult to press the need for vaccination in the absence of an
immediate threat, he again urged firmer measures to entrench a practice which,
if it could be made more general, would safeguard 'these unhappy lands from

[64] Rehmann, 'Schutzpocken in Siberien', p. 221.
[65] Rehmann, 'Schutzpocken in Siberien', p. 218; *BB. S&A*, 34 (1807), 295–6.

this dangerous enemy'. Ending in an optimistic note, he looked forward to the time when 'this triumphant discovery would freely make its path on our hemisphere from England to the edge of northern Asia'.[66]

Putting down Roots in Russia

In the Russian empire, vaccination spread widely but not so deeply. The court, the aristocracy and the urban elite warmly received the new practice, and the lay intelligentsia were eager to promote it. To maintain the practice in the provinces, institutional support and constant attention were required. Foundling houses and other charities were indispensable as vaccine depots in regional centres. Along with charity children, the children of members of the armed services and cadets in the army and navy were conscripted for vaccination. In October 1803, Admiral Chichagov approved the vaccination of children in the lower ranks of the Admiralty College in St Petersburg and, after vaccinating over 600 of them, Dr Rogers recommended further sessions every three months.[67] The Free Economic Society, a non-government organisation, published a paper encouraging vaccination in 1801 and used its network to promote the practice.[68] Vilnius, the capital of Lithuania, was a lively centre of vaccination activity. From its establishment in 1805, the Vilnius Medical Society had a strong focus on smallpox prevention, issuing instruction and disseminating vaccine, conducting its own experiments and maintaining foreign correspondence. At meetings over the winter of 1806–7, for example, a letter from Jenner was read out, Lobenvein gave a paper on popular prejudices against vaccine, Ferdinand Spitsnagel discussed his experience using vaccine crusts, and Rehmann's work in Siberia was reported.[69] On Jenner's birthday in 1807, the Society established a vaccine institute that offered free vaccination twice a week, kept careful records and issued certificates, supplied vaccine to practitioners at a modest charge and used the proceeds to induce poor parents to have children vaccinated.[70] In many provincial capitals and country towns, the practice was doubtless less well-supported. In the countryside, vaccination depended largely on the philanthropy or enlightened self-interest of the aristocracy. In 1802, for example, Dr Hakenszmit brought vaccine from Paris to use on the estates of Count Markov in Podolia and Valhynia, Ukraine, and in 1803 Dr Keir was employed to vaccinate the serfs of Count Vorontsov.[71]

[66] *BB. S&A*, 34 (1807), 299–300.   [67] Gubert, *Ospa i ospoprivivanie*, 1, pp. 507–8.
[68] Pratt, 'Free Economic Society', 563.
[69] Bagenskii, *Vilenskago Meditsinskago Obshchestva*, p. 6.
[70] Bagenskii, *Vilenskago Meditsinskago Obshchestva*, pp. 7–10.
[71] *Gaceta de Madrid*, 19 February 1802; Cross, *Banks of Neva*, p. 420, n. 103.

Among the urban proletariat and the peasantry, prejudices, old and new, had to be overcome before vaccination could be fully accepted. The practice made most headway in the Baltic provinces. The Lutheran pastors were supportive and the German townsmen generally well-disposed. In Russia itself there was more deep-seated hostility. In 1803, the peasants in Nizhnedevitsk and Voronezh Districts refused to allow their children to be vaccinated.[72] Dr Rehmann, who found the Buryats receptive to vaccination, claimed that the Russians themselves rarely submitted to the practice voluntarily, but only when ordered by a superior and then with much trembling and making the sign of the cross.[73] In addition to the Old Believers who were resolutely hostile, some Orthodox priests fuelled the prejudices of their flocks. In the report of the Podolsk Medical Office dated July 1803, Dr Kobtse claimed that the clergy in Baltiysky District condemned the new prophylaxis as 'unheard-of freemasonry', raised doubts 'by various forms of philosophizing, which not only twisted the truth but even offended against all probability', and were so successful in their fear-mongering that peasants fled with their children into the woods and fields.[74] The church authorities were enlisted to counteract this negative influence. The Holy Synod called on the bishops and clergy to impart the right attitudes to vaccination. In an edict of October 1804, it pronounced that the 'life-saving discovery of cowpox inoculation' had already saved the lives of countless young people across Europe and that, since its introduction into Russia, its value in preserving the lives of all who embraced it had been amply demonstrated. It asked parish priests to remind the people of the ravages of smallpox, convince them of the harmlessness of the procedure by giving examples of children who had been safely vaccinated and to do all that they could to persuade them to allow their children to be immunised.[75] There was some evidence that many people found the idea of infecting a child with an animal disease wholly repugnant. By 1811, the use of the expression 'pox of surety' was mandatory.[76]

More direct promotional strategies were also employed. In the last quarter of the eighteenth century the printing press was widely used to provide information and shape public opinion. Dr Kilwein, the chief physician of the Foundling House in St Petersburg, published a broadsheet containing instructions for inoculation, an illustration of the smallpox pustule and a depiction of two Russian families, one in misery because of smallpox, the other healthy and prosperous through vaccination.[77] During the reign of Alexander I, the *lubok* came into its own as a means of entertaining and instructing the masses. Mass-produced in St Petersburg and Moscow, *lubki* combined lively pictures with a

---

[72] Gubert, *Ospa i ospoprivivanie*, 1, p. 508.   [73] *BB, S&A*, 34 (1807), 287–91.
[74] Gubert, *Ospa i ospoprivivanie*, 1, p. 508.   [75] Gubert, *Ospa i ospoprivivanie*, 1, p. 509.
[76] Baron, *Life*, 2, pp. 183–7.   [77] Gubert, *Ospa i ospoprivivanie*, I, facing p. 498.

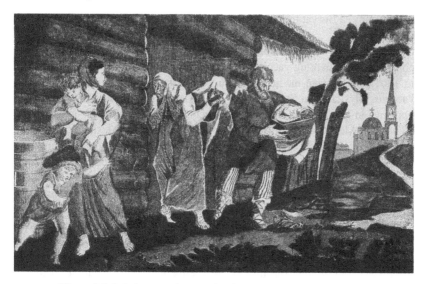

Figure 9.2 *Lubok* promoting vaccination
(V. O. Gubert, *Ospa i ospoprivivanie* (St Petersburg, 1896))

simple text and quite a number took vaccination as their theme.[78] In one a
mother with an infant in her arms and a toddler playing by her side sees a
distraught family, visibly infected with smallpox, leaving their house with a
dead child in a cradle. 'Thank God', she says, 'I listened to good people and so
saved my children through cowpox. Disease and pox kill other children. Mine
frolic and they are not pocked, and know no illness. No, they frisk and spin
their tops! God save the gentlemen who save the people from their ruin'
(Figure 9.2).[79] The *lubki* were intelligible to people with little or no education.
The texts were in verse for easy recitation and the largely self-explanatory
pictures made them accessible, too, to the empire's other language communities. Promoting vaccination in the ethnically and religiously diverse southern
and eastern provinces of the Russian empire presented further challenges.
From his base in Kazan', Mr Volkov vaccinated among the Tartars and
planned to translate a vaccination manual into the Tartar language. In 1805,
a medal, with inscriptions in Russian and Tartar, was issued to Mullah Hassan
Daud Ajiev for his assistance with vaccination.[80] The welcome given to
vaccination by the Buryats may be attributed to their prior experience of
smallpox inoculation and the employment of Buryat practitioners.[81] Damba

---

[78] Eight *lubki* on vaccination are printed in Gubert, *Ospa i ospoprivivanie*, 1, facing pp. 494–510.
[79] Gubert, *Ospa i ospoprivivanie,* I, facing p. 502 (transl. Dr Glynn Barratt).
[80] For the medal, see Gubert, *Ospa i ospoprivivanie*, 1, p. 511.   [81] *BB, S&A*, 34 (1807), 293–4.

Choreganov, a Buryat trained in western surgery, vaccinated some 393 people at Balangansk.[82]

Though drawing inspiration from western Europe, Russia charted its own course in implementing vaccination. Once the procedure had been established in 1801, the Russian medical men succeeded in maintaining the supplies of vaccine. Physicians in St Petersburg and Moscow kept up-to-date with developments in prophylaxis from western colleagues and foreign journals. In 1804 Tsar Alexander recruited the Scottish clinician Dr Alexander Crichton, who brought the latest ideas from Edinburgh and London, and Dr Bekiu went to Britain in spring 1805 to meet Jenner and other British vaccinators. Still, it is the self-sufficiency of the Russian system, especially after Napoleon's victory at Austerlitz severed communications with Britain, and the government's strong support of the new prophylaxis that are most impressive. The expedition led by Dr Buttats, introducing vaccination in the *gubernias* of European Russia in 1802–3, was unprecedented in its ambition. Overseen by the philanthropic committee of the Academy of Medicine, it may have served, in part, as an inspiration and model for the Spanish Philanthropic Vaccine Expedition approved in 1803. The orders to governors and medical officers in the provinces to support the establishment of vaccination anticipate the orders to institute *comités de vaccine* in Napoleonic France and the *juntas de vacunación* in the Spanish empire. Professor Mukhin's organisation of a school in Moscow in 1804 for people wishing to learn about the new prophylaxis proved a valuable initiative in the vast and sparsely populated empire. He wrote about the 'philoprogenitive fathers, rulers of their subordinates, and even the subordinates themselves who had come from the remotest places in Russia, in the name of others, to the Imperial Moscow Foundling House'.[83] The mobilisation of the nation for war in 1805 gave a boost to vaccination. By the end of 1806, the official tally of people vaccinated exceeded a quarter of a million. News of the success of vaccination in Russia was filtering through to western Europe. Dr Rehmann's account of his mission in Siberia was published in the *Bibliothèque Britannique* and was sent to inform the review of vaccination by the Royal College of Physicians in London in 1807.[84]

The Russian authorities did not rest on their laurels. In 1807, there was some loss of momentum, with the annual tally of vaccinations falling by 30 per cent.[85] A number of measures were introduced to promote practice, including a requirement that all wards of state should be vaccinated. The annual totals increased from 1808 onwards, with almost a quarter of a million people vaccinated in 1810 alone. By this time, the number of people vaccinated in

---

[82] *BB, S&A*, 34 (1807), 298–9.   [83] Gubert, *Ospa i ospoprivivanie*, 1, p. 497.

[84] MS. 2321. Vaccination Committee, Letters 3, no. 134, RCP.

[85] Gubert, *Ospa i ospoprivivanie*, 1, p. 513.

the Russian empire since the introduction of the practice in 1802 exceeded one million.[86] In May 1811, Tsar Alexander sought to consolidate this achievement by issuing a *ukase* to make vaccination generally available and mandatory. To this end, vaccination committees, comprising government officials and churchmen as well as physicians, were established in all *gubernias* and districts. The clergy were enjoined to co-operate 'with the beneficent views of the Emperor in destroying the prejudices which exist among the people against the inoculation of the cow-pox, or as it was now to be called the pock of surety'. The committees were instructed to maintain the supply of vaccine, to support and promote the practice, to record the vaccination status of individuals, to distribute promotional literature, and to keep a register of vaccinations. Above all, the entire population, except the newborn, was to be vaccinated within three years.[87]

A rare insight into the impact of this *ukase* is provided by the memoir of Dimitrii Ivanovich Rostislavov who lived in a village in the *guberniia* of Riazan.[88] He recalled that most mothers at this time were reluctant to have their children vaccinated and only did so 'after extensive urging and even coercion, and, of course, amidst weeping and wailing', and that the priests were 'virtually ordered by imperial edict to set an example for their parishioners by allowing their own children to be vaccinated'. The memoirist, the son of a priest, continued:

I did not know whether it was by coincidence or in response to the governmental instructions I just mentioned, but my vaccination and that of my two sisters was public, indeed almost a ceremony. It was Sunday, and many village women and men had gathered in the log cabin (*izba*) where we lived [. . .] Some of the women had started crying even before the operation. Most likely I felt shy because I was confused by the whole situation, for when the medical attendant started rolling up my right sleeve, someone said about me, 'He's scared and wants to cry'. To help me be brave, my dad answered, 'Come on, I know he's not scared and would never cry – he's not a little girl'. These words aroused my ambition and, as I recall today, I gathered up all my courage, so that I neither screamed nor cried, which of course won me praise from all sides. On the other hand, of course, my sisters (Natal'ia was two years younger than I, and Elizaveta was still an infant) did cry and fight back against the danger threatening them, so they had to be restrained.

Rostislavov's vaccination, which took place in Palishchii, a hundred miles southeast of Moscow, around 1813, was clearly etched in his memory.

By 1811, Tsar Alexander was seeking to break out of the geo-political straitjacket imposed by the French alliance. It was believed that Napoleon

---

[86] Gubert, *Ospa i ospoprivivanie*, 1, p. 513.   [87] Baron, *Life*, 2, pp. 184–6.
[88] Alexander M. Martin (ed.), *Provincial Russia in the age of Enlightenment: the memoir of a priest's son, Dimitrii Ivanovich Rostislavov* (DeKalb, IL, 2002), pp. 14–15.

was intent on rolling back Russian influence in Europe, making Russia 'a purely Asiatic power'.[89] Russia eased restrictions on Anglo-Russian trade and, after Napoleon began to mobilise in 1812, made a formal alliance with Britain. From St Petersburg, Dr Crichton took the opportunity to write to Jenner about the progress of vaccination. He enclosed the Emperor's *ukase* of 1811 and a table of the vaccinations, *guberniia* by *guberniia*, since 1802. The cumulative total was 1,235,597. He drew special attention to the half-yearly report from Irkutsk, 'one of the most distant and least civilised governments', where one of the most zealous vaccinators was 'a priest of the great Lama'. He also included in the package a case of the instruments that he had approved for use and some 'caricature prints in favour of vaccination', presumably *lubki*, that, he believed, 'operate as much on the mind of the poor peasants as the most eloquent discourses of the clergy'. Crichton acknowledged that the order for all Russians to be vaccinated within three years could not be executed. He referred to the adherents of 'a peculiar religious sect', presumably the Old Believers, who regarded it 'a damnable crime' to propagate a disease or take medicine and were wholly unmoved by threats of dire punishment. Crichton's letter, dated 12 September 1812, was remarkably upbeat, given the crisis looming in Russia.[90] It was written four days after the Battle of Borodino and two days before the French army entered Moscow.

War and Peace

After leading the *Grande Armée*, the largest and best organised army in recorded history, across northern Europe, Napoleon entered Moscow in the hollowest of triumphs in September 1812. Rather than attempting to defend the old capital, the Tsar's council of war had taken the decision to abandon it. Thousands of inhabitants loaded wagons with food and valuables and moved to villages away from the frontline. The Russians were aiming to deny the enemy shelter and sustenance. The French were stunned to find Moscow empty and unnerved when, a few days later, the city was in flames. Among the few buildings standing when the smoke cleared was the grand but grim-faced Foundling House, still home to fifty infants who had been left behind. By coincidence, Count I. A. Tutolmin, its director, was the highest-ranking officer remaining in Moscow. At the meeting, Napoleon questioned him about the institution, and probably its vaccination programme. He concluded by asking the Count to send his regards to the Dowager Empress Maria and assure her that he had placed the Foundling House under his personal protection.[91]

---

[89]   Saunders, *Russia*, p. 51.   [90]   Baron, *Life*, 2, pp. 184–7.
[91]   Paul Britten Austin, *1812. Napoleon in Moscow* (London, 1995), p. 56.

Amid all the destruction and loss in Moscow, the cradle of vaccination in Russia survived.

Emperor Alexander held his nerve. Short of food and supplies, Napoleon had little option other than to withdraw, and with the approach of winter the withdrawal became a retreat. Defenceless against the biting cold, the *Grande Armée* was also ravaged by disease. Several months before the invasion, typhus had appeared in its ranks and began to sap its strength. On their return, many thousands fell ill and died.[92] One consolation was that smallpox did not add to the misery of the cold, famished and diseased soldiers, who were largely protected by cowpox. In 1813, Tsar Alexander led a large Russian army westwards and in spring 1814 entered Paris in triumph. In May, he crossed the English Channel to join other leaders of the victorious allies in celebrating victory and beginning to make plans for Europe after Napoleon. He was interested in meeting Jenner and honouring his role in a discovery that had saved more lives than had been lost in the wars. Count Orlov, the Russian ambassador, was already in touch with Jenner and Dr Hamel, a Russian physician, came to Cheltenham to pay homage. In the English capital, the Tsar found himself overwhelmed by the political intrigue, social niceties and public attention.[93] The meeting with Jenner, who came reluctantly to London, proved hard to schedule. The Grand Duchess of Oldenburg, his sister, spent over an hour with Jenner, who described her to a friend as 'by far the finest woman of a royal race I have met with'.[94] Count Matvei Platov, Hetman of the Don Cossacks, over a jar of snuff, told Jenner that he had 'extinguished the most pestilential disorder that ever appeared on the banks of the Don'.[95] When he finally met Jenner, the Tsar spoke about the success of vaccination in Russia, where 'the vaccine had nearly subdued the small-pox', and observed how happy Jenner must feel in winning 'the thanks, the applause and gratitude of the world'. He was surprised to hear Jenner quibble that he had received 'the applause, but not the gratitude of the world' and then hastily acknowledge the Dowager Empress's gift of a diamond ring. It was all too embarrassing. In a kind gesture, the Tsar took the tongue-tied Jenner 'by the hand, with a good-natured smile, and held it till [his] embarrassment had disappeared'.[96]

The heroic phase of the history of vaccination in Russia ended in 1812. The plan instituted in 1811, not least the requirement for universal vaccination within three years, delivered an increase of 25 per cent in the annual total. The vaccination of 369,061 people in 1812, bringing the formal tally since 1802 to

---

[92] Stephan Talty, *The illustrious dead. The terrifying story of how typhus killed Napoleon's greatest army* (New York, 2009).
[93] Alan Palmer, *Alexander I. Tsar of war and peace* (London, 1974), pp. 293–6.
[94] MS. 5240/52, WLL.   [95] *Letters of Jenner*, ed. Miller, p. 86.
[96] Fosbroke, *Berkeley manuscripts*, pp. 238–40; Cf. Baron, *Life*, 2, pp. 206–7.

over 1.6 million vaccinations, is all the more remarkable in view of Napoleon's invasion in the second half of the year. The disruption to the programme was most evident in 1813. Although there was some increase in the numbers vaccinated east of the Urals, there were no returns at all from Moscow and neighbouring *gubernias*. More generally, there was a pulling back from the authoritarian measures of 1811, seemingly associated with a change of ministers in March 1812.[97] Tsar Alexander's spiritual crisis and mystical turn may have inclined him to resile from compulsory vaccination.[98] 'There is a power greater than sovereignty, namely the conscience or religious opinions of men', Dr Crichton wrote to Jenner in 1812, perhaps reflecting the Tsar's sentiments. After reporting the refusal of the Old Believers to accept vaccination, he noted that 'the government has come to the wise resolution of leaving this dispute to time'.[99] In April 1815, when Crichton published another report on vaccination in Russia, he had good data for 1811–13, but still lacked hard figures for 1814.[100] Although vaccination remained in good repute in governing circles, there was evidently some relaxation of the measures to promote and enforce it. Tsar Alexander's new minsters were modernisers of a liberal stamp. Count Mordvinov, for example, was sceptical and suspicious of measures that involved state intervention.[101] Appointed President of the Free Economic Society in 1823, he proposed the government's transfer of responsibility for vaccination, along with an annual budget, to this institution in 1824. For the next forty years, prophylaxis in Russia depended more on professional and philanthropic networks than on state power.[102]

---

[97] Orlovsky, *Limits of reform*, pp. 21–6; Marc Raeff, *Michael Speransky, statesman of imperial Russia, 1772–1839* (The Hague, 1957), ch. 5.

[98] Hartley, *Alexander I*, pp. 185–9.   [99] Baron, *Life*, 2, pp. 184–7.

[100] *Report of the National Vaccine Establishment for the year 1814* (London, 1815), pp. 5–6.

[101] Susan P. McCaffray, 'What should Russia be? Patriotism and political economy in the thought of N. S. Mordvinov', *Slavic Review*, 59 (2000), 572–96.

[102] Pratt, 'Free Economic Society', 563–6.

10 Passage through India
Vaccination in South Asia

In April 1802, Harford Jones, British Resident in Baghdad, received a curious parcel by courier. He had earlier written to Dr Jean de Carro in Vienna to request a sample of cowpox. Aware that it would lose its effectiveness on the long journey, de Carro sealed the vaccine virus for use on the 'banks of the Tigris' between glass plates and enclosed the package in a large ball of wax.[1] After a month on the road, and with temperatures rising, Jones knew there was no time to waste. His surgeon used cowpox to inoculate an Armenian child, 'the first whose parents we have been able to persuade to suffer the operation to be performed', and subsequently confirmed a vaccine response.[2] The immediate aim was to produce fresh lymph for onward transmission to the East India Company surgeon in Basra, John Milne, and through the Persian Gulf to India. In Basra, Milne succeeded in propagating a further supply of vaccine and arranged for its transport both in dried form and through successive vaccinations on board ship to Bombay (Mumbai).[3] On 14 June, Dr Helenus Scott of Bombay used vaccine from Basra on dozens of children, only one of whom, Anna Dusthall, took the infection. A little over a week later, he observed a true vaccine vesicle on her arm and took lymph to inoculate other children. On 2 July, he and a colleague wrote to the *Bombay Courier* to announce the beginning of vaccination in the subcontinent, declaring grandly 'We have it now in our power to communicate the benefit of this important discovery to every part of India, perhaps to China and the whole eastern world'.[4]

The passage of cowpox through Baghdad to Bombay reflected Britain's expanding interests in the Levant, the Middle East and India. The loss of the American colonies and the global conflict with France drove a perceptible 'swing to the East' in Britain's strategic priorities in the last decades of the

---

[1] AL40/6497–8, Herefordshire Record Office, Hereford; De Carro, *Histoire*, pp. 21–24.
[2] De Carro, *Histoire*, pp. 23–4.
[3] George Keir, *Account of the introduction of the cowpox into India* (Bombay, 1803), pp. 106–8.
[4] Keir, *Introduction*, pp. 19–25, at 19–20. This chapter draws on and expands Michael Bennett, 'Passage through India: global vaccination and British India, 1800–05', *Journal of Imperial and Commonwealth History*, 35 (2007), 201–20.

eighteenth century.[5] In addition to the French colonies in the Indian Ocean and India, the Dutch colonies in the East became targets for takeover. Napoleon's invasion of Egypt in 1798 revealed the geographical scope of French ambitions and underlined the seriousness of the threat to British interests in the East. The British government, however, did not directly concern itself with the introduction of smallpox prophylaxis in the Levant. The commanders of the British expedition to Egypt recognised the potential of vaccination, but the extension of the practice around Marmaris Bay was entirely attributable to the missionary zeal of Dr Walker. In relation to India, too, private initiatives were centrally important. Jenner attempted to send cowpox on threads early in 1800. News of its success in England inspired members of the expatriate community in India to take steps to introduce it. The directors of the East India Company were happy enough to hear of the progress of vaccination but largely left the business of introducing the practice to the men on the ground. It was a request from Elgin's brother in Bombay that prompted Lord Elgin to send samples from Istanbul, and it was Company men in the Middle East who enlisted the assistance of de Carro, who succeeded in delivering vaccine in the first stage of its passage to India.

Vaccination arrived in South Asia at a time of increasing British power. From 1798, Governor-General Richard Wellesley conducted diplomatic and military offensives that brought large areas of southern, central and northeast India under British control or influence. By the time of his recall in 1805, he had eliminated the French threat that appeared menacing after Napoleon's invasion of Egypt and laid the foundations of a new British empire in India.[6] The arrival of Frederick North as Governor of Ceylon (Sri Lanka) in 1799 likewise signalled Britain's interest in permanently replacing Dutch rule, and British military operations in the interior from 1803 led to the subjugation of the independent kingdom of Kandy. From the outset, the introduction of vaccination was associated with war and imperial expansion. Beginning in Bombay in June 1802, it was firmly established in British India and in the new colony of Ceylon during 1803, and more than a million Indians and Sri Lankans had been vaccinated by 1807. The history of smallpox prophylaxis in India subsequently became a significant focus of scholarship on relations between western medicine and the imperial enterprise.[7] According to David Arnold,

---

[5] Michael Duffy, 'World-wide war and British expansion, 1793–1815', in P. J. Marshall (ed.), *The Oxford history of the British empire. Vol. II. The eighteenth* century (Oxford, 2008), pp. 184–207, esp. 184–5, 195–8.

[6] Christopher A. Bayly, *The new Cambridge history of India. Vol. II, Part 1. Indian society and the making of the British empire* (Cambridge, 1988), esp. ch. 3.

[7] P. R. Greenough, 'Variolation and vaccination in south Asia, c. 1700–1865: a preliminary note', *Social Science and Medicine*, 14 (1980), Part D, 345–7; David Arnold, *Colonizing the body. State medicine and epidemic disease in nineteenth-century India* (Berkeley, CA, 1993);

vaccination came to be 'construed as a site of conflict between malevolent British intent and something Indian, something sacred, that was under threat of violation and destruction'.[8] As revisionist studies of vaccination in India have shown, however, it is necessary, to take into account the complex interplay of agencies and agendas, local conditions and logistical problems.[9] If vaccination in India created space for an interventionist state concerned to control colonial bodies and minds, it needs to be borne in mind that its introduction was driven by the same sorts of impulses, hopes and fears, visions of improvement and humanitarian concern evident in Britain and elsewhere. Although the sharpness and scale of the drive created tensions in Anglo-Indian relations, there is much evidence that many Indians and Sri Lankans embraced the new prophylaxis. Though the early success in vaccinating large numbers of people in South Asia was not be sustained, it laid firm foundations, and provided lessons and inspiration for the practice worldwide.

Smallpox and Inoculation in India

In spreading eastwards, cowpox came to lands long habituated by smallpox. Although endemic in most parts of the Middle East, the lack of statistical information makes it impossible to quantify smallpox's contribution to mortality and morbidity. In British India, a higher level of documentation makes it possible to obtain a clearer picture. In densely populated regions, especially the Ganges delta, it was endemic, but markedly seasonal, appearing in early spring and at its height in the middle of summer. In the more serious epidemics that occurred at intervals of around four to seven years, death-rates could rise dramatically. Most people caught the disease sooner or later, and it was the cause of around 6–10 per cent of deaths.[10] In southern India and Ceylon, smallpox was largely epidemic and characterised by high mortality rates among young people. Travelling through Mysore in 1800, Francis Buchanan visited a smallpox-ravaged village in which a hundred people had died, 'a very terrible mortality in so small a place!'[11] In Ceylon, there were severe

Mark Harrison, *Public health in British India: Anglo-Indian preventive medicine 1859-1914* (Cambridge, 1994); J. Banthia and T. Dyson. 'Smallpox in nineteenth-century India'. *Population and Development Review*, 25 (1999), 649–80.

[8] Arnold, *Colonizing the body*, p. 144.

[9] N. Brimnes, 'Variolation, vaccination and popular resistance in early colonial south India', *MH*, 48 (2004), 199–228; Sanjoy Bhattacharya, Mark Harrison and Michael Worboys, *Fractured states: smallpox, public health and vaccination policy in British India 1800–1947* (London, 2005), ch. 1.

[10] Banthia and Dyson. 'Smallpox in India', 676–8.

[11] Francis Buchanan, *A journey from Madras through the countries of Mysore, Canara and Malabar*, 3 vols. (London, 1807), 2, pp. 285–6.

epidemics in 1754–5, 1786 and 1796.[12] In an epidemic that spread through the island in 1800–2, the death-rate exceeded 22 per cent.[13] Spreading into the Sinhalese heartland, with the Raja of Kandy only narrowly surviving an attack in 1803, smallpox played its part in the downfall of the kingdom of Kandy.

Where smallpox was a relatively rare scourge, a common response to its appearance was to take flight. In Ceylon in 1800, the Rev. James Cordiner came across villages near Batticaloe where smallpox cases had been left to fend for themselves: forty had died, including three who had been taken by cheetahs.[14] In the afflicted town in south India observed by Dr Buchanan, the community held together by attempting to propitiate Mariamma, the goddess of smallpox and to ease the suffering of patients by applying leaves from a tree sacred to her.[15] In northern India, long familiarity with smallpox encouraged some recourse to inoculation (variolation). The practice was associated with the cult of Sitala, the goddess associated with smallpox and highly ritualised (Figure 10.1).[16] In Bengal, it was conducted on some scale by specialists who were members of a small and tightly knit caste. Known as *tikadors* (inoculators), they operated in spring using matter preserved from the previous season. Seeing its relevance to debates about the practice in Europe, J. Z. Holwell wrote an account of it in 1767 that attested to its standing and effectiveness, and its use of light incisions and the cooling regimen.[17] Elsewhere in India, however, inoculation seems to have not been a regular practice. It was little known in Dravidian India. Buchanan's informants in Mysore were horrified by the idea of it.[18]

Europeans who went to India were mainly smallpox survivors and found far greater health threats in the new environment. They had much to learn from Indian medicine and its rich pharmacopeia, especially in relation to diseases that were new to them. In relation to smallpox prophylaxis, some of the Englishmen who had not had the disease availed themselves of the services of the *tikadors*. Improvements in British inoculation practice, the growth of the expatriate community, including women and locally born children, and an expanding medical establishment, increased the demand for western-style inoculation. In 1787, the government in Bengal established an inoculation

---

[12] C. G. Uragoda, *A history of medicine in Sri Lanka* (Colombo, 1987), pp. 201–3.

[13] Banthia and Dyson, 'Smallpox in India', 652.

[14] James Cordiner, *A description of Ceylon, containing an account of the country, inhabitants and natural productions, with narratives of the island in 1800, the campaign in Candy in 1803, and a journey to Ramisseram in 1804*, 2 vols. (London, 1807), 1, pp. 254–5.

[15] Buchanan, *Journey*, 2, p. 286.

[16] Lauren Minsky, 'Pursuing protection from disease: the making of smallpox prophylactic practice in Colonial Punjab', *BHM*, 83 (2009), 164–90, at 170–2.

[17] [Holwell], *Account of inoculating*, pp. 16, 21–2.   [18] Buchanan, *Journey*, 2, p. 286.

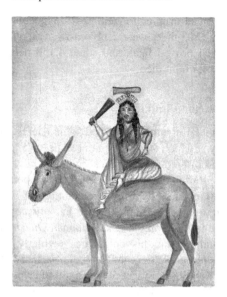

Figure 10.1 Sitala, goddess of smallpox and other epidemics, watercolour
(Wellcome Collections)

hospital outside Fort William (Calcutta (Kolkata), India).[19] At the same time,
the authorities in Madras recommended the inoculation to all East India
Company soldiers who had not had smallpox. After safely inoculating some
sepoys in Trichinopoly (Tiruchirappalli) in 1788, Surgeon Nicol Mein
expressed the hope that he would be able to introduce prophylaxis more
generally among Indians. In 1793, the Zamindar of Chintapally, in the northern
districts of the presidency of Madras, accepted inoculation in his own family.
A major smallpox epidemic in Madras in the late 1790s prompted Governor
Clive to institute an inoculation programme that provided training for Indian
practitioners and promotional material in the community languages. In 1802, it
was claimed that some 26,000 people had been inoculated.[20] In Ceylon,
Governor Frederick North offered free inoculation in response to a smallpox
epidemic in 1799, but only a few dozen natives in the army heeded the call. In
1800, he provided funds for a plan, drawn up by Dr Thomas Christie, to
establish hospitals in each of the four districts for the reception of patients, take

[19] S. P. James, *Smallpox and vaccination in British India* (Calcutta, 1909), p. 47.
[20] Brimnes, 'Variolation, vaccination', 202–3; N. Brimnes, 'The sympathizing heart and the
healing hand: smallpox prevention and medical benevolence in early colonial south India', in
H. Fischer-Tiné and M. Mann (eds.), *Colonialism as civilizing mission. Cultural ideology in
British India* (London, 2004), pp. 191–204, at 198 and 331 n.35.

firm measures to prevent the spread of infection and provide inoculation on a large-scale. Between 1800 and 1803 there were 2,110 cases of smallpox, 473 (around 22.5 per cent) of which proved fatal, and some 4,158 people were inoculated, 108 (2.6 per cent) of whom died.[21]

Cowpox and Its Passage to India

Though he never travelled outside England, Jenner had some interest in India, and long recalled a dinner party at which General Smith had been so impressed by his scientific brio that he had offered to help him secure a lucrative posting in the East India Company.[22] From the 1790s, he had the opportunity to discuss the potential of cowpox in India with the large number of East India Company men on leave or in retirement in Cheltenham.[23] In a private initiative in spring 1800, he sent vaccine to India on the East Indiaman *Queen* that was wrecked off San Salvador and he and his colleagues regularly supplied samples to officials and medical men setting out for India.[24] Henry Dundas, Minister for War and the Colonies and President of the Board of Control of the East India Company, commended the introduction of vaccination in India in March 1801, but committed no resources to make it feasible.[25] Frustrated by the lack of action, Jenner proposed raising a subscription to charter a vessel and allegedly declared his willingness to contribute £1,000.[26] In meetings with Lord Hobart, Dundas's successor in the ministry, he presented a plan to deliver fresh vaccine through successive inoculations on board a ship, claiming that all that was required was an experienced practitioner and ten people who had not previously been exposed to smallpox.[27] In January 1803, the Board of Ordnance approved a plan using men in an artillery train setting out for Ceylon to carry vaccine.[28] The plan was probably shelved with the arrival of the news of the successful propagation of cowpox in Bombay.

By 1802, British India was impatient for the introduction of vaccination. After reading of its endorsement by leading physicians and surgeons in London, Dr Helenus Scott of Bombay wrote to Sir Joseph Banks seeking his

---

[21] Thomas D. Christie, *An account of the ravages committed in Ceylon by small-pox previous to the introduction of vaccination; with a statement of the circumstances attending the introduction, progress and success of vaccine inoculation in that island* (Cheltenham, 1811), pp. 7–15.

[22] [John Lettsom], *Memoir of Edward Jenner from Dr Lettsom's oration before the Medical Society of London on the 8th March 1804* (London, [1804]), pp. 2–3.

[23] Mark Harrison, *Medicine in an age of commerce: Britain and its tropical colonies, 1660–1830* (Oxford, 2010), pp. 214–15.

[24] Christie, *Ravages in Ceylon*, p. 17n; Baron, *Life*, 1, pp. 410–12.   [25] CO 55/61, 364. TNA.

[26] [Lettsom], *Memoir of Jenner*, p. 5.   [27] Baron, *Life*, 1, p. 409; CO 54/12, 12r–13v. TNA.

[28] Baron, *Life*, 1, 408–10. CO 54/12, 1r–v. TNA; Christie, *Ravages in Ceylon*, 17n; P. E. Pieris, *Sinhale and the patriots 1815–1818* (New Delhi, 1950), pp. 505–6.

assistance in sending out vaccine and pointing out that inoculation in the hot
Indian climate was very dangerous, with a fatality rate of 'not less than one in
fifty'.[29] In response to a request from Jonathan Duncan, Governor of Bombay,
Lord Elgin dispatched dried vaccine lymph, propagated in Istanbul on his own
daughter, through Basra to Bombay, but it proved inert on arrival.[30] In his tour
of Ceylon early in 1802, Governor North made the examination of local cattle
for cowpox 'a principal object of enquiry'.[31] It was Harford Jones's direct
address to de Carro that prompted him to send the vaccine through Istanbul to
Baghdad whence, after a successful vaccination 'on the banks of the Tigris',
vaccine was sent on to Basra. After propagating vaccine lymph in Basra, John
Milne adopted a series of measures to secure the delivery of viable matter in
India, including vaccinating sailors and a boy on ships setting out for Bombay
and sending dried vaccine on threads, sealed between glass plates, one of
which produced the desired outcome.[32] On 14 June 1802, the vaccination of
the three-year-old Anna Dusthall, whose 'quietness and patience in suffering
the operation' contributed in some measure to its success, marked an epoch.
Her patience was further tested when the vesicle on her sore arm was squeezed
to obtain lymph to vaccinate five others.[33]

After announcing the introduction of vaccination in India on 2 July, Scott
and his colleagues began to dispatch samples of vaccine to other British bases.
A month-long passage brought vaccine to Trincomalee in Ceylon on
11 August, where bribes were offered to parents to allow their children to
be vaccinated.[34] Matter sent inland from Bombay to Hyderabad survived the
enervating August temperatures, and after a successful trial the local surgeon
was able to send threads imbued with vaccine to his colleagues. In September,
Dr Keir dispatched three lots of vaccine matter from Bombay along the coast
to Cochin (Kochi), one on an ivory lancet, another between glass, and a third
on thread. His colleague at Cochin conducted an experiment in which he
vaccinated twelve patients, four from each source, and reported that the
samples sealed between glass plates delivered the best results.[35] The British
authorities in Bombay approved the dispatch of two recently vaccinated Indian
children, accompanied by a Brahmin trained in the procedure, to Pune, the
capital of the so-called Maratha Confederacy. Dr Keir also sent two children
under vaccination from Bombay to Tellicherry, where the surgeon used lymph
from their arms to inoculate twenty-three children, some of whom were then
taken to seed the practice along the Malabar coast.[36] In late September, a boy
was vaccinated in Chingleput (Chengalpattu), south of Madras, to carry the

---

[29] Additional MS. 35,262. fos. 22 r-v, BL.   [30] Keir, *Introduction*, pp. 10–12.
[31] Christie, *Ravages in Ceylon*, pp. 17–18.   [32] Keir, *Introduction*, pp. 17, 106–8.
[33] Keir, *Introduction*, p. 18.   [34] Christie, *Ravages in Ceylon*, pp. 26–7.
[35] Keir, *Introduction*, pp. 26–7, 32–3.   [36] Keir, *Introduction*, pp. 31–2, 35–6.

virus on the final stage to Madras. In mid-October, Dr James Anderson, physician-general in the presidency of Madras, began his career as a champion of the new prophylaxis. After making several unsuccessful attempts to send vaccine to Calcutta, he seized the opportunity presented by the arrival of a Calcutta-bound ship from New South Wales. Prior to its departure, he arranged for the propagation of fresh lymph during the voyage by the successive vaccination of four children, including two boys from Botany Bay.[37] By the end of November, the Medical Board of Bengal reported to Governor-General Wellesley the inauguration of vaccination in Calcutta and presented plans for its establishment.[38]

The Establishment of Vaccination in India and Ceylon

The British delivery of cowpox to South Asia reflected a desire to protect the expatriate community from smallpox but involved a recognition of the needs of the indigenous population. The speed of the transmission and the rapidity with which the new practice was established owed much to the recent growth in the European population in India, the massive expansion of its military establishment, including medical men, and the building up of a network of communications to serve British needs. Once vaccination became available, European parents responded rapidly to the opportunity for their families. Sir George Barlow, Deputy Governor in Bengal, set an early example in Calcutta in having his children vaccinated and Dr Scott vaccinated his three young children in Bombay in the first months of the practice.[39] Colonel Arthur Wellesley, military governor of Mysore (Mysuru), requested Mr Gourlay, surgeon at Angadipuram, a hundred or so miles to the south, to send two children inoculated with cowpox to Seringapatam, as he wanted to have his 'godson' Arthur Freese vaccinated.[40] The authorities had many reasons to wish to extend the benefits of vaccination to non-Europeans, beginning with servants and sepoys. Most immediately, the maintenance of the vaccine supply depended on vaccinating a larger number of children than were available in the expatriate community. On the British side, there appear to have been few qualms about the passage of bodily matter across lines of race, colour or caste. Anna Dusthall was black: the areola around her vaccine pustule was reportedly 'very distinct, in spite of the blackness of her skin'.[41] Indian children were

---

[37] Christie, *Ravages in Ceylon*, pp. 28–9; Shoolbred, *Report 1802–3*, p. 4.
[38] Shoolbred, *Report 1802–3*, pp. 4–5, 85–91.   [39] Baron, *Life*, 1, p. 413.
[40] *Supplementary despatches and memoranda of Field Marshal Arthur Duke of Wellington, K.G. India. 1797–1805, Vol. 3 (Dec 1801–Feb 1803)*, ed. A. R. Wellesley (London, 1859), pp. 497–501; Rory Muir, *Wellington. The path to victory, 1769–1814* (New Haven, CT, 2013), pp. 102–3.
[41] Christie, *Ravages in Ceylon*, p. 22.

systematically used to carry vaccine from place to place. An Indian boy provided Madras with its first vaccine in October 1802 and three 'half-caste' children helped re-establish supply in November.[42] The use of children in propagating and disseminating lymph cannot have been entirely consensual. It was the norm, though, to obtain the consent of parents, some of whom were happy for their children to receive what was presented as 'a safe and certain antidote' to smallpox.[43] The first 'counter-proof' in South Asia occurred in October 1802, when Lieutenant Thiel, a Dutch officer in Jaffnapatnam, Ceylon, 'with a zeal for truth and an anxiety for his offspring', asked to have his recently vaccinated children inoculated with smallpox.[44] In the case of children used to transport vaccine, there is reference to mothers being paid to travel with their children.[45]

The British authorities made immediate moves to promote vaccination among all the peoples of South Asia. 'An address to the natives of Ceylon', published in September 1802, explained its benefits in Dutch, Malabar and Sinhalese as well as English, and urged them not to neglect through prejudice 'a duty they owe to themselves, to their families, and to society at large'.[46] In late 1802, Dr Scott reported that two or three thousand people were vaccinated in Bombay and that Indians were beginning 'to acquire confidence' in the practice.[47] The Brahmin who accompanied the children under vaccination to Pune presumably commended the practice in Indian circles. James Achilles Fitzpatrick, British resident of Hyderabad, who had his children by his Indian consort vaccinated, was hopeful that it would be accepted by the Nizam and his Chief Minister.[48] In January 1803, the Madras government circulated posters in the community languages explaining 'the very beneficial conse-quences which had resulted to mankind from this discovery'.[49] The hope that the Hindus would receive cowpox as a 'gift from Heaven through the medium of that highly favoured and long venerated animal' was soon found to be false.[50] Early in 1803, Dr Anderson concluded that it would be preferable to use a term other than cowpox in India and suggested that the Sanskrit word *amurtum*, which connoted both immortality and cow's milk, would be appro-priate as a substitute.[51] Many Indians and Sri Lankans, however, readily accepted the new prophylaxis. The recent experience of smallpox and inocu-lation in Ceylon must have made the Sinhalese and Tamils more responsive to the promise of protection. At the end of 1802, the government in Ceylon

[42] IOR/P/255/53, 4025–32, OIOC, BL.   [43] Christie, *Ravages in Ceylon*, pp. 29–36.
[44] Christie, *Ravages in Ceylon*, pp. 42–3.   [45] IOR/F/4/153/2613, pp. 99–100, OIOC, BL.
[46] Christie, *Ravages in Ceylon*, pp. 36–42.   [47] Baron, *Life*, 1, p. 413.
[48] William Dalrymple, *White mughals. Love and betrayal in eighteenth-century India* (London, 2002), p. 337.
[49] IOR/F/4/153/2613, pp. 1–2, OIOC, BL.   [50] IOR/F/4/153/2613, esp. p. 52, OIOC, BL.
[51] Keir, *Introduction*, pp. 94–5.

advertised the success of cowpox inoculation, reporting that 'upwards of ten thousand people of all ages and descriptions' had been vaccinated; that none had subsequently taken smallpox; and that the procedure was freely available in clinics each morning.[52] In the Presidency of Madras, too, the new practice also took off on the back of the recent inoculation campaigns, with 3,000 people vaccinated in the first months.[53]

Doctors in civilian and military employment familiarised themselves with the new prophylaxis and worked to extend the practice. It was hard to maintain a supply of good vaccine. Despite his best efforts, Dr Anderson was disappointed by the loss of vaccine along the Malabar coast during the hot season in 1803.[54] He explored, without success, the idea of inoculating a cow in the gardens of Government House in Madras to serve as a source of vaccine.[55] Learning from experience, John Shoolbred, superintendent of vaccine in Bengal from April 1803, took care to stagger vaccinations to assure supply over a longer timeframe.[56] The colonial governments made provision for vaccine depots in the administrative districts into which the presidencies of Bombay, Madras and Bengal and the colony of Ceylon were divided. In Ceylon, vaccine was to be maintained in each of the eight districts.[57] In the presidency of Madras, the programme was centralised under the oversight of the chief physician, Dr Anderson.[58] A more devolved system was set in place in the larger presidency of Bengal in May 1803. In addition to the establishment in Calcutta, subordinate stations, each with salaried staff, were established at Dacca, Murshidabad, Patna, Benares (Varanasi), Allahabad, Cawnpore (Kanpur) and Faruqabad.[59]

In its first two years in South Asia, vaccination made significant headway. By the end of 1802, Bombay was itself free from smallpox. To test Anna Dusthall's insusceptibility to smallpox, it was necessary to bring variolous matter on threads from Hyderabad as Dr Keir felt he could not justify bringing someone with smallpox into 'this populous island, which for so many months past has been exempt from it'.[60] In Ceylon, Dr Christie acted with great energy, issuing his subordinates with instructions in September 1802 to vaccinate free of charge, provide training in the practice, and keep records and issue certificates.[61] The prohibition of inoculation and the vaccination of tens

[52] Christie, *Ravages in Ceylon*, pp. 49–51.   [53] IOR/F/4/153/2613, 23–6, OIOC, BL.
[54] James Anderson, *Correspondence for the extermination of small-pox* (Madras, 1804), pp. 18–19.
[55] IOR/F/4/153/2613, pp. 48–9, 52, 93, 126–7, OIOC, BL.
[56] Shoolbred, *Report 1802–3*, p. 10.   [57] Christie, *Ravages in Ceylon*, pp. 30.
[58] Whitelaw Ainslie, 'Observations respecting the small-pox and inoculation in eastern countries; with some account of the introduction of vaccination into India'. *Transactions of the Royal Asiatic Society of Great Britain and Ireland*, 2 (1830), 52–73, at 61.
[59] IOR/F/4/169/2985, pp. 27–8, OIOC, BL.   [60] Keir, *Introduction*, p. 89.
[61] Christie, *Ravages in Ceylon*, pp. 33–6.

of thousands of people in 1803 cleared Colombo of smallpox for the first time in eight years.[62] The campaign in Madras, assisted by native inoculators, produced the most impressive statistics.[63] In April 1804, Surgeon Alexander Mackenzie reported 111,715 vaccinations in the presidency and 34,125 in the dependencies and ceded districts.[64] In Bengal, the achievement was more modest. In his report on 1802–3, penned in 1804, Shoolbred recorded only 4,456 persons vaccinated under the official scheme and around 4,000 by freelancers at the civil stations.[65] Still, he was able to point out that, since the advent of vaccination and the ban on variolation, the city was free of smallpox for a second time in the first months of the year, when the disease generally appeared and the *tikadors* plied their trade.[66] Governor-General Wellesley reported that 'many of the native inhabitants of Calcutta have already consented to the inoculation of their children according to the improved mode', but it is likely that most of the vaccinees were associated with the British colony.[67] According to Shoolbred's cooler assessment, the Indians, 'naturally averse to all innovation', had 'no affection for the new practice'.[68]

Embedding and Extending Vaccination

British medical men worked hard to embed and extend the new prophylaxis. They themselves had a steep learning curve in respect to identifying a vaccine response and maintaining a supply of genuine lymph. Aware of the problems associated with 'spurious' cowpox, they saw the importance of carefully inspecting the pustule and taking lymph at the recommended time. The pioneers of the practice in India found Jenner's print depicting the development of the vaccine pustule invaluable. In March 1803, the medical board in Bengal wisely made provision for the preparation of simple manuals with plates to show 'representations of the true and false disease in the common gradations of native colour', obviating the need for 'the more laborious and fallible process of verbal discrimination'.[69] Learning from experience elsewhere, they vaccinated children in batches to provide lymph over a longer timeframe. The growing volume of vaccinations provided opportunities for medical men, including Indian assistants, to observe the procedure and gain practical experience in it. In Madras, there was provision for formal training with certificates to attest the proficiency. Dr Anderson was an inspiration to his younger colleagues, one of whom wrote that his 'cheerful and active

---

[62] Christie, *Ravages in Ceylon*, pp. 31–3, 60.　[63] IOR/F/4/153/2613, 75, 91–2, OIOC, BL.
[64] IOR/P/255/53, 4016–19, OIOC, BL.　[65] Shoolbred, *Report 1802–3*, pp. 10–15.
[66] Shoolbred, *Report 1802–3*, pp. 64, 68.　[67] IOR/F/4/169/2985, 4, OIOC, BL.
[68] Shoolbred, *Report 1802–3*, pp. 12, 18.　[69] IOR/F/4/169/2985, 17–23, OIOC, BL.

benevolence' and awareness of 'the inestimable value of the newly-discovered preventive' allowed 'no man to sleep at his post' in pursuing all means to persuade Indians to adopt the practice.[70] The medical men in India kept up-to-date with and contributed to developments in the practice. After reading about James Bryce's success with vaccine crusts in Scotland, Shoolbred and his colleagues made their own trials late in 1804, finding them a useful means of maintaining supply in remote stations.[71]

The British authorities largely underwrote the establishment of vaccination. The large contingent of medical men employed by the government and the army took on the new practice as part of their duties. Furthermore, early moves to vaccinate orphans and children in public institutions and to encourage the vaccination of soldiers and their families helped to build a supply of vaccine. The orphan school in Calcutta served a central role in the Bengal government's vaccination programme. The order in Bombay in April 1803 to vaccinate sepoys who were susceptible to smallpox was not unusual.[72] The offer of free vaccination was by no means always sufficient to maintain the supply of vaccine locally. Funds were available to provide doles of rice for mothers and trinkets for children as inducements.[73] The surgeon at Allahabad reported his dependence on street children presenting themselves in return for 'trifling rewards'.[74] In addition to the salaries of the British surgeons who vaccinated as part of their official duties, there was provision for the payment of Indian vaccinators. In the presidency of Bengal, they were employed on salaries of eight rupees a month.[75] In Madras, they were paid premiums, at first twenty pagodas per hundred patients, probably the rate for variolation. Early in 1803 the premium was reduced to ten pagodas, still the equivalent of 35 rupees.[76] The system encouraged corner-cutting and inflation of the numbers vaccinated. Still, Dr Anderson, who was keen to make sure that returns were submitted and payments made, evidently had some confidence in the figures. The high tally of vaccinations – almost 145,000 in Madras and its dependencies by April 1804 – certainly made the practice a significant budget item.[77] Alexander Mackenzie was a critic of the system, believing it to be 'a field for abuse'. In March 1805, he reported that the vaccinations had cost 18,232 pagodas, but expressed concern that their validity had not been verified. He

---

[70] Ainslie, 'Observations', 61.

[71] John Shoolbred, *Report on the state and progress of vaccine inoculation in Bengal during the year 1804* (Calcutta, 1805), pp. 27–37.

[72] *A compilation of all the ... orders ... or regulations ... from 1750 to 1801, that are now in force and operating on the discipline and expenditure of the Bombay army*, ed. Edward Moor (Bombay, 1801), p. 32.

[73] IOR/F/4/169/2985, 5–9, OIOC, BL.   [74] Shoolbred, *Report 1804*, pp. 18–19.

[75] IOR/F/4/169/2985, 24–6, 29–33, OIOC, BL.   [76] IOR/F/4/153/2613, 2–3, OIOC, BL.

[77] IOR/P/255/53, 4016–19, OIOC, BL.

argued for a system of salaried vaccinators, who would be more conscientious and attentive to the needs of the district they served. In June 1805, the medical council accepted his recommendations and appointed him the new superintendent of vaccination.[78]

In the Presidency of Madras, too, there was some success in extending the new prophylaxis beyond the British enclaves. A major factor in the success of the programme was its ability to draw on a body of expertise and an administrative system built up in the recent campaigns to introduce variolation. The inoculators included a cadre of Indian practitioners, some from a military background, who had been trained in the European system. In 1805, there were no less than sixty-six native practitioners on the pay-roll, including ten Brahmins, twenty-three Telugus, twenty Tamils, three Muslims and even one low-ranking 'Pariayan'.[79] Sawmy Naik (Swami Naick), 'black doctor' of the 2nd Madras Regiment, rapidly established his prowess in vaccination. Needless to say, it was not simply a matter of mastering the procedure, especially the crucial problem of confirming a true vaccine response, but also persuading villagers to allow their children to be vaccinated and then serve as a source of vaccine for other children, even in other districts. On one occasion, Sawmy Naik had to face down an angry crowd in Black Town in Madras, 'who were ignorant of the beneficial effects of the cow-pox'.[80] The promotion of variolation and then vaccination proved a little confusing. The British Resident in Tanjore (Tanjur) observed that the shift in policy from promoting variolation to seeking to inhibit it weakened 'confidence in the reasoning' of the Europeans.[81] It may have invited invidious comparison between the certainties and transparency of the old method and the uncertainties and oddity of the new. Given all the problems, the scale of vaccination activity was little short of remarkable. Despite his doubts about the early vaccinations, Mackenzie blithely reported a rise in the tally of people vaccinated in Madras and its dependencies from 146,000 in April 1804 to more than 429,821, all 'successfully vaccinated', by May 1805.[82] For all the debate over the system of premiums in 1804–5, the British medical men recognised the contribution of Indian practitioners and the capacity of the best of them to live up to the responsibilities that the new system would impose. By 1807, the number of Indian vaccinators had risen to 156.[83]

In Bengal, the practice was much more reliant on European medical men. In Calcutta, there was provision for the training of Indian assistants who

---

[78] Brimnes, 'Variolation, vaccination', 206.   [79] Brimnes, 'Variolation, vaccination', 214.
[80] W. G. King, 'The introduction of vaccination into India', *The Indian Medical Gazette*, 37 (1902), no. 10, 413–14.
[81] Brimnes, 'Variolation, vaccination', 206.
[82] Abstract of persons vaccinated, Madras, 1805–6, Jenneriana BF, item 6 'Smallpox', WLL.
[83] Brimnes, 'Variolation, vaccination', 206, 224–7.

undertook most of the routine work. Outside the capital, however, the British civil officers who oversaw the practice must often have lacked the competence to train native assistants. The British collector at Tamluk in west Bengal, who sniped at 'the stupidity and apathy of the natives . . . which must ever disqualify them as practitioners on whom any reliance can be placed for keeping up the genuine disease', may or may not have had himself a full mastery of the practice.[84] The reservations about native practitioners made it harder for vacciination to compete with the *tikadors* who were well positioned in the medical market-place in Bengal and offered a procedure that, with its ritual trappings and record of success, was familiar and acceptable in their own communities. In Calcutta, the *tikadors* were naturally aggrieved by the police ban on their practice and even won some British sympathy. For his part, Shoolbred insisted that it was a 'mistaken humanity' to be more concerned for them than for the public good, pointing out Calcutta's newfound security from smallpox and that, if the inoculators were willing to seek instruction, they could make a living from vaccination.[85] Early in 1805, he persuaded two leading inoculators, Joydeb and Birjoo Paul, to participate in a public trial in which vaccinated children would be challenged by variolation. In March, the Pauls and twenty-four other *tikadors* signed a declaration in support of vaccination which was published, translated and distributed at government expense. In July, the Pauls and their assistants were given monthly pensions to vaccinate.[86]

In all parts of South Asia, vaccination struggled to find acceptance among the local population. In Ceylon (Sri Lanka), the Buddhist Sinhalese in the southwest were more amenable to vaccination than the Hindu Tamils in the northeast.[87] In Bombay and the Malabar coasts, the indigenous Christians appeared the most receptive. The Parsees were initially hostile but subsequently embraced the procedure.[88] In south India, some Muslim communities appear to have been more welcoming than the Hindus. The cults of Sitala and Mariamma - associated with smallpox in north and south India, respectively – generally disposed Hindus towards the traditional form of inoculation if not fatalism.[89] Among the Hindus, of course, there was variation according to region and caste.[90] In Madras, a quarter of the people vaccinated in 1802–4 were low-ranking or 'untouchable' Paraiyans.[91] The position was especially confused with respect to Brahmins and higher-caste Indians, with some embracing the practice and others leading resistance. In Bengal, high-caste Brahmins

[84] Shoolbred, *Report 1802–3*, p. 14.   [85] Shoolbred, *Report 1802–3*, pp. 66–9.
[86] IOR/F/4/186/3906, 2–4, OIOC, BL; Shoolbred, *Report 1804*, pp. 44–6.
[87] Christie, *Ravages in Ceylon*, p. 69.
[88] J. Banthia and T. Dyson, 'Smallpox and the impact of vaccination among the Parsees of India', *The Indian Economic and Social History Review*, 37 (2000), 27–51, at 36–7.
[89] Arnold, *Colonizing the body*, pp. 121–33.   [90] Brimnes, 'Sympathising heart', 200–2.
[91] Brimnes, 'Variolation, vaccination', 214.

were initially ill-disposed and the pilgrimage centre of Benares (Varanasi) became an influential centre of opposition.[92] In Calcutta, Shoolbred and his assistant vaccinated 1,500 people in 1804, including 1,200 Moslems, but only 105 Hindus. In the Presidency of Bengal, there were over 14,000 vaccinations, but only around half of the vaccinees whose religion was recorded were Hindus.[93] A significant number of Indians and Sri Lankans nonetheless accepted and even sought out the new prophylaxis. At Patna, for example, Mr Macnab persuaded 2,460 Hindus to accept vaccination.[94] Some Brahmins, like Alep Coby from Oude, took up vaccination behind the lines of British influence.[95] The hope was always that community leaders would set an example by adopting vaccination. In Bombay and Ceylon, the interest and approval of Brahmins and Buddhist monks were noted.[96] In the presidency of Madras, Indian practitioners were to the fore in extending vaccination. After observing the practice in his own district, Mooperal Streenivasachary, a scholarly Brahmin, wrote exuberantly in praise of English cowpox.[97] Although some vaccinators expressed disappointment that the only people who accepted vaccination were the poor, community leaders did sometimes set an example. In reporting his success in southeast Ceylon, Ludovice noted that he vaccinated an infant child of the chief *mudaliyar* of Matara and received assistance from the village headman at Dondra.[98]

The spread of vaccination outside the British enclaves was slow. Indian princes, who employed both European and indigenous doctors, showed some interest in the new prophylaxis. In 1803 Dr Anderson applauded the Dewan of Travancore for being the first Indian potentate 'to submit his own person to so great a novelty' as vaccination.[99] Expanding British influence led to the introduction of the practice into some client states. After the conquest of Mysore in 1799, for example, the restored Wadiyar dynasty ruled under British tutelage. At the end of 1802, Arthur Wellesley, the future Duke of Wellington,

---

[92] Shoolbred, *Report 1804*, pp. 14–16.   [93] Shoolbred, *Report 1804*, pp. 1–2.

[94] Shoolbred, *Report 1804*, p. 2.

[95] Dominik Wujastyk, 'A pious fraud: the Indian claims for pre-Jennerian smallpox vaccination', in G. J. Meulenbeld and Dominik Wujastyk (eds.), *Studies on Indian Medical History*, vol. 2 (Groningen, 1987), 131–67, at 137–8.

[96] Keir, *Introduction*, pp. 35–6; Christie, *Ravages in Ceylon*, p. 58.

[97] *The Asiatic Annual Register for the year 1805* (1807), 76; James Forbes, *Oriental memoirs: selected and abridged from a series of familiar letters written during seventeen years residence in India*, 4 vols. (London, 1813), 3, pp. 423–4; Debbie Lee and Tim Fulford, 'The beast within: the imperial legacy of vaccination in history and literature', *Literature and History*, 9 (2000), 1–23.

[98] Christie, *Ravages in Ceylon*, p. 66; *Selections from Calcutta Gazettes of the Years 1798, 1799, 1800, 1801, 1802, 1803, 1804, and 1805: showing the political and social conditions of the English in India upwards of sixty years ago*, ed. W. S. Seton-Karr, vol. 3 (Calcutta, 1868), p. 365.

[99] Anderson, *Correspondence*, p. 18.

sought vaccine and the practice seems to have expanded rapidly, with 42,000 people reportedly vaccinated during 1804.[100] In August, he observed 'that the expenses attending the general inoculation of the natives with the cow pox are greater than were expected; and that they are likely to increase in proportion to the success of the endeavours to propagate this mild disease'.[101] In embracing the new practice, the royal family of Mysore helped to legitimise it among their people. The vaccination of the young raja's second wife in July 1805 reportedly 'produced a salutary influence upon the minds of the inhabitants' who then sought to 'avail themselves of the benefit'. The event appears to have been commemorated by Thomas Hickey in an enigmatic group portrait that focuses on the young rani's upper arm and the hole in the sleeve through which she had been vaccinated.[102] The Abbé Jean Dubois, a French missionary in Mysore, took up the practice on a heroic scale, arranged translations of vaccination manuals into Canara and Tamil, and disseminated vaccine through south India. Liaising with Dr Anderson in Madras, he established a vaccine depot outside Seringapatam and was appointed superintendent of vaccination in Mysore.[103] William Ingledew, his successor, integrated the Seringapatam station more fully into the British system and wrote his own treatise for translation into Telagu and other languages.[104] Thomas Coats was another British surgeon who promoted vaccination in an Indian client-state. Appointed surgeon at the court of Peshwa Bajirao II at Pune in 1806, he offered medical services to the poor, re-established vaccination, and learned Marathi. In 1812, he wrote a work in Marathi entitled *The book of the origin and qualities of the bovine form of the Goddess* presenting an account of cowpox and its benefits.[105]

Imperious Vaccine

Within a few years of the arrival of cowpox in Bombay in 1802, vaccination was well established in British India and Sri Lanka, with all the major centres maintaining a supply of vaccine and superintendents overseeing vaccine

[100] Thomas Pruen, *A comparative sketch of the effects of variolous and vaccine inoculation, being an enumeration of facts not generally known or considered, but which will enable the public to form its own judgment on the probable importance of the Jennerian discovery* (Cheltenham, 1807), p. 39.

[101] *The dispatches of Field Marshal the Duke of Wellington, K.G., during his various campaigns in India, Denmark, Portugal, Spain, the Low Countries and France from 1799–1818*, ed. John Gurwood, new ed., vol. 3 [India, 1794–1805] (London, 1837), pp. 437–8.

[102] Nigel Chancellor, 'A picture of health: the dilemma of gender and status in the iconography of empire. India *c.* 1805', *Modern Asian Studies*, 35 (2001), 760–82, at 775 and 776.

[103] Tim Fulford (ed.), *Romanticism and science, 1773–1883*, 2 vols. (London, 2002), 1, p. 129. IOR/F/4/345/8031, OIOC, BL.

[104] IOR/F/4/276/6165, pp. 1–2, 8–10, OIOC, BL.

[105] Sumit Guha, *Health and population in South Asia from earliest times to the present* (London, 2001), pp. 143–54.

stations that supplemented or superseded the more informal practice undertaken by individual enthusiasts. The tally of vaccinations officially reported in the presidency of Madras reached 607,895 in September 1806.[106] Though there is reason to doubt the validity of some of the vaccinations, the figures appear to be broadly indicative. The Abbé Dubois claimed on his retirement in 1811 that he and his assistants had completed almost 99,000 vaccinations in Mysore since 1802.[107] Adding together estimates of the more modest tallies in the three presidencies, in the colony of Ceylon and in some of the princely states, it is likely enough that the overall tally exceeded a million by the end of 1806. Early in 1806, Jenner was informed that 800,000 people had been vaccinated in India, and in the following years he received gifts of £2,000, £1,300 and £4,000 raised by subscription in Bombay, Madras and Bengal, respectively.[108] From the outset, vaccine served as a balm to the British conscience about empire. 'If our influence in India, has ever entailed evils on the native', Governor Duncan wrote in 1802, 'this one important act of kindness on our part, ought to be viewed as no inconsiderable or inadequate compensation'.[109] A quarter of a century later, Dr Whitelaw Ainslie declared that vaccination in Asia has 'at length happily convinced millions, that if, from a powerful empire in the west came an inordinate thirst for dominion and the sword of the conqueror, thence also came the sympathizing heart and the healing hand'.[110]

The new prophylaxis certainly served the ends of empire. The links between the expansion of British power in south Asia and the spread of vaccination are all too apparent. The new prophylaxis helped to secure the expatriate communities and the native people working most closely with them from the scourge of smallpox. Along with sanitary measures, large-scale vaccination in the British enclaves created *cordons sanitaires*. Protection from smallpox allowed British magistrates and businessmen to travel with more confidence and enhanced British military capacity on the frontier. The authorities doubtless found the expenditure on the practice a worthwhile investment. Epidemic smallpox could involve considerable loss of life, devastate regional economies, reduce revenue to the government, and create instability. The systems established at a district level for revenue-collection and the maintenance of law assumed a new role that involved closer oversight of the lives of the Indian subjects. The promotion of vaccination provided the British regime with opportunities to present itself as a benevolent power. In the princely states of the subsidiary alliance system, like Hyderabad and Mysore, the new

---

[106] Abstract of persons vaccinated, Madras, 1805–6, Jenneriana BF, item 6 'Smallpox', WLL.
[107] IOR/F/4/345/8031, OIOC, BL; *Asiatic Journal*, 6 (June–December 1818), 388–9; Kenneth Ballhatchet, *Caste, class and Catholicism in India 1789–1914* (Oxford, 2013), p. 17.
[108] Baron, *Life*, 2, p. 352; Fisher, *Jenner*, p. 183.   [109] Keir, *Introduction*, p. 109.
[110] Ainslie, 'Observations', 72.

prophylaxis was a source of soft power. The empire of vaccine grew with British military expansion. In the war-zones, the armies were accompanied by surgeons with cowpox. Princely vaccinations were sometimes presented as acts of surrender to British magnanimity. After the conquest of Delhi, the Mughal emperor Shah Alam reportedly expressed an 'anxious desire to have his grandchildren vaccinated as smallpox was raging in city'. In June 1805, the son and daughter of Akbar Shah, the emperor's eldest son, were vaccinated and lymph from their arms was used to safeguard 'four more of the house of Timur'.[111] Recalcitrant rulers refused vaccine at their peril. Early in 1805, Sri Vikrama Rajasinha, the beleaguered king of Kandy, caught smallpox, 'a calamity which was said never before to have happened to a ruler of Lanka, and [which] was regarded as a token of divine displeasure'. Though he recovered, the demoralised king was deposed ten years later.[112] From Delhi, vaccination spread through Hindustan. It was observed that 'one advantage' of the British to the banks of the Sutlej River in 1809 was 'the introduction of vaccination to the Punjab', where the Singhs and Sikhs, 'whose religious prejudices are far less inveterate than elsewhere in India, have received it gladly and are likely to maintain it, making it feasible that we will soon hear of its spread to [Kashmir]'.[113]

The cowpox discovery was initially presented more as a divine gift to mankind than a symbol of the superiority of western science. Established as a practice in Britain and made available in India by the agents of empire, vaccination nonetheless had a strong ideological dimension. The peoples of South Asia, of course, had cause to doubt imperial benevolence, and the Indians who used the services of *tikadors* had no reason to regard western methods of inoculation as superior.[114] Even British medical men acknowledged that the Indian form of variolation was as safe as the European mode. It was certainly more culturally acceptable. The use of variolous matter mixed with holy water, and embedding the procedure in a range of ritual and propitiary practices, made it a holistic therapeutic experience.[115] In contrast, the western style of smallpox prophylaxis, often involving the direct transfer of bodily matter from one person to another by lancet, was surgical, secular, and unsettling.[116] The advantage of vaccination over variolation, of course, was that it could be used without risk to the broader community. Its appeal in India, though, was limited by its association with a cattle disease in England and its necessary reliance on matter passed from arm to arm. Aware of Hindu

[111] Shoolbred, *Report 1804*, pp. 50, 66–7.

[112] P. E. Pieris, *Tri Sinhala. The last phase 1796–1815*, 2nd ed. (New Delhi, 2001), pp. 82–3.

[113] *Asiatic Annual Register*, 11 (1809), 50–1.   [114] Christie, *Ravages in Ceylon*, p. 16.

[115] Harish Naraindas, 'Care, welfare, and treason: the advent of vaccination in the nineteenth century', *Contributions to Indian Sociology*, 32 (1998), 67–96, esp. 70–2.

[116] Arnold, *Colonizing the body*, p. 144; Brimnes, 'Variolation, vaccination', 208–10.

concerns about pollution, the British authorities in Bengal moved rapidly to secure a statement from Hindu magistrates and scholars that 'no person can be legally deprived of caste either for having undergone or performed the operation'.[117] At the outset, there was hope that Hindus, with their veneration of the cow, might be well disposed towards the new prophylaxis. It soon became apparent, however, that the association with the cow was not a strong selling point, especially when cowpox was translated as foot-and-mouth disease. British scholars who had some expertise in Indian languages and cultures nonetheless warmed to the challenge of making the new prophylaxis culturally acceptable. In late 1802, Thomas Colebrooke prepared a Sanskrit text presenting the procedure as having 'the blessing of Surahbi, the Bountiful Cow of Hinduism', publishing it as a pamphlet and, unusually for a Sanskrit text, as a supplement to the *Calcutta Gazette*.[118] Early in 1803, Francis Whyte Ellis, a notable philologist, composed a work in Tamil entitled *Aramavara Vilaccam* ('The legend of the cowpox'). It comprised a dialogue in antique style between the physician of the gods and the goddess Sakti, who reveals that she has created for a mankind a new beneficent product of the cow that purifies the body and 'prevents the fatal effects of smallpox'.[119] While there is no evidence that Ellis sought to pass off his work as authentic, his compatriots applauded it as a 'pious fraud', a deception for a worthy purpose. When some Brahmins presented an old Sanskrit text alluding to the prophylactic virtue of cowpox, implying that it was long known in India, the British authorities were less forgiving. They referred it to Jacob Blacquire, a Sanskrit scholar, who after comparing it to the same text in another manuscript, proclaimed that the allusion was an interpolation and dismissed it as an 'impudent forgery'.[120]

For British medical men in India, ignorance, prejudice and fatalism appeared the major obstacles to the growth of the practice among the native population. Practitioners in Britain itself, of course, saw themselves as contending with very similar problems and attitudes in sections of the population. Shoolbred's condemnation of the *tikadors* in Calcutta as profiteering at the expense of public safety can be set alongside Jenner's even harsher denunciation of inoculators in London. Still, there is little doubt that religious beliefs and cultural preferences in South Asia presented formidable barriers to the reception of smallpox prophylaxis. After all, the traditional Indian practice made little headway in large parts of India prior to the nineteenth century.

---

[117] IOR/F/4/186/3906, p. 3, OIOC, BL.
[118] Rosane Rocher and Ludo Rocher, *The making of western Indology: Henry Thomas Colebrooke and the East India Company* (Abingdon, 2012), p. 83.
[119] Thomas R. Trautmann, *Languages and nations: the Dravidian proof in colonial Madras* (Berkeley, CA, 2006), pp. 231–42; Rocher and Rocher, *Making of western Indology*, pp. 83–4; Wujastyk, 'Pious fraud', pp. 131–67.
[120] Shoolbred, *Report 1802–3*, pp. 54–6.

In specific regard to vaccination, of course, there were additional grounds for distaste for cowpox inoculation and suspicion of British intentions. A major problem, however, was the sheer imperiousness of the system needed to support it. A fundamental requirement of vaccination, after all, was a steady stream of people, usually children, to generate and maintain a supply of fresh lymph. The extension of the practice outside the European enclaves depended on hustle and regimentation, the corralling of children and the recording of names and ages and the pressure on parents and sometimes offers of payment to have their offspring vaccinated and serve on vaccination chains. Acknowledging popular apprehensions in 1803, William Horsman wisely counselled that 'every precaution should be taken, to prevent a greater alarm seizing them' and proposed that effort 'should be directed rather towards keeping up the disease, than diffusing it until they are more favourably disposed towards receiving it than they are at present'.[121] It was indeed the relentless and seemingly sinister nature of the system that prompted thousands of people in Trevatoor to confront John Dalton late in 1804 and declare that they would fight to the death to resist vaccination in their district. As he subsequently observed, 'no argument can persuade them that either a capitation tax hereafter or transportation will not be the fate of those that are vaccinated'.[122] The surgeon at Muzaffarpur likewise found it difficult in 1805 to convince people that the government was acting 'from benevolent motives'.[123]

There is a danger in presenting vaccination too exclusively in imperial terms and overlooking some success in naturalising the practice in India. The initial level of government support for the new prophylaxis was not meant to be permanent. The assumption that, once vaccination became generally available, it would become self-supporting, was perhaps not wholly unreasonable. After all, the *tikadors* were able to maintain their practice commercially in Bengal. Observing that vaccination had spread with 'unparallelled success', Dalton lamented in 1805 that it was 'not yet in requisition by the natives'. While the threat of smallpox prompted people 'to solicit [vaccination] for their families', he observed, they otherwise showed little interest.[124] The challenge in India and Sri Lanka, as elsewhere, was to make the practice routine so that the supply of vaccine could be maintained by a steady stream of children being presented for vaccination. Even in England, it was soon recognised that the practice required a level of support, organisation and oversight that could not be realised in the medical marketplace. From the outset, there was some variation in systems of managing and delivering vaccination and indeed some competing agendas that were to remain a feature of the practice in India.[125]

---

[121] IOR/F/4/153/2613, 126–7, OIOC, BL.   [122] IOR/P/255/53, 4096–7, OIOC, BL.
[123] Shoolbred, *Report 1804*, p. 23.   [124] IOR/P/255/53, 4096–7, OIOC, BL.
[125] Bhattacharya, Harrison and Worboys, *Fractured states*, pp. 6–12, 34–40.

One set of variables in South Asia was the use of native vaccinators, the training provided them, and the responsibilities accorded them. In Madras, Dr Anderson built up a strong team of Indian vaccinators that reaped dividends in terms of the expansion of the practice. In 1804–5, the system of remuneration was reviewed and the system of payment per capita was replaced by salaried positions.[126] The need for adaptation to local circumstances was recognised. As Anderson observed, 'one mode or system will not answer equally for all parts of the country; and therefore it seems advisable to attend to the proposals of persons of local residence, that what is most practicable for each district, may be distinctively known'.[127] Given the close networking among the pioneers of vaccination in South Asia, however, the variation in practice was perhaps not as great as it later became. Amid the variables, the vaccine itself appears to have been a constant. It was observed in 1803 that all of it was derived from Anna Dusthall, the first vaccinee in Bombay, 'the mother of all our poison, the beneficent Medea of India'.[128] Though other samples of vaccine presumably arrived from Britain, there is no evidence of their successful propagation, let alone their circulation. According to Dr Christie, the strain introduced from Bombay in 1802 was still in service in Ceylon on his departure in 1810 and, though it had passed through 399 persons in succession, it had not lost its character or 'preservative capacity'.[129]

The large number of vaccinations in South Asia in the first decade of the practice attests the energy and enthusiasm of the medical men, the solid support given by the British authorities, and the readiness of sections of the local population to embrace the new prophylaxis. Indians who promoted or took up the new prophylaxis made major contributions. 'In the humane undertaking', declared James Forbes in 1810, 'the Brahmins have risen superior to prejudice, and under their extensive and powerful influence all other castes have adopted the practice'.[130] It is known that some Brahmins in Hindustan incorporated vaccination into their practices.[131] While the activity of Indian vaccinators outside the British system is almost entirely undocumented, their achievement in the presidency of Madras is a matter of record. Among practitioners worldwide, there are few that can compare with Sawmy Naik, who vaccinated 777,712 people between 1802 and 1828.[132] Still, the scale of the task of containing smallpox in British India was daunting. In Madras in 1803, Dr Anderson observed that 7,000 vaccinations a month were insufficient to 'extinguish smallpox' and that a third of the people still lacked

---

[126] Brimnes, 'Variolation, vaccination', 224–7.
[127] Fulford (ed.), *Romanticism and science, 1773–1883*, 1, p. 129.
[128] Keir, *Introduction*, p. 90.   [129] Christie, *Ravages in Ceylon*, p. 98.
[130] Forbes, *Oriental memoirs*, 3, pp. 422–3.   [131] Wujastyk, 'Pious fraud', 137–8.
[132] King, 'Introduction', 414.

any sort of immunity.[133] The population of the presidency of Madras alone has been estimated as around fourteen million.[134] Even the million or so vaccinations in British India in the first decade of the practice fell very far short of protecting the population. In regard to vaccination in India, the adage that the European impact at this time was no more than a pin prick on the hide of an elephant is irresistibly appropriate. Still, the new prophylaxis made it possible to bring smallpox under control in the major European enclaves which, as centres of commerce and communication, would have normally acted as foyers of infection. To Dr Scott in Bombay in 1806, it was a wonder that in an island 'swarming with mankind' there had been no deaths from smallpox since the introduction of vaccine.[135] Dr Christie took pride in the fact that Ceylon (Sri Lanka) was free from smallpox from February 1808, when an infected fishermen communicated the disease to several people in Galle, to October 1809, when the disease was brought to Jaffnapatnam by boat and passed to a man in the prison where 'its progress was immediately arrested by the indiscriminate vaccination of all the other prisoners'.[136] The record of vaccination in South Asia in the early nineteenth century should not be assessed solely by reference to progress towards smallpox eradication. It was no mean feat to establish a firm foundation for the practice. Even as early as 1805 it is fair to assume more than 100,000 vaccinations annually in India. There is substance and solidity to vaccination in South Asia in the early nineteenth-century that have been too easily overlooked.[137] It is perverse not to acknowledge the quantum of suffering avoided and saved. A contemporary observer had every reason to report with satisfaction around 1810 that, through vaccination, 'the lives of thousands perhaps tens of thousands [of people in India] are annually preserved'.[138]

Vaccine Hub in the East

Remarkably, too, British India rapidly emerged as a hub for the wider dissemination of vaccination. The early passage of cowpox through Mesopotamia and the Persian Gulf bore little fruit. In Baghdad, even the Christian community lost confidence in the procedure when a recently vaccinated child died in 1803.[139] After propagating vaccine in Basra to send to Bombay in 1802, John Milne continued vaccinating for a time and sent samples to other East India Company surgeons around the Persian Gulf.[140] Subsequently based in Goa, he

---

[133] Anderson, *Correspondence*, pp. 6–7.
[134] Guha, *Health and population in South Asia*, pp. 39, 51.   [135] Baron, *Life*, 2, p. 92.
[136] Christie, *Ravages in Ceylon*, pp. 92–5.
[137] Banthia and Dyson, 'Smallpox in India', 676–8.   [138] Forbes, *Oriental memoirs*, 3, p. 422.
[139] *MPJ*, 31 (December 1813–June 1814), 520.   [140] *MPJ*, 12 (June–December 1804), 452.

vaccinated on some scale and took a keen interest in the fortunes of the new prophylaxis in the Middle East. Early in 1805, he received and forwarded to Dr Anderson at Madras a letter from Andrew Jukes reporting on his work in promoting the practice in Persia. After obtaining vaccine from Milne in 1802, Jukes began vaccinating in Bushire (Bushehr) and even took samples with him on a mission to Tehran. Late in 1804 he received a new supply of vaccine from Vienna and soon found himself busy vaccinating children brought to him by anxious mothers. Alarmed by reports of the activity, the Sheikh of Bushire took steps to close it down, casting 'aspersions on a practice emanating from the impure hand of an unbeliever'. In a bid to restore its credit, Jukes demonstrated the procedure to a Persian physician from Shiraz who, though impressed, made no move to endorse it.[141] In 1808 and 1810, Jukes accompanied embassies to Tehran, had some success in demonstrating the value of the practice, but felt defeated by 'the apathy of the government [in Persia] towards the general good of the community'.[142] Around this time, too, there were signs that vaccination was not wholly a lost cause in Mesopotamia. In 1810, a merchant from Istanbul was able to kindle new interest in Baghdad by staging the vaccination of his infant son.[143]

Even as cowpox was finding footholds in British India, there were moves to introduce it elsewhere in the East Indies, with vaccine dispatched to Fort Marlborough (Bengkulu) in Sumatra, Prince of Wales Island (Penang) and to the East India Company factory at Canton (Guangzhou). In a scheme organised by Dr Christie in Colombo early in 1804, a medical assistant on board a ship bound for Fort Marlborough succeeded in maintaining the vaccine virus over seven weeks by vaccinating in succession six Sinhalese sailors and a slave, only to find, on arrival in Sumatra, that Fort Marlborough had been recently suppled with vaccine, kept alive in a similar fashion, from Madras.[144] There was even a plan, promoted by Governor-General Wellesley but set aside as impracticable, for the delivery of vaccine by serial vaccination to New South Wales. Portuguese and French merchants, too, carried vaccine from India to seed the new prophylaxis in like manner in Mozambique, Mauritius and Cape Colony in 1803–4.[145] Meanwhile, British surgeons continued to extend vaccination through northern India. From 1811, William Moorcroft, a veterinarian, sought to enlist a Kashmiri trading house with agents in Nepal, Tibet and on the Chinese border to assist in the expansion of vaccination into

---

[141] Anderson, *Correspondence*, pp. 43–4; *BB, S&A*, 30 (1805), 83–7.

[142] John Malcolm, *The history of Persia from the most early period to the present time*, 2 vols. (London, 1815), 2, p. 532n; Willem M. Floor, *Public health in Qajar Iran* (Washington, DC, 2004), pp. 39–41.

[143] *MPJ*, 31 (December 1813–June 1814), 520.   [144] Christie, *Ravages in Ceylon*, pp. 75–81.

[145] See Chapter 13.

the Himalayan kingdoms and across the border into China.[146] A smallpox epidemic in 1816 prompted the rulers of Nepal to request the newly arrived British Resident to introduce the new practice. Once vaccine arrived, vaccination began in earnest, but it was too late to save Raja Girvana from the contagion.[147] Christian missionaries used India as a base for missions to Burma and the Himalayan states that often associated vaccination with evangelisation. In 1813, the Reverend Felix Carey enjoyed some success as a vaccinator at the Burmese court in Rangoon.[148] In 1818, the *Missionary Herald* made an object lesson of the recent death of the Raja of Nepal, claiming that, through 'superstition or a dislike to innovation', he had stubbornly resisted the procedure.[149]

By 1800, India was the cornerstone of an expanding British empire in the East, an assemblage of 'networks, complex threads of correspondence and exchange that linked distant components together and ensured a steady, but largely overlooked cultural traffic'.[150] Cowpox played a significant but largely neglected role in the construction of this world, materially and symbolically. The vaccine virus was not simply delivered from the metropolis to the margins, but was transmitted through old and new webs of exchange in the Indian Ocean and a complex set of regionally-based networks. At the same time, vaccination activity in South Asia – the observations, experiments and achievements – added new strands of information, technology and biomatter to the web of exchange, and informed and shaped the global history of the new prophylaxis. Most strikingly, the success of the practice in South Asia was a source of inspiration in Britain, heartening Jenner and strengthening the claims made on behalf of vaccination in Britain.[151] On his return home in 1810, Dr Christie was astonished to learn that the practice still had detractors in England and, in retirement in Cheltenham, wrote an account of its success in shielding Ceylon from the ravages of smallpox.[152] To the champions of vaccination, its history in the East showed what could be achieved through a combination of administrative and medical expertise. As Jenner observed, ruefully comparing the limited support for vaccination in Britain with Wellesley's ambition for the eradication of smallpox in India: 'What pygmies we look like!'.[153]

---

[146] *Papers regarding the administration of the Marquis of Hastings in India* (London, 1824), p. 86; Christopher A. Bayley, *Empire and information: intelligence gathering and social networks in India 1780–1870* (Cambridge, 1999), p. 107.

[147] Susan Heydon, 'Death of the king: the introduction of vaccination into Nepal in 1816', *MH*, 63 (2019), 24–43, at 37–40.

[148] IOR/F/4/490/11883, OIOC, BL.   [149] *Missionary Herald*, 14 (1818), 8–9.

[150] Tony Ballantyne, 'Empire, knowledge and culture: from proto-globalization to modern globalization', in A. G. Hopkins (ed.), *Globalization in world history* (London, 2002), pp. 115–40, at 133.

[151] Baron, *Life*, 2, pp. 344–5.   [152] Christie, *Ravages in Ceylon*, pp. i–ii.

[153] Saunders, *Cheltenham years*, pp. 162–3.

11 'This New Inoculation Is No Sham!'
Vaccination in North America

In summer 1800, *Foxwell* struggled across the Atlantic. Leaving Bristol on 3 May, it entered Boston harbour on 4 July, in time for homecomers to celebrate Independence Day.[1] Dr Benjamin Waterhouse, professor of physic at Harvard, soon had in his hand a packet of vaccine from Dr John Haygarth. A Rhode Islander, Waterhouse had gone to Britain for medical training prior to the American War of Independence. Through Dr John Fothergill, his mother's cousin, he was introduced to Dr John Lettsom, a fellow Quaker, and Dr Haygarth, both noted for their work on smallpox prevention.[2] After surgical training in Edinburgh and London, and a doctorate of medicine at Leiden, he returned to New England in 1782 unusually well qualified and internationally networked. Although he was appointed to a chair at Harvard, he found it difficult to break into the clannish medical community in Boston. His marriage in 1788 to Elizabeth Oliver brought a formidable companion and useful connections, but his salary and income from private practice never seemed sufficient to maintain his growing family, social position and professional obligations. On reading Jenner's book on cowpox early in 1799, he was 'struck with the unspeakable advantages that might accrue to this country, and indeed to the human race at large' and published an account of the new inoculation in the *Columbian Centinel* under the heading, 'Something Curious in the Medical Line'.[3] For over a year, he was disappointed in his efforts to secure viable vaccine. Over two months old on arrival, Haygarth's sample had been carefully sealed in a corked vial.[4] Waterhouse took immediate steps to make a trial of it. Since his wife and two older children had been inoculated in the old style, he experimented on his four younger children and several servants.[5] After observing the early progress of the vaccine infection, he was called out of town, leaving Elizabeth to check on the patients and show friends 'the first vaccine pustules raised in the New World'. To test the effectiveness of the prophylaxis a month later, he wrote to William Aspinwall, who ran an inoculation hospital at Brookline, asking him, 'on philanthropic principle', to

---

[1] Cash, *Waterhouse*.   [2] Cash, *Waterhouse*, pp. 48–9.   [3] Cash, *Waterhouse*, pp. 122–3.
[4] *MPJ*, 9 (January–June 1803), 65.   [5] Cash, *Waterhouse*, pp. 124, 127, 397.

attempt to infect three of the subjects with smallpox. Elizabeth spent ten days with the children in the hospital and allowed herself to be re-inoculated so that her response could be compared with her children's. According to a memorialist who praised her life as 'one bright commentary on all the female virtues', Elizabeth ever recalled the 'agony and suspense' following the experiment.[6] The children's health was not the only issue: 'the lady, her family, and her nearest connexions would sink in the public estimation if her children, after all that had been said and done, should not resist the small pox'. Happily, they were shown to be insusceptible to smallpox. 'This new inoculation of yours is no sham!' Aspinwall declared, 'As a man of humanity, I rejoice in it, although it will take from me a handsome annual income'.[7]

The relative ease and regularity of the Atlantic passage had brought early news of the cowpox discovery and the trials in London to North America. From spring 1799, samples of vaccine began to arrive in some profusion, and Waterhouse was probably not the first to propagate vaccine successfully. There were no major linguistic and cultural barriers to the transmission of information about the new practice between the former British colonies. Still, the scale of the land mass and dispersal of settlement on the continent presented significant challenges for the extension of the practice. Newfoundland was nearer, and politically closer to Britain, than New England. Jenner had a good friend at Trinity who received a copy of the *Inquiry* on publication and early samples of vaccine virus.[8] Vaccination began in Boston, Massachusetts, two years before it found a firm footing in some of the southern states. The advance of the new prophylaxis along the St Lawrence and across the Appalachians would be relentless but slow. The advent of vaccination on the cusp of the new century, however, took place at a crucial juncture in the history of the American Republic. The presidential election of 1800, a contest between John Adams and Thomas Jefferson, decisively shaped the nation's destiny. In Salem, Massachusetts, the first vaccinations took place in the interstices of the election. In his journal, William Bentley recorded in late October the unprecedented zeal for electioneering and the election itself in early November. In between times, on 30 October, he went to Beverly 'to see the first example of the kine pox in our neighbourhood' and the inoculation of his own four children with it.[9] The election came close to destroying the Union, with the northern states backing Federalist Adams and the southern states supporting Republican Jefferson, but vaccination was not an election issue. Both

---

[6] *Niles' Weekly Register*, 9 (September 1815 to March 1816), Supplement (1816), 181–2.

[7] Cash, *Waterhouse*, pp. 126–7.

[8] John W. Davies, 'A historical note on the Reverend John Clinch, first Canadian vaccinator', *Canadian Medical Association Journal*, 102 (1970), 957–1.

[9] *The diary of William Bentley, Vol. 2: 1793–1802* (Salem, MA, 1907), pp. 354–5.

presidential candidates had been variolated as young men and encouraged its use but, aware of the dangers of the old practice, were early and strong champions of the new prophylaxis. It can be claimed that vaccination played some role in stitching together the new nation.

Smallpox and Inoculation in North America

Smallpox appeared in the European colonies of North America in the 1600s and was a regular visitor to Atlantic ports from the early eighteenth century, with major outbreaks in Boston, New York and Charleston. After a severe epidemic in 1738, Charleston, South Carolina, was ravaged again in 1760: the tally of 650 deaths suggests that most of the population of 8,000 took the disease.[10] Around 1775 a more general epidemic welled up along the Atlantic seaboard. The movement of soldiers and fugitive slaves in the War of American Independence increased its range, velocity and ferocity. Over the following years it found its way along the Mississippi and Missouri river systems and spread through the Prairies. On coming through a devastated district on the Assiniboine River, an explorer was informed that smallpox had spread its 'desolating power, as the fire consumes the dry grass of the field' and 'destroyed with its pestilential breath whole families and tribes'.[11] By 1781–2 it was responsible for a terrible mortality among Native Americans along the Saskatchewan River, and the Hudson's Bay Company imposed rigorous quarantine to protect the Lowland Crees living around its trading posts.[12] Around the same time, too, it crossed the Rockies to the Pacific Coast. When George Vancouver visited the northwest coast in 1791 he found dozens of recently depopulated villages.[13] A conservative estimate is that there were some 130,000 smallpox deaths across North America in the epidemic of 1775–82.[14] In Philadelphia and elsewhere, smallpox became endemic. Even at the height of the yellow fever epidemic, smallpox was a major killer, responsible for more than 10 per cent of children's deaths in the working-class district of Southwark.[15]

---

[10] Suzanne Krebsbach, 'The great Charlestown smallpox epidemic of 1760', *The South Carolina Historical Magazine*, 97 (1996), 30–7, at 37.

[11] Alexander Mackenzie, *Voyages from Montreal on the River St Lawrence through the Continent of North America to the frozen and Pacific Oceans in the years 1789 and 1793* (London, 1801), pp. 21–3.

[12] Paul Hackett, 'Averting disaster: the Hudson's Bay Company and smallpox in Western Canada during the late eighteenth and early nineteenth Centuries', *BHM*, 78 (2004), 575–609, esp. 577–8, 585–8.

[13] Fenn, *Pox Americana*, pp. 227–31.   [14] Fenn, *Pox Americana*, pp. 263–75.

[15] Simon Newman, 'Dead bodies: poverty and death in early national Philadelphia', in Bill Gordon Smith (ed.), *Down and out in early America* (University Park, PA, 2004), pp. 41–62, esp. 52–3.

First used in Boston in 1721, smallpox inoculation was used on a larger scale in the American colonies than in Britain until the 1730s. Its deployment on slave plantations gave some colonial practitioners considerable experience and encouraged adaptations that made it cheaper and safer than the more invasive and medicalised mode in England. The 'American mode of inoculation', as it was termed, paralleled and probably informed some of the technical improvements associated with the Suttons in the 1760s.[16] Still, there was no general enthusiasm for variolation. Although many people acknowledged its utility during smallpox outbreaks, they sought to inhibit it once the immediate danger passed. With the spread of the 'new inoculation', attitudes became more favourable in some places. In Philadelphia prophylaxis became generally available from the 1750s. In New York in the 1770s, John Lathom offered inoculation in the Suttonian mode, leasing houses along the Hudson River and taking on partners in New England and even Canada.[17] For many people, though, inoculation houses were foyers of infection and an affront to neighbourliness. In and around Boston, plebeian hostility was fuelled by class resentment: after all, only the wealthier families could afford to have their children inoculated. Inspired by the Boston Tea Party, men from Marblehead in 1774 blackened their faces, laid siege to the inoculation hospital on Cat Island and set about the destruction of 'Castle Pox'.[18] Among the leaders of the American struggle for independence, however, inoculation was regarded positively. Although George Washington was a smallpox survivor, both Thomas Jefferson and John Adams were inoculated as young men. Several delegates to the Continental Congress in Philadelphia in 1775, including Josiah Bartlett, John Hancock, Patrick Henry, George Wythe and Francis Lightfoot Lee, had themselves inoculated in the city, forging a new bond among the men who signed the Declaration of Independence.[19]

The epidemic that spread across North America during the War of Independence gave inoculation a new profile.[20] In 1775, Philadelphia was a hot house of infection and prophylaxis as well as revolutionary politics. Epidemic smallpox posed a real dilemma with the mobilisation for war. As John Adams wrote to his wife, smallpox is 'ten times more terrible than

---

[16] Henry Lee Smith, 'Dr Adam Thomson, originator of the American method of inoculation for small-pox: an historical sketch', *The Aesculapian* (1909), 1 (3–4), 151–5.

[17] Gronim, 'Imagining inoculation', 267–8.

[18] Andrew M. Wehrmann, 'The siege of "Castle Pox": a medical revolution in Marblehead, Massachusetts, 1764–1777', *New England Quarterly*, 82 (2009), 385–429.

[19] Stephen Coss, *The fever of 1721: the epidemic that revolutionized medicine and American politics* (New York, 2016), p. 272; *Founding Families: Digital Editions of the Papers of the Winthrops and the Adamses*, ed. C. James Taylor (Boston, 2016).

[20] Fenn, *Pox Americana*, ch. 3.

Britons, Canadians and Indians together'.[21] The problem was that, while most British soldiers had been exposed to smallpox or inoculated, the overwhelming majority of Americans lacked resistance to the disease. The presence of smallpox in Boston thus gave the British garrison a further line of defence against the Americans seeking to dislodge it. The American strike against the British in Quebec was likewise broken by the spread of smallpox among the besiegers. In February 1777, General Washington took the bold decision to order the inoculation of the Continental Army and over the course of the year some 40,000 men went through with the procedure, with 300–400 deaths.[22] While the inoculation of statesmen and soldiers was accompanied by wider recourse to prophylaxis in the late 1770s, it did little to change the perception that it should be subject to strict control and countenanced only when smallpox was an immediate threat. Containment measures were certainly more useful in North America, with its more dispersed population, than in western Europe. As Dr Waterhouse informed Dr Haygarth, Rhode Island kept itself free from smallpox by imposing strict quarantine and banning inoculation.[23] Even so, when smallpox struck, quarantine could be extremely costly and disruptive for communities highly dependent on trade, and the removal and lodgement of infected children in pest-houses seemed to many parents too cruel to contemplate. It was the cause of some wonder that in New England, 'the most democratical region on the face of the earth', the people had 'voluntarily submitted to more restrictions, and abridgments of liberty, to secure them against this terrific scourge, than any absolute monarch could have enforced'.[24] Still, smallpox all too often found its way into even the most isolated districts. In 1799, soldiers brought smallpox to Salem, North Carolina, resulting in the infection of a third of the small community of Moravian Brethren and three deaths.[25] Early in 1801, Simeon Perkins in Liverpool, Nova Scotia, prepared himself for the approach of smallpox by calling in the doctor to inoculate his family, 'all on the left hand, between thumb and forefinger'.[26] When smallpox broke out in New Orleans early in 1802, there was widespread recourse to smallpox inoculation, which in turn played a role in spreading the disease along the Mississippi, with First Nations peoples dangerously exposed.

---

[21] *Adams family correspondence. Vol. 2. 2 June 1776–March 1778*, ed. Lyman H. Butterfield, Wendell D. Garrett and Margorie Sprague (Cambridge, MA, 1963), p. 23.

[22] Ann M. Becker, 'Smallpox in Washington's Army: strategic implications of the disease during the American Revolutionary War', *Journal of Military History*, 68 (2004), 381–430, at 425n.

[23] Haygarth, *Inquiry*, pp. 138–46.

[24] Benjamin Waterhouse, 'Narrative of facts concerning the inoculation of the kine-pock', *Medical Repository*, 5, (1801–2), 373–81, at 374.

[25] Mary Lou Moore, 'Bright spot in the eighteenth century', *American Journal of Nursing*, 69 (1969), 1705–9, at 1707.

[26] *The diary of Simeon Perkins, 1797–1803*, ed. Charles B. Fergusson (Toronto, 1967), pp. 269, 279–80, 282.

Cowpox to Kinepox

News of Jenner's successful trial of cowpox crossed the Atlantic as early as autumn 1796. Soon after his experiment on James Phipps, Jenner wrote to his old friend, the Rev. John Clinch in Trinity, Newfoundland, about his 'discovery'. In response, Clinch asked for 'a sketch of your idea in print'.[27] After the publication of the *Inquiry* in 1798, Jenner sent copies to Clinch and his nephew, the Rev. George Jenner, who was then minister at Harbour Grace. He may have sent samples of cowpox as early as 1799. A letter to Clinch in July 1800 indicates that he had already sent cowpox on threads as he explains that he is sending more in case they had not proved effective.[28] Though it is sometimes claimed that Clinch was the first to vaccinate in North America, there is no evidence that he did so successfully before October 1800, when he and Dr McCurdy were vaccinating in Trinity.[29] Admiral Pole, Governor of Newfoundland, supported their endeavours. On hearing of smallpox at St John's, he requested McCurdy to extend 'the blessing' of cowpox, at his expense, 'to all who are not obstinately determined against it'.[30] Feeling the full force of epidemic smallpox over winter 1800–1, with over 800 smallpox deaths at Halifax, residents of the neighbouring colony of Nova Scotia looked in vain for the early arrival of cowpox.[31]

If British Newfoundland had a slight head start with the new prophylaxis, the United States were not far behind. Dr David Hosack of New York was aware of cowpox late in 1798, when he received a copy of George Pearson's *Inquiry* and began asking about local knowledge of cowpox. The first public notice of Jenner's discovery appeared in the second issue of North America's first medical journal, the *Medical Repository*, early in 1799. On receiving cowpox in summer 1799, Hosack obtained permission from the authorities to use it to inoculate two prisoners, but it proved inert.[32] Dr John Chichester of Charleston, South Carolina, who also received vaccine from Pearson around this time, may have had more luck, but certainly did not maintain the practice.[33] After publishing his article on cowpox in March 1799, Dr Waterhouse had to wait until July 1800 before securing viable vaccine. After his experiments over the summer, he moved to the forefront of the practice, publishing

---

[27] Baron, *Life*, 1, pp. 115–17.   [28] Baron, *Life*, 2, pp. 324–5.

[29] Davies, 'Historical note on John Clinch', 959–60.   [30] MS0016/6, RCS.

[31] Robert H. Halsey, *How the President, Thomas Jefferson and Doctor Benjamin Waterhouse established vaccination as a public health procedure* (New York, 1936), p. 19.

[32] John Redman Coxe, *Practical observations on vaccination: or inoculation for the cow-pock; embellished with a coloured engraving, representing a comparative view of the various stages of the vaccine and small-pox* (Philadelphia, 1802), pp. 128–9.

[33] T. J. Pettigrew, 'On the introduction of vaccine matter into America', *Annals of Philosophy*, 9 (1817), 404–17.

an account of Jenner's discovery and his own practice in Boston in a book boldly entitled *A Prospect of Exterminating the Small-pox*.[34] By late autumn, however, he found that his supply of vaccine was becoming less reliable and observed that much of the vaccine obtained by other operators was also failing to deliver satisfactory results. Advertising his concern about the circulation of spurious vaccine, he expressed doubts about the security of many people who believed themselves to be vaccinated. Confident that he would be resupplied from Britain in the spring, he announced that he was suspending his vaccinations over the winter, claiming that 'very cold weather is unfavorable to the kinepox'.[35]

Waterhouse looked to make a financial return from vaccination. In late August, Dr John Warren, a Boston colleague, wrote to his son in London, informing him that 'the cow or kine pox is making some noise here' and that Waterhouse had the only local supply, and asked him to send him some in 'a closely sealed phial'.[36] Given his efforts to introduce vaccination in Boston, Waterhouse felt justified in seeking to keep the business in his hands for as long as possible, and was charging his private patients $5 for the procedure. He was not pleased when Dr Samuel Brown, a recent graduate, placed a notice in newspaper under the heading '*Pro bono publico*' announcing his readiness to vaccinate at no charge if anyone under vaccination would allow him to take lymph. Another threat was Dr James Jackson who, after paying ten guineas for instruction in London, returned to Boston with cowpox and up-to-date knowledge of the practice. 'If I had matter enough I could make a mint of money in a bit of time', he informed a friend in London, from whom he sought a fresh supply, 'Everybody here is in a rage to have [it]'.[37] Waterhouse was happy enough to make vaccine available, at a price, to practitioners outside Boston. He made franchise arrangements with over a dozen colleagues in towns across New England.[38] In return for vaccine and a monopoly of the practice in Portsmouth, New Hampshire, for example, Dr Lyman Spalding offered 10 per cent of his vaccination income, but Waterhouse countered that he had recently declined an offer of 25 per cent. Both men were concerned to prevent patients from allowing other practitioners to take lymph from them and their negotiations were informed by an awareness that the practice was becoming widespread. In the end, Waterhouse agreed to supply vaccine to Spalding and

---

[34] Benjamin Waterhouse, *A prospect of exterminating the small-pox, being the history of the variolæ vaccinæ, or kinepox, commonly called the cow-pox: as it has appeared in England: with an account of a series of inoculations performed for the kinepox, in Massachusetts* (Boston, MA, 1800).

[35] Waterhouse, *Prospect*, p. 38.   [36] Halsey, *Jefferson and Waterhouse*, pp. 15–16.

[37] J. J. Putnam, *A memoir of Dr James Jackson, with sketches of his father Rev. Jonathan Jackson, and his brothers ... and some of their ancestry* (Boston, 1906), pp. 220–3.

[38] Cash, *Waterhouse*, pp. 138, 150, n.21.

no one else in the district for a flat sum of $150.[39] During 1801, Waterhouse's grip on the practice in New England was broken. For his part, Jackson secured good vaccine from England and earned enough to 'maintain me and a wife in a snug way'. He was initially able to earn $150 from vaccination in one month alone, but the business fell away as more practitioners entered the field. Still, 'cowpox gave me notoriety', he observed, 'and that is a great advantage to a young man if it comes to him fairly, without any tricks'.[40]

Waterhouse was not wholly mercenary in wanting to keep control of vaccination. Dubious vaccine and careless practice damaged its reputation. For a time, there was an unseemly scramble for cowpox by all and sundry. 'I have known the shirt sleeve of a patient, stiff with the purulent discharge from a foul ulcer', he recalled, 'cut into small strips, and sold about the country as genuine kinepox, coming directly from me. Several hundred people were inoculated from this caustic animal poison'.[41] Even medical men were caught up in scams. Dr James Carrington persuaded his wife to be inoculated with matter obtained from 'a kine pock peddler' that turned out to be smallpox.[42] Over the winter of 1800–1, there was a major calamity in the port of Marblehead when Dr Elisha Story took matter from a sailor who claimed to have been vaccinated in London. After using it on his children and others, it became apparent that it was smallpox. Another local doctor who had used vaccine supplied by Waterhouse but had not realised that it had not elicited a true vaccine response, was embarrassed to find that the children he had treated caught smallpox. To make the calamity a perfect storm of contagion and confusion, the two doctors conducted an old style general inoculation of over a thousand residents, with sixty-nine deaths. The disaster impacted badly on 'the credit of vaccination' and, as Waterhouse observed, prompted 'not a few execrations of the original promoter thereof'.[43]

As the first American physician to propagate cowpox, and to explain and promote its use, Waterhouse was accepted for a time as the local authority in the field and had some success in putting his own stamp on the practice. Finding that many people, 'especially ladies', were put off by the name 'cowpox', he proposed 'kinepox' (singular 'kinepock'), using the old word for cattle but also hinting at the 'kind' nature of the pox, as an alternative.[44] His Bostonian colleagues were not impressed: Dr Warren regarded the innovation as vain and the term ridiculous.[45] Still, in a letter to a colleague in April 1801, Waterhouse pronounced it to be the standard American term,

---

[39] Cash, *Waterhouse*, pp. 140–2.   [40] Putnam, *James Jackson*, pp. 220–3.
[41] Waterhouse, 'Narrative of facts', 375–6.
[42] H. Carrington Bolton, *Life and writings of Elisha North, M.D.* (1887), p. 5.
[43] Cash, *Waterhouse*, pp. 147–9.
[44] Harvard Medical Library MS, c. 75 2, Countway Library of Medicine, Boston.
[45] E. Warren, *The life of John Collins Warren, M.D.*, 2 vols. (Boston, MA, 1860), 2, p. 78.

and indeed the neologism was already coming into general usage.[46] During 1801, there were reports of local sources of kinepox, none really substantiated.[47] Dr Elisha North of Goshen, Connecticut, for example, used matter from a local cow to inoculate a man travelling to New York, instructing him to present his pustule to a colleague in the city. By this means, he claimed, rather fancifully, 'the first genuine kine pock that was ever introduced into the city of New York originated from an American source'.[48] It was Waterhouse, however, who provided the vaccine that established the practice properly in New York. In May 1801, Dr Valentine Seaman performed the first successful vaccination in the city with matter taken from a patient vaccinated for this purpose by Waterhouse in Boston.[49] To aid his work in distributing vaccine, dispensing advice and addressing concerns, Waterhouse saw the need for institutional support. In the wake of the debacle at Marblehead, he looked to the Massachusetts Medical Society to help to restore confidence in the practice, and raised the possibility of collaborating with them in a vaccine institute, but his Bostonian colleagues were not disposed to fall in line behind him. In June 1801, in an address to medical men across the United States, Waterhouse pressed the need 'to collect and lay before the American public' all cases of people who 'after having gone through the kine pox' had been exposed to smallpox without infection.[50] Expressing disappointment that no medical society was prepared to act as 'a central point, to which everything relating to this new inoculation may be directed', he stated that he had no other option than 'to go on in this business as he began it – *alone*' and invited all practitioners who had conducted trials to send him details by post so that they could be put 'before a scrutinizing public' to 'establish the credit of this most precious discovery'.[51] The medical men in New York at least showed capacity for collaboration. In January 1802, Seaman and some colleagues set up the New York Institution for the Inoculation of the Kine-Pock, electing Jenner and Waterhouse as honorary directors. Its mission was to vaccinate the poor at set hours, maintain a stock of fresh vaccine, and promote the practice locally.[52]

Waterhouse delighted in his status as Jenner's chief disciple in America. In 1801, he was described in print in London as the 'Jenner of America'.[53] He was delighted to receive from his 'Magnus Apollo' copies of hand-painted

---

[46] Harvard Medical Library MS, c. 75 2, Countway Library of Medicine, Boston.
[47] *Medical Repository*, 5 (1802), 477.   [48] Bolton, *Elisha North*, pp. 6–8.
[49] *Medical Repository*, 5 (1802), 236–8.   [50] Halsey, *Jefferson and Waterhouse*, p. 29.
[51] Halsey, *Jefferson and Waterhouse*, pp. 28–30.
[52] *Constitution for the government of the New-York Institution for the inoculation of the kine-pock* (New York, 1802).
[53] Ring, *Treatise*, 1, p. 443.

prints depicting the stages of the vaccine pustule, distributing them to select colleagues.[54] He commended to the public the 'golden rule' that Jenner had vouchsafed him. 'I don't care what British laws the Americans discard', Jenner had written, 'so that they stick to this – never to take the virus from a vaccine pustule for ... inoculation after the efflorescence is formed around it'.[55] He pestered Dr Lettsom for information about Jenner and late in 1801 received a print of his portrait which he put on display in Boston's leading coffeehouse. 'I sought your life in England and failed in the attempt', he joshed in a letter to Jenner, but 'our worthy friend Lettsom can inform you that I *hung* you in America, and that too in a very public place!'[56] Above all, he treasured the silver snuff-box sent from Jenner in 1802 with the words 'From the Jenner of the Old World to the Jenner of the New' engraved on it.[57] If he had long lost his monopoly of vaccination, he retained for some time his status as the American Jenner. By this stage, he was also engaged in a gratifying correspondence with the future President of the United States.

President Jefferson and the New Prophylaxis

In autumn 1800 Dr Waterhouse sent an early draft of *A Prospect of Exterminating the Small-pox* to his President John Adams, who acknowledged his 'zeal and industry', meriting 'the thanks of all the friends of science and humanity'.[58] After the presidential elections in November, Waterhouse sent the book to the President-elect Thomas Jefferson, which arrived at Monticello, Virginia, on Christmas Eve. On Christmas morning, Jefferson was at his desk writing to thank Waterhouse and inform him that he deserved 'well of his country' for his work in introducing and promoting Jenner's cowpox. 'Every friend of humanity', he wrote, 'must look with pleasure on this discovery by which one evil more is withdrawn from the condition of man; and contemplating the possibility that future improvements and discoveries may still more and more lessen the catalogue of evils'.[59] Soon after his inauguration, Jefferson asked Waterhouse to send him some kinepox. After failing with the first sample, he asked for it to be sent 'two or three times successively until we can inform you that it has at length taken'.[60] To assist its survival in the summer heat and humidity, he suggested that it be placed in

---

[54] Benjamin Waterhouse, *A prospect of exterminating the small-pox. Part II. Being a continuation of a narrative of facts concerning the progress of the new inoculation in America* (Cambridge, MA, 1802), p. 78n.

[55] Halsey, *Jefferson and Waterhouse*, p. 43.

[56] Harvard Medical Society, H MS c 16. 1, Countway Library of Medicine, Boston.

[57] Cash, *Waterhouse*, p. 185.   [58] Halsey, *Jefferson and Waterhouse*, p. 15.

[59] Waterhouse, *Prospect. Part II*, p. 22.

[60] *The papers of Thomas Jefferson*, vol. 34, ed. Barbara B. Oberg (Princeton, NJ, 2007), p. 462.

'a phial of the smallest size, well corked and immersed in a large one filled with water and well corked'.[61] On 8 August, he inoculated 'six persons of my own family' with matter sent in late July and a week later repeated the procedure with matter sent on 1 August.[62] A fortnight later, he reported his success with the lymph propagated in Monticello. 'We have now twenty of my family', he declared, 'on whom the disease has taken'.[63]

Jefferson had a longstanding interest in smallpox prophylaxis. As a young man he arranged his own inoculation in Philadelphia and as a lawyer defended the right of people to inoculate. As a parent and slave-owner, he may have been frustrated by the laws inhibiting variolation in Virginia. The epidemic that raged during the Revolution left Virginia very exposed. Large numbers of slaves who decamped in response to the British emancipation proclamation fell victim to smallpox. Among the casualties were around fifteen runaways from Monticello whose value Jefferson included in claiming compensation from the British government.[64] Jefferson was probably able to arrange the inoculation of family members and slaves who travelled on business outside the plantation in other jurisdictions. Sally Hemings, a domestic slave to whom he was especially attached, was inoculated in Paris in 1787.[65] Given his background and beliefs, it is not hard to explain Jefferson's immediate recognition of the potential of vaccination. It is telling, though, that he saw the extermination of smallpox as a more realisable prospect than the eradication of slavery. In June 1801, Waterhouse made a somewhat presumptuous pitch to Jefferson. He sent him an illustration of the appearance of the vaccine pustule on black skin, declaring that 'an exertion to preserve this wretched people from the horrors of small-pox cannot but be agreeable to the beneficent *Ens Entium*, who has seen fit to make that enviable distinction between the situation and faculties of this helpless race and us!'[66]

In his first year as president, Jefferson spent a surprising amount of time on kinepox inoculation. His household accounts indicate that the practice became routine at Monticello.[67] He was not the first to make a trial of the new prophylaxis in Virginia. When his children caught smallpox after vaccination in spring 1801, Joseph Prentis, a judge of the High Court of Virginia, dismissed kinepox inoculation as a 'chimera'. Jefferson's adoption

[61] *Papers of Jefferson*, 34, pp. 629, 640.
[62] *The papers of Thomas Jefferson*, vol. 35, ed. Barbara B. Oberg (Princeton, NJ, 2008), pp. 8, 47.
[63] Halsey, *Jefferson and Waterhouse*, pp. 35–6.
[64] Cassandra Pybus, *Epic journeys of freedom: runaway slaves of the American Revolution and their global quest for liberty* (Boston, MA, 2006), pp. 48–50.
[65] Annette Gordon-Reed, *The Hemingses of Monticello: an American family* (New York, 2008), pp. 215–16.
[66] Cash, *Waterhouse*, p. 202.
[67] M. D. Peterson, *Thomas Jefferson and the new nation. A biography* (New York, 1970), p. 683.

of the new prophylaxis thus had more than a symbolic significance. From the autumn of 1801 to the spring of 1802 he and his physician Dr Gantt served as a sort of informal vaccine institute. He even made substantive technical contributions to the practice, proposing a means of preserving vaccine and calculating more precisely the optimal time for taking lymph from a pustule.[68] According to Waterhouse, Jefferson advanced the cause of vaccination in Virginia and the southern states by two years. Dr John Spence of Dumfries, Virginia, for example, began vaccinating with vaccine supplied from Monticello. In November, he reported that he had vaccinated over a hundred patients and that the practice was receiving a 'liberal reception'. He was pleased to announce too that he had been able to enlighten Judge Prentis, who had been speaking 'of the Jennerian discovery with some indignation', by showing him a true vaccine pustule, so different from what he had earlier observed. He also offered the cautionary story of a young gentleman, 'not bred to physic', who took up the practice with enthusiasm but little expertise, and vaccinated 'three children of a poor family, from the arm of a mulatto girl', with unfortunate outcomes.[69]

Jefferson provided vaccine to both Washington and Philadelphia. Sending vaccine to Philadelphia, he asked in return for 'fresh variolous matter' to test the resistance of his patients, as none was available in Virginia.[70] In private initiatives, he encouraged the spread of vaccination southwards and westwards, making it a national as well as a philanthropic cause. He was especially concerned to make the new prophylaxis available to Native Americans. Late in 1801, he welcomed Little Turtle and other leaders of the Miami nation in Washington. According to Waterhouse, he explained to them that the 'Great Spirit had lately made a precious donation to the enlightened white men over the great water' that had the power to protect people from smallpox. Little Turtle, who had been inoculated with smallpox on an earlier visit, accepted vaccination on behalf of his people and around ten warriors were vaccinated. On their departure, the Miami leaders took home kinepox and instructions for its use.[71] In February 1802, Jefferson likewise arranged the vaccination of delegates of the Shawnee and Delaware nations.[72] In 1803, he requested the leaders of the Lewis and Clark expedition setting out across the continent to 'carry with you some matter of the kinepox; inform those of them with whom

[68] Halsey, *Jefferson and Waterhouse*, pp. 48–9.   [69] *Medical Repository*, 5 (1802), 381–7.
[70] *Papers of Jefferson*, 35, pp. 572–3; Coxe, *Practical observations*, pp. 120–2.
[71] Silvio A. Bedini, *Thomas Jefferson. Statesman of science* (New York, 1990), pp. 313–14.
[72] J. Diane Pearson, 'Medical diplomacy and the American Indian. Thomas Jefferson, the Lewis and Clark Expedition, and the subsequent effects on American Indian health and public policy', *Wicazo Sa Review*, 19 (2004), 105–30, at 108.

you may be, of its efficacy as a preservative from the smallpox; & encourage them in the use of it'.[73]

'The City of Brotherly Love': Vaccine Philanthropy

The largest city in the new republic, Philadelphia aspired to national leadership.[74] The heart of the independence movement in the 1770s and constitution-making in the 1780s, it was the nation's capital in the 1790s. Continuing as a major centre for business, banking and brokerage, it retained some centrality in the intellectual and cultural life of the new nation. The 'City of Brotherly Love' was more ethnically diverse than Boston and New York, and renowned for its philanthropy. The medical school of the University of Pennsylvania was intellectually livelier, more socially engaged, and recruited more widely than its two rivals, Harvard and Columbia. A place of continental concourse, the crowded city was also a foyer of infection. In the 1790s, yellow fever proved an even deadlier scourge than smallpox and its aetiology a matter of acrimonious debate in the medical fraternity. Dr Benjamin Rush, Philadelphia's most celebrated physician and public figure, found himself out on a limb in refusing to accept the role of contagion. In a letter to Jenner in the spring of 1801, Dr Waterhouse drew attention to Philadelphia's tardiness in taking up the new prophylaxis and passed on gossip that 'the leading physician there pronounces it too beastly and indelicate for polished society!'[75] There were many Philadelphians, however, who were following the cowpox saga with interest. In October 1799, Mrs Elizabeth Drinker wrote a note in her journal about Jenner's cowpox and Woodville's corroboration of its prophylactic value.[76]

During 1801, Philadelphians were making serious efforts to introduce the practice. Among the physicians, Dr John Redman Coxe was the most eager in the cause. The son of a British Loyalist who returned to England, he had been brought up by his maternal grandfather, Dr John Redman (Redmond) in Philadelphia. After the war, he visited his father in London and attended lectures in the teaching hospitals. On his return, he obtained a medical degree from the University of Pennsylvania, found a mentor in Dr Rush, and secured positions in the hospital and the dispensary. A member of the American Philosophical Society, he found an ally in the vaccination cause in the Society's secretary John Vaughan, and indeed the Society's president,

---

[73] *Letters of the Lewis and Clark Expedition, with related documents, 1783–1854*, vols. 1–2, ed. Donald Dean Jackson (Urbana, IL, 1978), p. 64. Pearson, 'Medical diplomacy', 109–12.

[74] Gary B. Nash, *First City. Philadelphia and the forging of historical memory* (Philadelphia, 2002), ch. 4.

[75] Baron, *Life*, 1, p. 442.

[76] Cecil K. Drinker, *Not so long ago. A chronicle of medicine and doctors in colonial Philadelphia* (New York, 1937), p. 101.

Jefferson himself. Aware of Jefferson's vaccination experiments, Vaughan wrote to ask him to procure some vaccine for them.[77] On the arrival of a package of vaccine, Coxe vaccinated himself and four others.[78] In detailing his own case he reported that he remained fit enough for work and, seven days after the procedure, to respond, late at night, to an urgent call from a patient twenty-five miles away. To add to the drama, his carriage overturned on the road at four in the morning, he stood 'in mud and rain for half an hour before it was righted', and he spent the day attending his patient. Happily, his vaccine vesicle remained intact and, on his return home, he drew lymph from it to inoculate a group of patients.[79] He was soon called on to demonstrate the procedure on a medical student from Kentucky, providing material for Dr Rush's lecture on kinepox in January 1802.[80] Over the winter of 1801–2, he continued his experiments, detailing fifty-one cases, including some using new matter from England.[81] By 1 March, he had vaccinated several hundred people, including his newborn son, Edward Jenner Coxe, and two black children, Lewis Calansalingo and his sister.[82] He had also made vaccine available to one hundred practitioners.[83] Still, anxious that vaccine supply might be lost over the summer, he urged the need for a vaccine institution. He also felt that a public endorsement of the new practice by 'our oldest physicians would strongly tend to accelerate its progress'.[84] If he had once considered cowpox 'too beastly', Dr Rush certainly was now a great advocate. In February 1802, he informed Jefferson that 'vaccination, as you have happily called it, has taken root in our city and will shortly supersede the old mode of inoculation'.[85] In the meantime, Coxe consolidated his leadership of the practice locally by publishing *Practical Observations on Vaccination*, a useful compendium of European and American accounts of the practice, including his own. Through his father, he sent a copy to Jenner, who sent his compliments through the same channel.[86]

Behind the scenes, John Vaughan, a merchant, philanthropist and scholar, played a significant role in promoting vaccination in America. As secretary of the American Philosophical Society, he was at the centre of a web of men of science and humanitarian concern. He was probably involved in moves to introduce vaccine as early as 1800 when his father, a London merchant, sent a

[77] *Papers of Jefferson*, 35, pp. 490–1.   [78] Coxe, *Practical observations*, p. 122.
[79] Coxe, *Practical observations*, p. 139.
[80] *Papers of Jefferson*, 35, pp. 698–9; *Letters of Benjamin Rush*, ed. L. H. Butterfield, 2 vols. (Princeton, NJ, 1951), 2, p. 845.
[81] Coxe, *Practical observations*, pp. 135–48.
[82] *Philadelphia Medical Museum*, 1 (1805), pp. 224–5; Coxe, *Practical observations*, p. 149.
[83] Coxe, *Practical observations*, p. 123.   [84] Coxe, *Practical observations*, pp. 57–8, 150.
[85] *Letters of Rush*, 2, p. 840.
[86] Gilbert Collection of MSS. Letters, pp. 383–4, College of Physicians, Philadelphia.

sample to his eldest son Benjamin in Maine.[87] In a letter to John in December 1801, Benjamin reported on his use of vaccine in Maine, referred to the important 'project' in which John was involved with Jefferson, Coxe and Rush and hoped that their exertions would meet with success.[88] Another letter from John Vaughan to Jefferson, requesting permission to publish the president's account of his vaccination activity, gives some indication of the nature of this 'project'. Dr Coxe and myself, he wrote, 'both conceive a very valuable purpose would be answered' by publishing the account, in stamping 'with authority and respectability, the evidences of a discovery, more important than has been made for centuries'. Such a publication, they felt, 'would have a very decided & extensive effect, thro' means of the medical students', and it was their hope that 'sufficient virus may soon be obtained to give them the means of spreading it thro' the Continent'.[89]

Jefferson was reluctant to use the presidential office to promote his views, but his endorsement of vaccination was probably well known. The three Philadelphians certainly showed energy and enterprise in the vaccination cause. Dr Rush was the doyen of the medical college at the University of Pennsylvania, which recruited students from all the middle, southern and western states. His students from out of town, like the young man from Kentucky on whom Coxe demonstrated the procedure, could return home trained in vaccination and with the vaccine to establish the practice in their own communities. Dr Rush published a local edition of Jenner's *Instructions on Vaccine Inoculation* to assist the extension of the practice.[90] Dr Coxe took on the business of propagating vaccine in Philadelphia, and making it available on request. In March 1802, he provided vaccine in dried form to Dr Ramsay of Norfolk County who, after a ten-day ride home by boat, used it successfully on a young gentleman and a female slave.[91] He likewise made vaccine available to Dr Chapman of Bucks County by vaccinating a young man sent to him for this purpose.[92] He supplied vaccine to many practitioners, sending samples as far afield as the Mississippi Territory and Martinique.[93] As the supplier of vaccine, he often received reports of its use, some of which appear in his *Practical Observations*, passing on useful tips like Ramsay's use of twisted cotton thread for collecting and administering vaccine.[94] For his part, Vaughan brought to the table business connections and an influential correspondence network. It was to him that Dr Brown of Lexington, Kentucky, reported in June 1802 that 'the Jennerian inoculation has gone on here with astonishing

---

[87] Benjamin Vaughan Papers, B V46p, APS.   [88] Benjamin Vaughan Papers, B V46, 13, APS.
[89] *Papers of Jefferson*, 35, pp. 698–9.
[90] Robert L. Brunhouse, 'David Ramsay, 1749–1815', *Transactions of the American Philosophical Society*, new series 55, no. 4 (1965), 1–250, at 154.
[91] Coxe, *Practical observations*, pp. 130–2.   [92] Coxe, *Practical observations*, p. 147.
[93] Coxe, *Practical observations*, pp. 140, 152.   [94] Coxe, *Practical observations*, pp. 130–2.

rapidity'.[95] It was through his good offices that Dr Ramsay received from Coxe an annual supply of vaccine.[96] 'To me the people of Charleston have been indebted annually for the disease', he wrote in 1807, 'and I have been indebted to you'.[97] There are other hints that Vaughan was contributing financially to the cause. He assisted in distributing and probably underwrote Coxe's *Practical observations*.[98] He was doubtless among the 'friends of humanity' who, according to the minutes of the General Assembly of the Presbyterian Church, held in Philadelphia in May 1803, paid for 250 copies of 'a publication on vaccine disease' for the use of delegates and some copies of Jenner's *Instructions* to be taken by missionaries 'to the frontiers of the country, and distributed for the caution and direction of those who have less opportunity of obtaining medical aid and advice on the subject of vaccine inoculation'.[99]

In Philadelphia, vaccination became a national enterprise. It was a time of rapidly expanding horizons for the new republic. Alongside the original thirteen states, three new states had been recognised in the 1790s, and a fourth, Ohio, was added in 1803. Beyond the Appalachians, there were vast territories under Federal administration: the Mississippi Territory, acquired from Spain in 1798 and largely unsettled, and Louisiana, purchased from Napoleon in late 1803. Though he had no wish to make vaccination the business of government, Jefferson was personally interested in seeing its expansion westwards as well as southwards. The 'friends of humanity' in Philadelphia evidently regarded themselves as well placed to further this enterprise, seeking to enlist missionaries in the distribution of vaccination tracts 'on the frontiers of the country'. The introduction of kinepox in Natchez, the small capital of the Mississippi Territory, is testimony to their reach. At the beginning of 1802, smallpox broke out in New Orleans, then still under Spanish rule. William C. C. Claiborne, the newly installed governor of the Mississippi Territory, was justifiably alarmed. He instructed merchants not to expose goods from Louisiana for sale, established a pest house outside Natchez, and prohibited recourse to variolation. Unsurprisingly for an ally and appointee of Jefferson, he was well disposed towards kinepox. Observing that it would be 'peculiarly unfortunate, if at this time, we should not be benefited by this important discovery', he proposed a subscription to send a reliable person to obtain it from Kentucky.[100] He may already have looked to Philadelphia for supply, as Coxe sent a sample to Natchez in the spring of 1802.[101] Happily, kinepox arrived in time to be put into service. At the end of the smallpox outbreak, the medical officer reported

---

[95] Coxe, *Practical observations*, p. 152.   [96] Brunhouse, 'Ramsay', 153–4.
[97] Brunhouse, 'Ramsay', 155, 160.   [98] Brunhouse, 'Ramsay', 155.
[99] *Minutes of General Assembly of Presbyterian Church, 1803*, pp. 17–18.
[100] Laura D. S. Harrell, 'Preventive medicine in the Mississippi Territory, 1799–1802', *BHM*, 40 (1966), 364–75, at 367.
[101] Coxe, *Practical observations*, p. 123.

eleven cases, with two fatalities, and the containment of the infection by
'a very general circulation' of kinepox, involving the vaccination of 'two
thirds of the inhabitants'.[102]

Vaccination was becoming known among Native Americans. On their
return from their embassy early in 1802, the Miami chieftains introduced
vaccination among their communities in the Indiana Territory. In spring, Little
Turtle's interpreter wrote to Dr William Thornton, informing him that 300 of
the Miami nation had been vaccinated and 'many more would receive the
matter before the letter could arrive' in Washington.[103] The Lewis and Clark
expedition that set out from Philadelphia in summer 1803 took packets of
vaccine westwards but seemingly had no opportunity to use them. The
Cherokee in Tennessee, who were familiar with smallpox inoculation, heard
reports of the advantages of vaccination. The appearance of smallpox in their
communities in 1805 prompted an American trader and two English-speaking
Cherokees to ask the Indian Agent to obtain kinepox for them. When Dr
McNiel arrived from Maryville, however, he played down the value of kinepox, perhaps because it was unavailable locally, and offered to undertake a
general inoculation in the old mode for $150. The Cherokee chieftains who
declined the offer may well have accepted vaccination.[104] Around this time,
Gideon Blackburn, a missionary who ran a school for Cherokee children in
Maryville, obtained kinepox from Dr Rush in Philadelphia and used it to
suppress a local outbreak.[105] Needless to say, it was not easy to deliver viable
vaccine on the frontier, and the problems arising from the use of ineffective
vaccine by inexpert hands can have done little to encourage Native American
confidence in the procedure or trust in the white men offering it.

Testing Times

In Boston, the original home of kinepox, vaccination experienced early setbacks. The difficulties with vaccine, the inexperience of the vaccinators and
the recklessness of hucksters who took up the practice, led to problems that
often only became manifest months or years later. After declaring that kinepox
was 'no sham' a year earlier, William Aspinwall reported seeing patients who,
though vaccinated, had taken smallpox naturally or through inoculation.[106]
The failures, real and alleged, fanned prejudice against the practice.

---

[102] Harrell, 'Preventive medicine', 371–2.
[103] *The European Magazine, and London Review*, 42 (1802), 178–9.
[104] Julie L. Reed, *Serving the nation: Cherokee sovereignty and social welfare, 1800–1907* (Norman, OK, 2016), pp. 23–7.
[105] *General Assembly's Missionary Magazine or Evangelical Intelligence*, 2 (1806), 137–8, 495–6.
[106] Cash, *Waterhouse*, pp. 174–7.

'The natives of America are skillful in bush-fighting!' Waterhouse reminded Jenner in November 1801, alluding to the backwoodsmen who had proved more than a match for the Redcoats. 'Had I not a kind of apostolic zeal', he continued, 'I should at times feel a little discouraged'.[107] In 1802, Waterhouse called on Boston's Board of Health to settle doubts about vaccination by organising a public trial. In one of the most thorough tests of the new prophylaxis to date, nineteen boys were vaccinated in August and, three months later, taken to Noddle's Island, about a mile from Boston, to be inoculated with smallpox. They were accompanied by one child who had been vaccinated in 1800 and, as controls, two children who were still susceptible. The panel of six physicians soon found that the twenty boys who had been vaccinated resisted smallpox and that the unvaccinated pair took the infection. After a further trial in which the twenty boys were inoculated with smallpox from the newly infected pair, the panel declared them to be healthy and unblemished. 'The decisive experiment', Waterhouse declared, 'has fixed forever the practice of the new inoculation in Massachusetts'.[108]

The pioneers in Boston, New York and Philadelphia, with their large populations, a critical mass of practitioners and medical schools and societies, laid the groundwork for the establishment of vaccination in North America. Even though they were able to learn from Waterhouse's experience in Boston, practitioners like Seaman in New York and Coxe in Philadelphia still found it a challenge to master cowpox inoculation, maintain a supply of vaccine and generalise good practice. The need for an institutional base for vaccination was well recognised. The Kine-Pock Institute in New York was the most promising initiative, but even a subvention from city hall to contract to vaccinate charity children could not guarantee its survival. Absorbed into the New York Dispensary in 1805, it managed to retain its identity as a centre for the practice in the city and its hinterland. In 1807, Dr Seaman usefully presented data that showed that the proportion of smallpox deaths had declined from one in ten in the fifteen years before vaccination to one in forty in the last two years.[109] Time and again, however, hopeful beginnings in other cities and towns were followed by disappointments. Dr Ramsay, who worked hard to maintain the practice in Charleston, depended on the supply of vaccine from distant Philadelphia. On one occasion, he was so desperate for vaccine that he responded to a rumour of its availability in Savannah, Georgia, by sending a black boy with a letter to a colleague there and asking him to vaccinate him, and once he was surely 'infected with the disease', to send him back 'by the stage or by water'.[110] The South Carolina Medical Society provided little assistance and its investigation of alleged vaccination failures in 1806 proved unhelpful. In

---

[107] Baron, *Life*, 1, p. 473.   [108] Cash, *Waterhouse*, pp. 189–93, at 193.
[109] *Medical Repository*, 10 (1807), 430–1.   [110] Brunhouse, 'Ramsay', 152.

defending the reputation of the practice in 1808, Ramsay found himself invoking the verdict of the Royal College of Physicians in London in 1807 that vaccination provided a level of protection against smallpox that 'if not absolutely perfect, is as nearly so as can perhaps be expected from any human discovery'. The sceptics may 'believe all the physicians in England are fools', he declared, 'but to all rational men the point is so satisfactorily established'.[111]

Smallpox itself put vaccination to the sternest test. After the epidemics at the turn of the nineteenth century, its profile seemed to diminish for several years. The new prophylaxis may have played some role in containing outbreaks. In 1805, Waterhouse expressed concern that a third of the population of Massachusetts were susceptible to the disease, but if indeed two thirds were insusceptible it would suggest a significant expansion of prophylaxis since 1800. Kinepox was reportedly used to suppress what might have been serious outbreaks of smallpox in Scotch Plains, New Jersey, in 1803 and Stamford, Connecticut, in 1804.[112] A great deal of anecdotal evidence attests the value of vaccination. In one case, a black freedman became ill on a visit to his mother, a slave, on a nearby plantation. The mother, who had arranged her own vaccination, avoided the contagion, and the circumstance persuaded all the plantation-owners in the district to vaccinate their slaves.[113] The quiescence of smallpox, however, encouraged complacency. 'The spirit of vaccination' spread rapidly, Dr Samuel Akerly of New York wrote, 'until the fear of small-pox vanished, and then it was suffered to decline'.[114] An epidemic along the eastern seaboard in late 1808 and early 1809 revealed neglect of prophylaxis. In Philadelphia, the number of smallpox deaths rose from 32 in 1807 to 145 in 1808.[115] In the summer of 1809, a 'very fatal species' of smallpox in Virginia spread 'in an alarming manner, through various parts of Maryland'.[116] In the course of the epidemic, people who believed that they had been properly vaccinated took the infection. In some places, there was recourse to variolation. Though he retained his faith in the new prophylaxis, Akerly felt that some of the failures could not be explained away and that the 'idea of annihilating the small-pox' was an 'enticing' but perhaps impossible dream. He declined to support a bill in the New York Legislature to prohibit variolation. 'Science is

---

[111] Brunhouse, 'Ramsay', 161–2; David Ramsay, *The history of South-Carolina: from its first settlement in 1670 to the year 1808*, 2 vols (Charleston, 1809), 2, p. 81.
[112] Sylvanus Fancher [Fansher], 'Progress of vaccination in America', *Massachusetts Historical Society Collections*, Series 2, vol. 4 (1816), 97.
[113] *Philadelphia Medical Museum*, 1 (1805), 401–3.
[114] *Medical Repository*, third series, 2 (1811), 32–3.
[115] *London Medical Repository and Review*, new series 4 (1827), 425.
[116] *The Papers of James Madison, Presidential Series. Vol. 1. 1 March–30 September 1809*, vol. 1, ed. Robert A. Rutland, Thomas A. Mason, Robert J. Brugger, Susannah H. Jones and Fredrika J. Teute (Charlottesville, VA, 1984), pp. 257–61.

not fixed', he reasoned, 'but is, and perhaps always will be, progressive. To clog it then with such a law, is laying it under restrictions from which it should ever be free'.[117]

More generally, though, the epidemic of 1808–9 brought new vigour to the vaccination cause. In Philadelphia, a group of physicians and 'public spirited gentlemen' formed a Vaccine Society in March 1809 to publicise vaccination and fund the vaccination of the poor in their homes.[118] In Baltimore, Dr James Smith, who began vaccinating in 1801 and distributing vaccine to colleagues in 1802, secured approval in 1809 for his scheme for a state vaccine agency in Maryland.[119] In Massachusetts, Dr Waterhouse applied himself again to the energetic promotion of kinepox inoculation. For some time, he had encouraged Sylvanus Fancher (or Fansher), an eccentric gentleman from Southport, Connecticut, in his vocation as a vaccinator. Attired in 'a faded blue cloak, slouched hat with overhanging green goggles', Fancher travelled around New England offering vaccination, using watch-chains and other trinkets to distract children while he injected them.[120] He won acclaim for a public trial of vaccination in Randolph, Vermont in 1808, in which seventy-five people vaccinated by him were exposed to smallpox in the pest-house and found to be immune. One mother 'heroically offered herself and her child' to a special experiment in which she was variolated and the baby at her breast vaccinated. While she had hundreds of pustules on her face, neck and breasts, the baby remained well, 'with one beautiful pustule, and playful'.[121] With Fancher as his partner, Waterhouse took on a major commission in the whaling port of New Bedford in late summer 1809. The town offered kinepox inoculation to all residents, and more than 1,500 people of all ages, from 'five days old to upwards of seventy years', were immunised 'without a single disagreeable accident'.[122]

The township of Milton, Massachusetts, won some celebrity for its approach to vaccination.[123] In July 1809, the selectmen appointed a committee, including Dr Amos Holbrook and John Mark Gourgas, a Genevan gentleman from

[117] *Medical Repository*, third series, 2 (1811), 30–5.

[118] John Thomas Scharf and Thomas Westcott, *History of Philadelphia, 1609–1884*, 2 vols. (Philadelphia, 1884), 2, p. 1476; James Thacher, *American medical biography: or memoirs of eminent physicians who have flourished in America*, 2 vols. in one (Boston, MA, 1828), 2, p. 211.

[119] Whitfield J. Bell, Jr, 'Dr James Smith and the public encouragement for vaccination for smallpox', *Annals of Medical History*, third series, 2 (1940), 500–16, at 503–5.

[120] Cash, *Waterhouse*, pp. 223–5; B. Riznik, *Medicine in New England 1790–1840* (Sturbridge, MA, 1969), p. 24; Fancher, 'Progress of vaccination', 97.

[121] Benjamin Waterhouse, *Information respecting the origin, progress, and efficacy of the kine pock inoculation* (Cambridge, MA, 1810), pp. 22–5.

[122] Waterhouse, *Information*, p. 25.

[123] *A collection of papers relative to the transactions of the town of Milton, in the State of Massachusetts, to promote a general inoculation of the cow-pox, or kine pock, as a never failing preventative of small pox infection* (Boston, MA, 1809).

London, who served as the committee's secretary, to consider measures for a general vaccination. After soliciting and publicising endorsements of the practice from physicians around Boston, the committee offered the procedure to residents for the token fee of 25 cents. Over three days in late July, Holbrook vaccinated 317 residents, over a quarter of the population, and subsequently organised a public trial in which a sample of the vaccinated children were shown to be immune. Satisfied as to the effectiveness of the practice, the selectmen resolved to conduct a general vaccination every year and publicise their proceedings for the benefit of other communities.[124] The president of the Boston Board of Health declared that Milton had set an example that has done it honour and hoped that 'it will be emulated in every town, not only of this, but of every State of the Union'.[125] With other townships following its lead, Milton presented a bill to the State Legislature in January 1810 'to make it obligatory, for every town in the Commonwealth, to organise, and offer annually, to their people a public inoculation of the cow pox, or kine pock, under proper regulations and restriction'. Though General Gore, Governor of Massachusetts, was supportive, the Senate was unwilling to do more than encourage townships to take prudential measures.[126]

Individual activism and collective self-help drove vaccination in the United States. Although he welcomed the revival of the practice in New England, Waterhouse felt frustrated by the lack of remuneration for his early endeavours and continuing his *pro bono* work. He was naturally concerned that 25 cents per vaccination, the nominal fee in the Milton experiment, might become normative. He favoured a model in which physicians were paid a modest salary by the state or private charity to vaccinate the poor for free and allowed to charge commercial fees to patients who could afford them. In January 1810, he likewise addressed the State Legislature outlining his contribution to vaccination, declaring his readiness 'to devote the remainder of his days' to the task 'of exterminating the small pox from the land', but making clear that, while working 'to preserve the offspring of *others*', he needed an income to support his own.[127] When nothing came of this approach, he advertised his own kine pock institution, using his own home and rooms in the Exchange in Boston, and even offering vaccination, for the convenience of sailors, on the Sabbath.[128] In Baltimore, more centrally positioned in the new nation, Dr James Smith had some success in scaling up his enterprise. As vaccine agent in Maryland in 1809, he engaged the interest of President Madison in his work,

---

[124] Cash, *Waterhouse*, pp. 245–8.
[125] John Ballard Blake, *Public health in the town of Boston, 1630–1822* (Cambridge, MA, 1959), p. 184.
[126] Cash, *Waterhouse*, pp. 249–51.   [127] Cash, *Waterhouse*, pp. 230–1.
[128] Cash, *Waterhouse*, p. 252.

submitted a proposal to Congress to supply vaccine to the District of Columbia, and addressed a circular letter to members of Congress offering to provide vaccine and advice on the practice to all citizens of the United States. It was a bold move, but very opportune. With the epidemic of 1808–9 still fresh in people's minds, the looming war with Britain underlined the nation's need for a secure supply of vaccine. In February 1813, Congress passed an act 'for the encouragement of vaccination', authorising the appointment of 'an agent to preserve the genuine vaccine matter, and to furnish the same to any citizen of the United States, whenever it may be applied for, through the medium of the post office'. President Madison duly appointed Smith as Vaccine Agent for the United States of America. Although he was not salaried, he was authorised to charge fees for vaccine and allowed free postage. In addition, he secured a contract from the State of Virginia, worth $600 per annum, to supply vaccine at no charge to its residents.[129] The war of 1812–14 brought some government support, too, to Waterhouse, who had been dismissed from Harvard in 1812. He was appointed to a series of salaried positions in military hospitals in Massachusetts until he was honourably discharged in 1821.[130]

The National Vaccine Agency represents a rare moment of Federal involvement in public health in the United States. Although it had less to offer in the northern states, where vaccination was well established, it provided vital support for the new prophylaxis in the southern states and the territories beyond the Appalachians. From 1813, Smith placed advertisements in provincial newspapers and journals, like the *Georgia Express*, stating his readiness, on receipt of $5 in banknotes, to provide vaccine matter and instructions that would 'enable any discreet person, who can read and write, to secure his own family' from smallpox.[131] He likewise appointed assistants, operating on commission, to go on the road to supply vaccine and vaccinate. He and his assistants reportedly vaccinated over 100,000 people. In 1816, he submitted a series of proposals to expand his agency's role, including a system by which physicians provided with vaccine were required to submit records of their cases. Congress was reluctant to expand the role of the Federal government at the expense of the states.[132] In 1818, Smith took a new tack by proposing a national vaccination institute in Washington, funded by subscription from participating states, corporations and individuals. Remarkably enough, he managed to raise some $26,000 in subscriptions.[133] In the autumn of 1821, however, his edifice came crashing down. A serious epidemic in Baltimore,

---

[129] Bell, 'Smith and vaccination', 504–5.   [130] Cash, *Waterhouse*, pp. 360–72.

[131] Robert Cumming Wilson, *Drugs and pharmacy in the life of Georgia, 1733–1959* (Athens, GA, 1959), p. 131.

[132] Bell, 'Smith and vaccination', 508.   [133] Bell, 'Smith and vaccination', 508–9.

Smith's home-base, proved highly embarrassing. The epidemic took 200 lives, including a young girl whom Smith had vaccinated two years earlier. To compound the misery, Smith mistakenly posted a sample of smallpox, set aside for tests, to Dr John Ward in Tarboro, North Carolina. When Ward's patients broke out in smallpox, Smith sought to cover up his negligence. This gave his critics ammunition to discredit his enterprise. After reading the report of the committee instituted to examine the affair, Congress repealed the act of 1813 in May 1824.[134]

Cowpox in Canada

In the British colonies of North America, there was a long struggle to establish vaccination. Although cowpox came early to Newfoundland, it was not until the spring of 1802 that Dr Joseph Bond, after receiving vaccine sent by his brother, an acquaintance of Jenner, achieved some continuity of practice in the maritime provinces. The advance of the new prophylaxis along the St Lawrence and the Great Lakes was fitful and slow. A British army officer in Quebec used vaccine from London to vaccinate children of a fellow-soldier in November 1801.[135] Dr Langmore of Quebec began vaccinating in the spring of 1802 and advertised free vaccination of the poor at the Hotel Dieu in August.[136] The supply of vaccine evidently dried up. In Montreal, Elizabeth Hale reported that in November she was she obliged to have her children inoculated with smallpox as 'every attempt of sending the vaccine matter' from England had failed. In the spring of 1804, cowpox was not only available but 'public opinion has undergone such a revolution' that she felt that there was sufficient demand for supply to be maintained.[137] As in the United States, there was official support to extend vaccination to the First Nations. Early in 1803, Father Le Noir, a missionary among the Abenaquis, wrote to Montreal seeking medical assistance in introducing vaccination.[138] Delighted by reports that large numbers of Native Americans were embracing the practice, Jenner sent a copy of *the Inquiry* to present to their chieftains. At a meeting at Fort St George in November 1807, Colonel Gore, governor of Upper Canada, formally presented it to the leaders of the Five Nations, who declared that they would teach their children 'to speak the name of Jenner' and 'to thank the

---

[134] Rebecca Fields Green, '"Simple, easy, and intelligible": Republican political ideology and the implementation of vaccination in the Early Republic', *Early American Studies: An Interdisciplinary Journal*, 12 (2014), 301–37.
[135] R. Cameron Stewart, 'Early vaccinations in British North America', *Canadian Medical Association Journal*, 39 (1938), 181–3.
[136] *MPJ*, 17 (January–June 1807), 546.   [137] Rusnock, 'Catching cowpox', 24–5, 31.
[138] John W. R. McIntyre and C. Stuart Houston, 'Smallpox and its control in Canada', *Canadian Medical Association Journal*, 161 (1999), 1543–7, at 1545.

Great Spirit for bestowing upon him such wisdom and so much benevolence', and presented a belt and string of Wampum to be given to Jenner.[139] In a remarkable initiative, obviously related to attempts to make similar provision in England and to the establishment of the National Vaccine Agency in the United States, the Legislature of Lower Canada passed an act in 1815 for the vaccination of the population at public expense, a move that, though it was not continued, significantly increased the social reach of vaccination.[140]

Democratic Vaccine

The seeds of the new prophylaxis could scarcely have fallen on more fertile ground than Anglophone America. There was no real barrier of language and culture to the transmission of new techniques and ideas and Americans had a good understanding of the advantages and disadvantages of smallpox inoculation. Few cities in Europe could rival Philadelphia as a centre for smallpox inoculation. Conversely, few places could rival New England in the careful regulation of the practice. The distances between major population centres made smallpox somewhat easier to avoid than in Europe, but isolated communities were necessarily much more vulnerable when *variola* finally struck. The potential of the new prophylaxis for North Americans was all too plain. It allowed individuals personal security, while not occasioning danger to the community. The great challenge in North America was in making vaccine available in remote districts and maintaining a supply of vaccine outside the few large cities.

Medical men led the way in promoting vaccination. Practitioners with transatlantic connections had a head start in acquiring cowpox and knowhow. In the early years, Waterhouse and other physicians sought to make their name and fortune from kinepox inoculation. As the challenges of the new prophylaxis became better understood, there was a growing emphasis on collaboration in maintaining the supply of good vaccine and the reputation of the practice. Aware of the progress of vaccination elsewhere in the world, medical men exhibited a high degree of consensus about the utility of the new prophylaxis and sought to keep informed about developments in the practice. As in Britain and elsewhere, the introduction of vaccination in North America coincided with the foundation of professional journals like New York's *Medical Repository*, which first informed Americans about the cowpox discovery, and Dr Coxe's *Philadelphia Medical Museum*, which included some thirty

---

[139] Baron, *Life*, 2, pp. 101–5.
[140] Barbara Tunis, 'Public vaccination in lower Canada, 1815–1823: controversy and a dilemma', in Jean-Pierre Goubert (ed.), *La médicalisation de la société française 1770–1830* (Waterloo, Ontario, 1982), pp. 264–78.

items on vaccination in its first issue in 1805.[141] Although sometimes stoking rivalry, the new prophylaxis generally served as a bond among medical men. In New York, leading physicians and surgeons supported the establishment of the kine-pox institution that continued under the auspices of the New York Dispensary. In Philadelphia, the vaccination cause may have helped to heal the divisions in the medical community arising from rival understandings and approaches to yellow fever. In April 1803, some fifty physicians, including many former adversaries, published a categorical endorsement of vaccination as 'a certain preventive of the Smallpox'.[142] While there was recognition of the need for collaboration in the propagation and distribution of vaccine in North America, however, there was always some concern that government support of vaccination would give a few practitioners undue advantage and bar others from the practice.

In terms of lay opinion, there was little entrenched prejudice against vaccination. Americans warmed to the quirky novelty and the slightly homespun nature of the practice. Once people were convinced that it was 'no scam', the new prophylaxis was well able to hold its own in the medical marketplace.[143] Although the endorsement of vaccination by President Jefferson assisted in establishing its reputation, elite sponsorship of the practice was less relevant in North America than in the Old World. In shaping public opinion, newspapers played an important role and were generally supportive of the new prophylaxis. More than most peoples, North Americans came to 'own' vaccination. For themselves and for their children, individuals, women as much as men, decided to accept or sometimes reject the practice, making their call on what they had read about the practice, heard from family, friends and neighbours or experienced themselves. Abigail Adams, the wife of John Adams, may have been disposed towards vaccination by her own experience of variolation, her observations of its progress in Boston and the decision of her son and daughter-in-law, then in Europe, to have her grandson vaccinated.[144] Elizabeth Drinker of Philadelphia took an early interest in the cowpox discovery and subsequently made it her business to see that her grandchildren were vaccinated rather than variolated.[145] John Duffy has identified 'rugged individualism' as the characteristic approach of the early Republic to public health.[146] In the towns and townships of the middle and northern states, citizens came together as individuals to make the decision to support vaccination. Grassroots activism can be seen in the use of ward-based committees in general vaccinations in

---

[141] *Philadelphia Medical Museum*, 1 (1805).   [142] Drinker, *Medicine and doctors*, pp. 101–2.
[143] For similar points about variolation, see Gronim, 'Imagining inoculation', 263–8.
[144] *A traveled First Lady. Writings of Louisa Catherine Adams*, ed. Margaret A. Hogan and C. James Taylor (Cambridge, MA, 2014), p. 191.
[145] Drinker, *Medicine and doctors*, pp. 102–3.
[146] John Duffy, *The Sanitarians: a history of American public health* (Urbana, IL, 1992), p. 53.

Boston and Philadelphia in 1816.[147] The 'friends of vaccination' in the south ward in Philadelphia resolved to obtain from each household a list of persons liable to smallpox and 'to exert their influence with such to be immediately *vaccinated*, and where they deem it expedient, to have it done for them', with John Vaughan finding time to door-knock in the block formed by Sixth and Seventh Streets.[148]

Formally at least religion played little role in framing responses to vaccination. The separation of church and state and the multiplicity of denominations make it hard to generalise about religious attitudes. Even if they did not assume the substantive roles assigned to state churches in Europe, the major churches were favourably disposed to vaccination. There is little substance to claim that Timothy Dwight, the Congregationalist 'Pope' of Connecticut, opposed vaccination. If he had some initial doubts, he supported the practice as early as 1801 and hailed it as a singular blessing of Providence.[149] The Assembly of the Presbyterian Church cooperated with the Philadelphia 'friends of humanity' in distributing literature on vaccination, and its committee for missions subsequently applied to Dr Rush to send vaccine for Cherokee children at Maryville.[150] There was a natural fit between denominational allegiances that encouraged humanitarian activism and the cause of vaccination. It is not surprising to see Quakers like Benjamin Waterhouse and Unitarians like John Vaughan active in smallpox prophylaxis. Members of the Society of Friends organised and bore the cost of the general vaccination at New Bedford in 1809.[151] Still, it is notable how generally the cause of vaccination was invested with religious significance. In congratulating the Boston Board of Health on its endorsement of vaccination in 1802, Abigail Adams told the members that their promotion and extension of 'so valuable a discovery are highly honorable to you as men and Christians assimilating you to the perfect pattern whom we are told went about doing good'.[152] In circulating their plan for vaccination, the selectmen of Milton, declared: 'Our souls are inflamed with the desire to have this undertaking pursued ... we wish for no praise nor reward, but to be suffered to proceed, that our dust may lay down in mercy, and a blessing repose on our families'.[153] There is little evidence of a cult of Jenner, but his name was greatly revered in North America. Dr Waterhouse came as close to

---

[147] Blake, *Public health in Boston*, p. 189.

[148] Harris, Reuben III, re. smallpox vaccination, 1816, The Wyck Papers, III, APS.

[149] Timothy Dwight, *Travels in New-England and New-York*, 4 vols. (London, 1821–3), 4, p. 1088.

[150] *Minutes of Presbyterian Assembly*, pp. 17–18; *General Assembly of the United Presbyterian Church in the United States of America, Minutes, 1959*, part 1 (1959), p. 242.

[151] Waterhouse, *Information*, p. 25.

[152] Adams-Hull Collection, Box 1, Folder 76, Massachusetts Historical Society, Boston.

[153] *Transactions of Milton*, p. 47.

idolatry as an American patriot could go, while Dr Coxe named his son Edward Jenner Coxe. Most Americans would doubtless have endorsed President Jefferson's high estimation of Jenner's providential role in the cowpox discovery.[154] There was perhaps some tendency to see Jenner as an honorary American, a man in the mould of Benjamin Franklin.[155] Many Americans sought him out in England and Jenner appears to have enjoyed their company. His last significant substantive publication on vaccination was a letter he wrote to an American friend.[156]

The United States made its own contribution to the global cause of vaccination. Waterhouse's experiments and reports on cases in the United States informed transnational discussion of the practice. Sylvanus Fancher pioneered the successful use of vaccine in crystalline form and his technique of using multiple incisions to accelerate the vaccination process to arrest a recent smallpox infection was published overseas.[157] Philadelphia was at the heart of the new nation's engagement with the wider world of knowledge, and rapidly emerged as an important centre for the dissemination of vaccine to the West Indies and Latin America and a clearing-house for information on vaccination worldwide. Two of the leading figures in vaccination in France, the former count of Larochefoucault-Liancourt and Dr Valentin, lived as exiles in Pennsylvania in the 1790s and on their return home kept medical friends in Philadelphia informed of developments in France. In June 1802 John Vaughan sought advice from the Spanish consul regarding the introduction of vaccination to Spain.[158] Alexander von Humboldt brought reports of indigenous cowpox in Peru and an account of the arrival of the expedition in Mexico to the city in 1804. In 1805, Léonard Clair Laborde, a French colonial physician visited the city and, at the request of his Philadelphia colleagues, wrote up an account of the introduction of vaccination in Mauritius.[159] Edward Cutbush, a Philadelphian naval captain, translated and published in Philadelphia Dr Calagni's Italian treatise on vaccination.[160] Jenner's last book on vaccination was published in the city in 1818.[161]

According to John Duffy, the 'success of vaccination in drastically reducing the incidence of smallpox' in the United States 'during the first thirty or forty

[154] Peterson, *Jefferson and new nation*, pp. 683–4.

[155] Halsey, *Jefferson and Waterhouse*, p. 39.

[156] Edward Jenner, *Letter from Doctor Edward Jenner, to William Dilwyn, Esq, in the effects of vaccination, in preserving from the small-pox. To which are added sundry documents relating to vaccination, referred to and accompanying the letter* (Philadelphia, 1818).

[157] Medical Repository, 10 (1807), 401; Sylvanus Fancher, 'Acceleration of the constitutional action of cow-pox', *The Lancet*, 2 (1828–9), 417–20.

[158] Ms. Comm. to APS [June 1802]. Archives, no. III, 1, APS.

[159] *Philadelphia Medical and Physical Journal*, part 1, vol. 2 (1805), 71–5.

[160] Calagni, *A letter on inoculation of vaccina*.   [161] Jenner, *Letter to Dilwyn*.

years of the nineteenth century proved almost self-defeating'.[162] In the early decades, the immediate threat of smallpox provided a major impetus for vaccination. An epidemic in 1815–17 prompted renewed action. When the infection appeared in Savannah, Georgia, in March 1816, the port's health officer urged people to have their families and slaves vaccinated, calling on his medical colleagues to support the campaign.[163] In Boston the Board of Health organised a successful general vaccination.[164] The authorities in New York allocated $1,000 for a vaccination campaign.[165] As the intervals between epidemics became longer, however, the number of susceptible people grew, adding to the danger of large-scale infection. It became apparent, too, that some of the people who had been previously vaccinated fell victim to the disease, underlining the need for some national oversight of the practice. The failure of the experiment with a National Vaccine Agency, however, discouraged further Federal involvement. Dr Waterhouse, who built a second career as the champion of public health in the United States army and navy,[166] continued to urge the necessity of a national approach to vaccination. He vested some hope in the election of his old friend John Quincy Adams, as sixth president of the United States, writing to him in 1826: 'I would leave the world contented could I be the means – the instrument of retaining and keeping alive this great prophylactic, this great blessing which Providence has put into our hands'. Observing that the individual practitioner, 'however zealous', can do little without the support of the government, he added pointedly: 'The U.S. has a department, *Le Bureau de la Guerre* [War Department] for the destruction of human life; and why not some benevolent establishment for the preservation of human life? – something that may apply the Jennerian discovery to its best purpose'.[167]

---

[162] Duffy, *Sanitarians*, p. 56.   [163] Wilson, *Drugs and pharmacy*, p. 131.
[164] Blake, *Public health in Boston*, p. 189.   [165] Duffy, *Sanitarians*, pp. 54–5.
[166] Harold D. Langley, *A history of medicine in the U.S. Navy* (Baltimore, MD, 1995), p. 131.
[167] Cash, *Waterhouse*, pp. 252–3.

12   A New Pox for the New World
Vaccination in Latin America

At the end of Lent 1804, the Royal and Philanthropic Vaccine Expedition approached Caracas, the capital of Venezuela. Setting out from La Coruña in November 1803 and Tenerife in early January 1804, the *María Pita* had crossed the Atlantic and made landfall in Puerto Rico in February. After finding that cowpox had already been introduced on the island and expressing his dissatisfaction with the management of the new practice, Dr Balmis left without securing the services of as many children as he would have liked to maintain the vaccination chain. Driven by a storm beyond La Guaira, the port for Caracas, the *María Pita* arrived at Puerto Cabello, 125 miles further west. Aware that success depended on the timely transfer of the lymph in Caracas, he found additional children to be vaccinated on the final stage of the journey. Arriving in Caracas shortly before Easter, Balmis and his party were warmly received by the Captain-General of Venezuela, the Archbishop of Caracas and the general populace.[1] The city boasted a cathedral, a university and an orchestra, but it lacked many of the amenities of civic life, including a printing press and newspaper. With a population of around 800,000, Venezuela was developing economically and, though deeply stratified by rank and status, wealth and race, it was beginning to embrace change.[2] As Humboldt observed on his visit in 1799, the younger generation was imbibing new ideas and looking to the future.[3] Simón Bolívar, the future liberator of Spanish America, was rounding off his education in Europe, but another young man, Andrés Bello, who would become the most distinguished man of letters in independent Latin America, was centrally involved in the reception of the new prophylaxis. The vaccination of children in Easter week assumed an almost sacramental quality and the inauguration of the practice led to a round of celebrations for which Bello wrote a poem and a theatrical piece.[4] Before Balmis left, he

---

[1] Smith, 'Real Expedición', 21–2; Ricardo Archila, 'The Balmis Expedition in Venezuela. Part II: founding of the Central Vaccination Board, 1804', in J. Z. Bowers and Elizabeth F. Purcell (eds.), *Aspects of the history of medicine in Latin America* (New York, 1979), pp. 142–77.

[2] John Lynch, *Simon Bolívar. A life* (New Haven, CT, 2006), p. 4.   [3] Lynch, *Bolívar*, pp. 4–5.

[4] Antonio Cussen, *Bello and Bolívar. Poetry and politics in the Spanish American Revolution* (Cambridge, 1992), pp. 7–8.

presided over the establishment of a vaccination board, with Bello as its secretary, to oversee the rapidly expanding practice.

It was a moment of triumph for Balmis and the expedition. Smallpox, introduced in Spanish ships three centuries earlier, had been a wildly destructive force in the Caribbean islands and Latin America. Once the prophylactic value of cowpox began to be recognised, the introduction of the benign pox into the New World came to appear a matter of urgency and indeed symbolic significance. The voyage into the tropics and the heat and humidity of the Caribbean, however, long frustrated attempts, beginning as early as 1799, to introduce and properly establish the vaccine virus in this part of the world. Awareness of the cost of smallpox in lives, labour and revenue and the logistical challenges in extending the prophylaxis through its dominions prompted the Spanish crown to set in train a grand expedition, not a little Quixotic, to take vaccine around the world. The introduction of vaccination in Venezuela represented its first significant success in extending the practice. Furthermore, since Balmis was charged to establish an administrative system that would enable the practice to thrive and spread, it represented the first stage in the realisation of a grand imperial vision. Aware of the magnitude of the task still before him, Balmis decided to split the expedition. One part, under the leadership of José de Salvany, the sub-director, was charged with introducing vaccination throughout South America. The main part, led by himself, would establish the new practice in Cuba, through the viceroyalty of New Spain (Mexico) and then across the Pacific to the Philippines. Even with a division of labour, it was a herculean undertaking. It would be two and a half years before Balmis would return to Spain. Salvany would remain in harness for another six years. During this time, the expedition would immunise over a million people, mainly non-European; devise measures for embedding vaccination in an empire on the point of dissolution; and provide inspiration to the global vaccination cause (Figure 12.1).

Massacres of the Innocents: Smallpox, Casual and Inoculated

Unknown before the early sixteenth century, smallpox hit the Americas with great ferocity, playing a significant role in destroying the indigenous cultures of the Caribbean and the ancient civilisations of Mesoamerica and South America. It remained an unusually destructive force among both the colonial and native populations. In the Caribbean, the movement of ships, commodities and people ensured that smallpox was never far away and serious outbreaks occurred with some regularity. In Barbados, a clergyman wrote in 1750, 'we are seldom free from [smallpox] in some part of the island or other'.[5] On the American

---

[5] Griffith Hughes, *The natural history of Barbados in ten books* (London, 1750), p. 39.

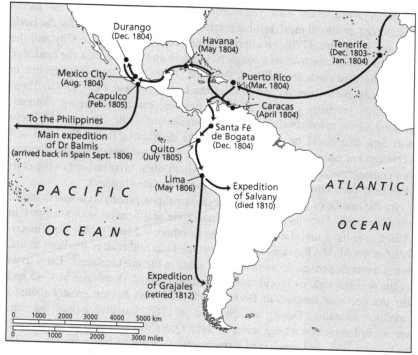

Figure 12.1 Map of the spread of vaccination in Spanish America: Route of the Royal and Philanthropic Vaccine Expedition (1803–12)

mainland, the colonies and their hinterlands were subject, every decade or so, to epidemics of some severity. The Portuguese empire in Brazil was especially exposed to new strains of smallpox by the large-scale importation of African slaves.[6] Though good demographic data is lacking, mortality levels were reportedly in excess of those in Europe. In Mexico City, smallpox allied with typhus was the cause of over 25,000 deaths in 1761–2.[7] An unusually virulent smallpox epidemic in Caracas in the late 1760s, during which over 6,000 people died, was commemorated in a painting in the Cathedral of the Virgin and the Company of Heaven offering consolation to the city.[8] In highland Ecuador, Espejo observed that smallpox, formerly appearing every twelve

---

[6] Alden and Miller, 'Out of Africa', 195–224.   [7] Cooper, *Epidemic disease*, pp. 53–4.
[8] José Esparza and Germán Yépez Colmenares, 'Viruela en la Venezuela colonial: epidemias, variolización y vacunación', in Susana Ramírez. Luis Valenciano, Rafael Nájera and Luis Enjuanes (eds.), *La Real Expedición filantrópica de la vacuna. Doscientos años de lucha contra la viruela* (Madrid, 2004), pp. 89–118, at p. 100; Alexander von Humboldt, *Voyage aux régions équinoxiales du Nouveau Continent: fait en 1799, 1800, 1801, 1802, 1803 et 1804* (Paris, 1817), 4, pp. 174–5.

years, returned every two years from 1764 onwards.[9] The West Indies constituted an almost inexhaustible reservoir of variolous infection for the lands around. In the late 1770s, smallpox returned in force to Mexico City and the epidemic spread northwards through New Spain and merged with the epidemic spreading westwards from British America. There were related epidemics in Guatemala, New Granada and Peru in the late 1770s and early 1780s. There were high mortality rates in all the provinces, especially among children, leading to its association with Herod's massacre of the innocents.[10] There was little that could be done to combat its destructive force. The civil and ecclesiastical authorities worked together to report and isolate smallpox cases, but containment and isolation measures, which often involved removing children from their families, were resented and sometimes resisted.[11]

By the middle of the eighteenth century, smallpox prophylaxis was in use in the Caribbean. The slaves who had undergone scarification with smallpox in Africa may have introduced the custom to others.[12] Many others were inoculated on the Middle Passage, often in response to an outbreak of smallpox at sea, but sometimes perhaps to increase their value in the marketplace.[13] Early trials of the western style of inoculation took place in Saint-Domingue in 1745 and the practice was credited in Barbados in 1750 with having greatly reduced smallpox mortality. During an epidemic in 1768, inoculation was put into service in Jamaica on a large scale. Dr John Quier was a pioneer of the practice at Worthy Park and conducted experiments to achieve better results.[14] The manager at Golden Park, near Kingston, did not wait for the owner's authorisation to inoculate 100 slaves, 'as every estate around did it, we were absolutely obliged out of self-preservation to do it'.[15] After his arrival in Saint-Domingue in 1774, Simeon Worlock inoculated slaves on a massive scale. By the mid-1780s, he and his associates had reportedly inoculated over 40,000 people.[16] Arguably, variolation was more routinely deployed in the Caribbean than in any other part of the world on the eve of the cowpox discovery.

[9] Suzanne Austin Alchon, *Native society and disease in colonial Guatemala* (Cambridge, 2001), pp. 106–7.

[10] Pedro Lautaro Ferrer, *Historia general de la medicina en Chile desde el descubrimiento y conquista de Chile, en 1535, hasta nuestros dias*, vol. 1 (Talca, 1904), p. 256.

[11] Paul Ramírez, '"Like Herod's massacre": quarantine, Bourbon reform, and popular protest in Oaxaca's smallpox epidemic, 1796–7', *The Americas*, 69 (2012), 203–35.

[12] Karol Kimberlee Weaver, *Medical revolutionaries: the enslaved healers of eighteenth-century Saint Domingue* (Urbana, IL, 2006), pp. 53–4.

[13] Stewart, 'Edge of utility', 54–70.

[14] Michael Craton and James Walvin, *A Jamaican plantation. The history of Worthy Park 1670–1970* (London, 1970), pp. 132–3.

[15] Betty Wood (ed.), 'The letters of Simon Taylor of Jamaica to Chaloner Arcedekne, 1765–1775', in *Camden Miscellany*, 35 (London, 2002), pp. 65–6.

[16] McClellan, *Colonialism and science*, pp. 144–5; Bennett, 'Curing and inoculating smallpox', 35–6.

In the Spanish empire, smallpox prophylaxis came into use more slowly. During an epidemic in Venezuela in 1766, the Captain-General instructed a medical man from the Canaries to inoculate his own children and following his example some 5,000 people were inoculated.[17] In the south of the continent, Father Chaparro, who began inoculating around 1765, inspired other clergy in the viceroyalty of Peru to take up the lancet when smallpox threatened.[18] In the mid-1770s, Dr Cosmé Bueno sought to promote inoculation and set it on a more professional footing in Lima.[19] When smallpox appeared in Mexico in 1779, after an interval of seventeen years, the authorities had reason to fear high mortality rates. For the first time, there were moves to introduce variolation. Dr Esteban Morel, who had written a thesis on the topic, began inoculating privately at home.[20] Martín de Mayoraga, Viceroy of New Spain, moved by the 'incalculable distress' in the city, gave his approval for the inoculation and a handbill advertised Morel's offer to inoculate free of charge. Despite the large number of cases and some 18,000 deaths, few people presented their children for inoculation.[21] In Guatemala, the authorities were better prepared. When smallpox arrived in summer 1780, the government authorised Dr José Flores to introduce inoculation. Over the autumn, he and his colleagues inoculated 'thousands' around the capital. In rural districts, so as not to alarm Amerindian children and parents, he set aside his lancet, used a poultice made from beetles and Spanish fly to raise a blister, made a small incision, and then applied a piece of fabric impregnated with smallpox matter.[22]

Epidemic smallpox at the turn of the eighteenth century intensified the focus on variolation in Spanish America, serving to highlight the advantages and disadvantages of the practice. As an epidemic began to build in Mexico in 1796, the Marquis de Branciforte, Viceroy of New Spain, took steps to stall the disease by imposing quarantine and ordering the isolation of infected people.[23] The measures were not wholly practicable. Amerindians often took to flight rather than risk being corralled in pest-houses where death usually followed. The separation of sick children from their families provoked riots in the province of Oaxaca.[24] Early in 1797, the viceroy called on the people to pray for divine mercy and protection, but gave some countenance to inoculation.[25] In Mexico City, the archbishop, some local notables and several medical men commended the practice. Dr Montaña inoculated his own daughter and the children of private patients. Once the infection became general, the risks

---

[17] Esparza and Yépez Colmenares, 'Viruela en Venezuela', 100–1; Humboldt, *Voyage*, 4, pp. 174–5.
[18] Barros Arana, *Historia de Chile*, 6, pp. 227–30; Ferrer, *Historia de la medicina*, pp. 270–2.
[19] Warren, *Medicine in Peru*, pp. 81–4.   [20] Cooper, *Epidemic disease*, pp. 56–63, 66.
[21] Cooper, *Epidemic disease*, pp. 64–8.   [22] Few, *For all humanity*, pp. 57–60.
[23] Cooper, *Epidemic disease*, pp. 97–8.   [24] Ramírez, 'Oaxaca's smallpox', 213–18.
[25] Cooper, *Epidemic disease*, pp. 99–102.

associated with the practice were less evident. In August, the Viceroy authorised public inoculation and conceded that patients need not be confined to lazarettos.[26] Around 3,000 people were inoculated, with a fatality-rate of less than 1 per cent. Many people, however, had reservations about the practice. A satirical poem presented it as a dangerous scam and described the *inoculados* as 'walking with death'.[27] Once the epidemic passed its peak, the number seeking inoculation fell away.[28] By the spring of 1798, the epidemic came to an end, with over 7,000 fatalities. Inoculation, which had saved several hundred lives, gained credit as a prophylactic measure. In the viceroyalty of Peru, however, where inoculation was a more familiar but less controlled procedure, the medical men were concerned about its tendency to spread the infection. As an epidemic began to build in Lima in 1802, the authorities backed away from variolation and vested their hopes in the early arrival of vaccine.[29]

Seeding the Caribbean: Cowpox, Kinepox, Vaccine and Vacuna

News of cowpox arrived in the British West Indies in 1799. From this time, most consignments of mail from England brought samples of vaccine lymph, usually inert on arrival. Learning of its success in the Mediterranean in 1800, Dr Simmons of Manchester noted that 'most beneficial consequences might be expected also from introducing it among the slaves in the West Indies'.[30] Plantation-owners and their agents were not slow off the mark. Early in 1801, Dr John Rooke of Montego Bay, Jamaica, received vaccine for use on the plantations of Charles Rose Ellis. Vaccinating himself and fifteen blacks, Rooke alone took the infection, leading him initially to 'suspect that people of colour were insusceptible of the disease'. His own 'singularly providential' infection, however, enabled him to continue vaccinating, suppress an outbreak on a neighbouring estate, and immunise some 4,000 people in his district.[31] After obtaining vaccine around April 1801, George Farquhar of Clarendon vaccinated 1,200 people in the parish of Trelawny.[32] During 1802, however, Jamaica lost its supply of vaccine. It was a personal concern for the Governor of Jamaica and his pregnant wife, who had heard about cowpox before leaving England. When Lady Maria Nugent gave birth to a healthy boy in October 1802, she was distraught that they would need, as she put it, to give her baby smallpox.[33]

Aware of its success in Europe, Spanish colonies were likewise seeking vaccine. Early in 1802, the Economic Society of Havana received a copy of

---

[26] Cooper, *Epidemic disease*, pp. 105–6, 112–17.   [27] Cooper, *Epidemic disease*, pp. 122–32.
[28] Cooper, *Epidemic disease*, pp. 136–7, 141–2.   [29] Warren, *Medicine in Peru*, pp. 84–6.
[30] *MPJ*, 5 (January–June 1801), 137.
[31] *MPJ*, 5 (January–June 1801), 543–4; *Annals of Medicine* (1801), 325–6.
[32] Coxe, *Practical observations*, pp. 61–2.   [33] *Nugent's journal*, p. 171.

Pedro Hernández's *Origen y descubrimiento de la vacuna*. On the advice of Dr Tomás Romay y Chacón, it arranged for its republication and offered a reward of 300 or 400 pesos to the first person to find cowpox locally or introduce it from overseas. Over the year, Romay received several samples from Spain and the United States that proved inert.[34] In Guatemala, there was likewise a well-informed constituency of interest. While Dr Flores, now in retirement in Spain, was to become involved in planning the vaccine expedition, Dr Narciso Esparragosa, his pupil, sought out and translated accounts of the new prophylaxis. The *Gaceta de Guatemala* kept its readers informed about developments. Premature reports of the arrival of vaccine in Mexico led to a subscription being raised for a courier to secure samples. Hopes were raised and disappointed again in August 1802, when vaccine from New Orleans proved inert, and in December, when vaccine from Spain failed in a trial on the son of a government official.[35] Severe smallpox epidemics in the kingdom of New Granada and the viceroyalty of Peru lent urgency to measures to introduce the new prophylaxis. In a petition to King Carlos IV late in 1802, the council at Santa Fé de Bogotá called for assistance. The Spanish government was very aware of the devastating impact of smallpox on the Spanish colonial economy, and recognised the potential of vaccination to serve its reformist agenda in the empire.[36] In the past, there had been no need for the metropolitan government to do more than oversee, from a distance, the initiatives taken locally. Conscious of the difficulties in delivering vaccine in good condition and establishing sound practice, the Council of the Indies sought advice from Dr Flores in March 1803 on the feasibility of a vaccine expedition. In June, King Carlos announced a royal expedition, headed by Dr Balmis, to deliver fresh vaccine to Spanish America and the Philippines by the successive vaccination of children, establish the new prophylaxis by training practitioners and maintaining a supply of good lymph, and promote the practice among the colonial and indigenous populations.[37]

The Truce of Amiens of 1802–3 reopened lines of communication between Europe and the Caribbean. An expedition from France to suppress the slave revolt in Haiti in 1802 brought vaccine, and the first vaccinations took place in Martinique around this time.[38] Samples of vaccine continued to arrive in some profusion in Jamaica and other British colonies, but the new prophylaxis does

---

[34] Tomás Romay, *Memoria sobra la introduccion y progreso de la vacuna en la isla de Cuba* (Havana, 1805), pp. 3–5.

[35] John Tate Lanning, *The eighteenth-century Enlightenment in the University of San Carlos de Guatemala* (Ithaca, NY, 1956), pp. 246–9; Smith, 'Real Expedición', 50.

[36] Warren, *Medicine in Peru*, pp. 88–9.

[37] Mark and Rigau-Pérez, 'World's first campaign', 63–94, at 66–9.

[38] Geneviève Leti, *Santé et société esclavagiste à la Martinique (1802–1848)* (Paris, 1998), pp. 412–13.

not appear to have been properly established until late in 1803.[39] In 1802, the Royal Vaccine Commission in Copenhagen took the initiative of sending sixteen vials of vaccine to the Danish colony of St Thomas (US Virgin Islands), none of which succeeded. Early in 1803, however, an enterprising medical man brought some kinepox from Philadelphia to St Thomas and built up a stock of vaccine by offering free vaccination for the poor, 'coloured as well as white'.[40] From the Danish colony, samples were made available to medical men in neighbouring islands, including Francisco Oller, a military surgeon in Puerto Rico. In November 1802, Ramón de Castro, Governor of Puerto Rico, presided over the first successful vaccinations. Over two months, Oller and a colleague vaccinated 1,557 people including Oller's own son, the governor's two daughters and Bishop Arizmendi.[41] Prior to leaving Puerto Rico for Cuba in February 1804, Doña María Bustamente decided to have her son and two mulatto maids vaccinated. In Havana, Dr Tomás Romay was delighted to learn of their arrival. Given the prospect of a prize, he had little trouble in persuading Doña Bustamente to allow him to collect lymph from her son and maids. Romay immediately vaccinated his own five children and some thirty others.[42]

Arms around the Caribbean

After setting out from Spain, Dr Balmis had established vaccination in the Canaries and maintained a chain of vaccine infection across the Atlantic. On his arrival in Puerto Rico in February, he can be forgiven for his querulous response to the news that the new prophylaxis had begun on the island. In the two months prior to Balmis's arrival, Oller and his team had vaccinated some 1,557 people. From the outset, Balmis behaved badly, disdaining gestures of good will, inspecting the surgeon's handiwork with suspicion and stoking negativity. He knew all too well the problems that inexpert and hasty practice could create and the need to limit the numbers vaccinated to maintain a reserve of non-immune children to assure the future supply of vaccine. The Governor showed himself willing to address Balmis's concerns and arranged for him to instruct local medical men and Oller was deferential. When it came to the

---

[39] *Nugent's journal*, pp. 171, 173–4, 232, 236, 240.

[40] Niklas Thode Jensen, 'Safeguarding slaves: smallpox, vaccination, and government health policies among the enslaved population in the Danish West Indies, 1803–1848', *BHM*, 83 (2009), 95–124, at 100; José G. Rigau-Pérez, 'The introduction of smallpox vaccine in Puerto Rico in 1803 and the adoption of immunization as a government function in Puerto Rico', *Hispanic American Historical Review*, 69 (1989), 393–423, at 400.

[41] Rigau-Pérez, 'Introduction in Puerto Rico', 393–423.

[42] Romay, *Vacuna en Cuba*, p. 5; Smith, 'Real Expedición', 22; José López Sánchez, *Tomas Romay and the origin of science in Cuba* (Havana, 1967), pp. 84–94, 237, n. 147.

substantive issue, the question of whether the vaccinations had been success-ful, Balmis was hoist on his own petard. When Oller's patients were tested, they were found to be immune. In a stormy meeting, at which the Governor, Bishop and other notables were present, however, Balmis declared that the trials were a piece of theatre 'designed to dupe the people' and that all the vaccinations needed to be repeated. Tempers were so enflamed by his insulting behaviour that violence was only narrowly avoided. For his part, Balmis made no apology for his behaviour, took no steps to build on Oller's work and brought forward his plans for departure. After securing minimal supplies and barely sufficient children for the vaccination chain, the expedition set out for Venezuela.[43]

Arriving in Caracas shortly before Easter, Balmis was well received. The populace welcomed the arrival of the expedition and the Captain-General of Venezuala accorded it the respect and assistance that Balmis believed it warranted. On Good Friday, Balmis vaccinated some sixty-four children and then, with the help of an assistant, some 2,064 people over the following week. The first in line was reportedly Luis Blanco, who retained a memory of the event until his death seventy years later.[44] The success of the vaccinations was celebrated in a great festival. There was a concert which involved, according to Balmis, everyone 'who had, or claimed to have, musical talent'. The literary tributes from Andrés Bello may have been more to his Balmis's taste. His *Oda de la Vacuna* described the devastation of smallpox, leaving both palace and hut in mourning, the old perishing with the young, and hailed the providential discovery of vaccine and the king's benevolence in sending the expedition to America.[45] His dramatic work on the same theme, *Venezuela Consolada*, was also presumably staged.[46] Balmis and his team conducted a further round of vaccinations, bringing the local total to over 12,000. He took some trouble to involve the local medical men on whom the future of vaccination would depend. José Domingo Díaz, Venezuela's most prominent physician, proved a strong supporter of the practice until his death in 1807. Vicente Salias, another local medical man, was accorded the honour of testing the patients vaccinated in Easter week.[47]

Sensible of the challenges in establishing vaccination, Balmis sought to set it on the firmest possible foundation. Rather than entrusting it to a hospital or charitable institution with other priorities, he drew up a plan for a high-level agency that would be specifically charged with the maintenance, oversight and

---

[43] Smith, 'Real Expedición', 21.
[44] Esparza and Yépez Colmenares, 'Viruela en Venezuela', 107.
[45] Cussen, *Bello and Bolívar*, pp. 7–8.
[46] Emilio Balaguer Perigüell and Rosa Ballester Añón, *En el nombre de los niños: la Real Expedición Filantrópica de la Vacuna (1803–1806)* (Madrid, 2003), pp. 181–6.
[47] Archila, 'Expedition in Venezuela, II', 176, n. 28.

promotion of the practice. He accordingly sought approval of a plan for a *junta*, a council or board, that would comprise key officials of the state, the church and the city, leading medical men, and prominent laymen. It would meet weekly, appoint two doctors to vaccinate in rotation and an executive secretary to handle the paperwork, collect data, provide information, conduct enquiries, and publicise the practice.[48] Amid some ceremony on 28 April, the Captain-General inaugurated the *Junta central de la vacuna* and the Archbishop of Caracas led the community in a service of thanksgiving. The junta wasted little time in getting down to business, appointing Bello as the first secretary. In June, it was collecting data on smallpox in Caracas; in July, it arranged for the routine vaccination of newly imported slaves on board ship; in August, it instructed mayors to call on people to seek vaccination and secured the Captain-General's agreement to impose fines for non-compliance; in autumn, it was investigating a report of cowpox on cattle near Villa del Calabozo. At the end of 1804, after collating returns from thirty-one cities and towns, it reported 12,450 vaccinations.[49]

While in Venezuela, Balmis received news from Quito. The vaccine that the Viceroy of New Granada had brought from Spain proved inert on arrival and Dr Berges, who was going to collaborate with the vaccine expedition, had died. Balmis accordingly decided to divide the expedition and send José Salvany, the sub-director, with a share of the personnel, equipment and supplies, to assume responsibility for introducing the practice in New Granada and the other southern viceroyalties of Peru and Rio de la Plata. Balmis drew up a new set of instructions, modified in the light of experience, that stressed the need to establish vaccination boards in provincial capitals. From the outset, Salvany was dogged by misfortune. A week after leaving La Guaira on the voyage to Cartagena, his ship capsized at the mouth of the Magdalena River, losing equipment, though fortunately no lives, in the accident. For three days the party, including children under vaccination, were stranded on a beach suffering from the unforgiving climate, hunger and thirst and insect bites. A local official happily came to their rescue and provided food and clothing and new children to vaccinate. On 24 May, Salvany and his bedraggled party arrived in Cartagena. They received a warm reception, found time to recuperate from their ordeal and were able to formally inaugurate their philanthropic mission. It was the first stage in a long, arduous and dangerous expedition through tropical rainforest and across high mountain-passes that would ultimately cost Salvany his health and life.

Prior to setting out for Cuba, Balmis knew that vaccine had preceded him. Arriving in Havana on 26 May, he found that Dr Romay had matters well in

[48] Archila, 'Expedition in Venezuela, II', pp. 145–7.
[49] Archila, 'Expedition in Venezuela, II', pp. 149–50, 155–7, 175, n.25.

hand. After vaccinating his own children, Romay used two of them in a public trial in which ten vaccinees were inoculated with smallpox. He developed a nine-point plan to maintain vaccine pending the arrival of the royal expedition, including setting up a clinic and routinely vaccinating slaves brought into the country.[50] Although he must have been aware that Romay was using vaccine propagated by Oller in Puerto Rico, Balmis raised no concerns about the validity of his vaccinations. He doubtless held the eminent Cuban physician in higher regard than the Puerto Rican surgeon.[51] Using his authority as director of the royal expedition to support Romay's work, Balmis largely restricted himself to public demonstrations of the procedure and training local practitioners. Romay himself was an eloquent advocate for the practice, addressing his fellow citizens both as fathers, who would want to secure their children from smallpox, and as patriots, who would bring their children back to the clinic to provide lymph for others. He had less difficulty than colleagues elsewhere in maintaining a supply of vaccine. The Economic Society served as an informal vaccine institute and the vaccination of slaves proved a reliable source of vaccine. Romay's only concern was that dependence on slaves bred complacency among the European population. When he found that 248 slaves had been vaccinated in November, but only fourteen white children, he asked rhetorically: 'Is it perhaps the case that the value of slaves is more appreciated than the lives of children?'[52] By this time, Balmis had long moved on to the next stage of his expedition. Prior to leaving in June, he congratulated the Governor of Cuba and Dr Romay on their achievement, presented his plan for a *junta central de la vacuna*, and recommended that Romay remain in charge until its formation.[53] Since he was unable to find Cuban children to carry vaccine to Mexico, he purchased four slaves for vaccination *en route*, planning to recoup the cost by selling them in Veracruz. Although he knew that vaccine had already been introduced in Mexico, he was resolved to maintain the strain of vaccine that he had brought across the Atlantic.

The New Prophylaxis in Central America and Mexico

In the four months since Balmis's arrival in Puerto Rico, the frontline of vaccination had moved from the Caribbean to Central America and Mexico. Since their arrival in New Spain late in 1803, Viceroy José de Iturrigaray and his physician, Dr García Arboleya, had sought opportunities to introduce

---

[50] Romay, *Vacuna en Cuba*, pp. 8–10.
[51] Adrián López Denis, 'Disease and society in colonial Cuba, 1790–1840', PhD thesis, University of California, Los Angeles, 2007, esp. pp. 123–4.
[52] López Denis, 'Disease in Cuba', p. 129.
[53] Romay, *Vacuna en Cuba*, p. 18; Smith, 'Real Expedición', 22–3.

vaccine in the viceroyalty. In April 1804, the breakthrough came with the arrival in Veracruz of two frigates of the Royal Armada from Cuba. One of the officers had brought with him vaccine dried on threads. Once ashore in Veracruz, the ship's doctor, Pérez Carrillo, under the oversight of José María Pérez, surgeon of the Royal Armada, used the vaccine to conduct the first successful vaccination in the viceroyalty. In late April, the *ayuntamiento* (governing council) wrote to the Viceroy to confirm the propagation of vaccine and inform him that Pérez was bringing four recently vaccinated soldiers to transmit the vaccine 'live' to Mexico City.[54] By this time, dried vaccine, dispatched by courier, was also well on the way to the capital. On its arrival, García Arboleya immediately vaccinated five children from the Royal Orphanage. Pausing in Jalapa to vaccinate army recruits and in Puebla to vaccinate twenty-four people, including the eight children of the Governor-Intendant, the Count of Cadena, Pérez arrived in time to join García Arboleya in certifying the success of the vaccinations in the orphanage. After demonstrating the practice in the viceregal palace, the physician and the naval surgeon vaccinated, amid some ceremony, five children in the Foundling Hospital, including the Viceroy's infant son Vicente. At the Viceroy's request, the *protomedicato* (a panel of three senior physicians) then drew up a plan for maintaining a supply of vaccine. It proposed that four children be vaccinated every nine days at the Foundling Hospital and that, since the number of foundlings was limited, each of the city's wards should present at least five children a year for vaccination. It further stipulated that, although practitioners would initially obtain vaccine from the central repository, they would need to maintain their own supply and not vaccinate infants under the age of one until their ward had provided its quota of children for the central repository. It likewise required practitioners to submit lists of names and ages of people vaccinated and details of the outcome of the operations to a clerk at the Foundling Hospital. The Viceroy approved the plan and took steps to extend the practice through the viceroyalty.[55]

From Havana, Dr Balmis had written to advise Viceroy Iturrigaray that he intended to cross to Sisal in Campeche, sail on to Veracruz and then take the road to Mexico City. Although he would have been informed about the beginnings of the practice in the capital of New Spain, he would have had no doubt that he still had work to do in reviewing the arrangements for the establishment of vaccination, making provision for the foundlings he had brought across the Atlantic, and preparing for the voyage across the Pacific. On arrival at Sisal on 25 June, however, he was persuaded that the situation in Campeche and Guatemala needed his immediate attention. The council in

[54] Smith, 'Real Expedición', 23–5.   [55] Smith, 'Real Expedición', 27–9.

Veracruz had dispatched a surgeon, Miguel José Monzón, with a group of young musicians, who would be successively vaccinated to transmit vaccine to Campeche. With the approval of the Captain-General of Yucatán, Monzón began vaccinating on some scale around Sisal, but a keen local physician, Dr Carlos Escoñet, who knew about Balmis's concerns in Puerto Rico, assumed that Monzón's vaccine, ultimately derived from Oller, was suspect and found fault with the vaccinations. Although the Captain-General intervened to censure Escoñet, the reputation of the practice was undermined. At the same time, a Guatemalan resident in Veracuz, aware of the demand for vaccine at home, secured a sample from the same stock, sealed it between glass plates and paid for a special courier to take it to Guatemala. On receipt of the package in Guatemala City, Dr Esparragosa broke the seal on the glass, moistened the vaccine, 'a little speckle the size of a fly's wing resting on a small piece of lint', and injected it into the arms of six children. By late May, he was sure that he had been successful and over the following three weeks he conducted 4,000 more vaccinations. On 17 June, a *fiesta* was held to celebrate the 'happy success of vaccination'.[56]

After hearing the allegations in Campeche and alarmed at the wide distribution of the allegedly suspect vaccine, Balmis instructed Antonio Gutiérrez to check on the vaccinations in Campeche and another assistant, Francisco Pastor, to follow up on the introduction of the practice in Guatemala. Although Gutiérrez approved the validity of Monzón's vaccinations, Balmis was not entirely convinced.[57] In the meantime Pastor had set out with four boys for the long journey to Guatemala, sailing along the Yucatán coast and then heading inland to Villahermosa, the provincial capital of Tabasco, where four more children were enlisted to take vaccine through the jungle to Ciudad Real de Chiapas. Finally arriving in Guatemala City in November, he rapidly ascertained that vaccination, strongly supported by the Captain-General, the Archbishop and the chief physician, had indeed made good progress in the city and was becoming available in several provinces.[58] Pastor assisted in the formation of a central vaccination board and in framing regulations to embed the practice, including the requirement that only a set proportion of children under one year of age was to be vaccinated to ensure a reserve of susceptible infants for the future propagation of vaccine. Provisions were made to keep records of birth, deaths and vaccinations, introduce vaccination in remote districts, and train local practitioners.[59] The central vaccine board, with Dr Esparragosa as its secretary, began its work in March 1805. It proved highly effective and its diligent record-keeping reveals the failures as well as successes of the practice.

---

[56] Smith, 'Real Expedición', 51–2; Lanning, *Enlightenment*, p. 256.
[57] Smith, 'Real Expedición', 31.   [58] Few, *For all humanity*, pp. 178–80.
[59] Smith, 'Real Expedición', 54–6; Few, *For all humanity*, pp. 174–8.

It was a herculean task to maintain vaccine supply, win acceptance of an alien and intrusive procedure, assure the quality of the vaccinations, establish the practice among a colonial population scattered over a vast territory, and introduce it to unreconciled indigenous peoples in remote districts.[60]

Finally arriving in Veracruz on 24 July, Dr Balmis was ill and exhausted. After a month in the enervating climate of the Yucatán, he felt that he might have contracted yellow fever. He was received by Governor Dávila, who handed him a letter from the Viceroy that briefed him on the progress of vaccination. Since the voyage from Sisal was longer than anticipated, Balmis was anxious to propagate lymph from the children he brought from Campeche and was frustrated to find that all the susecptible children had been vaccinated two months earlier. After vaccinating ten 'volunteers' from the garrison, he and his company took the road northwards. Declining to vaccinate in Jalapa and Puebla, as originally proposed, he headed straight for Mexico City. A former chief surgeon in the city's military hospital, Balmis was no stranger to the capital of New Spain. He can be forgiven if he imagined that, as director of the Royal and Philanthropic Vaccine Expedition, he would be returning to the city in triumph. He may have aimed to arrive for the festival of St Hippolytus (13 August) commemorating the conquest of Mexico and celebrating the Spanish monarchy.[61] It would have been a fitting day to deliver the king's gift of the life-preserving vaccine lymph. Arriving on the outskirts of Mexico City on 8 August, he sent a letter to the Viceroy. When there was no immediate response, he breached protocol, entered the city in the evening and pressed on directly to the Viceroy's residence. Far from being the high point of the expedition, there was embarrassment all round.[62]

The relationship between Viceroy Itirrugaray and Dr Balmis was to remain strained. The Viceroy and his medical men were understandably reluctant to have their work in Mexico subsumed in Balmis's grand enterprise. Mindful of his commission, Balmis stood on his dignity and insisted on his need to begin propagating his Spanish strain of vaccine. At his insistence, twelve people were conscripted to undergo the procedure. His supply of vaccine would again have been lost if an official had not rounded up twenty Indian mothers with children by threatening them with fines. According to Balmis, the mothers 'exclaimed loudly that they did not owe anyone anything', accepted the vaccination of their children 'only after a thousand entreaties', and afterwards 'went to the closest apothecary to get an antidote for the poison that had been introduced into their children's arms'.[63] Balmis presented the

[60] Few, *For all humanity*, pp. 178–91.
[61] Linda Ann Curcio-Nagy, *The great festivals of colonial Mexico City: performing power and identity* (Albuquerque, NM, 2004), pp. 78–9.
[62] Smith, 'Real Expedición', 33.   [63] Smith, 'Real Expedición', 35.

Viceroy with his plan for the management of vaccination, including a central vaccination board, with two salaried secretaries, one medical and the other administrative and a set of similarly constituted provincial boards.[64] The Viceroy leisurely sought advice as to its consistency with the arrangements he had made in conformity with the royal edict of May 1803. He evidently wished to maintain his own direct association with vaccination by making it the responsibility of the *Junta de Caridad* (charity board). In his progress through the city in October he gave coins to encourage children to accept the procedure and his wife assisted in the vaccination of hundreds of children in the *barrio* of Santiago.[65] In June 1807, long after Balmis's departure from Mexico, he clarified the administrative arrangements, announcing that the *Junta de Caridad* had approved five vaccine clinics in the capital and that the city's thirty-two mayors were required to deliver one child each a week for vaccination.[66]

Frustrated in the capital, Balmis applied himself to the diffusion of the practice in the provinces. On 18 September, he set out back along the road to Puebla with two recently vaccinated boys. Advised of his coming, the Count de Cadena and Manuel Ignacio Gonzalez del Campillo, the new Bishop of Puebla, joined the civic notables in according him a warm reception. In the cathedral, the bishop called on people to thank God for the blessing that He had given to mankind in the discovery of vaccine and the king who had sent it to them at great cost.[67] Balmis and his assistants vaccinated 230 children the next day and 10,209 more over the following three weeks. He instituted a vaccination board, *La Junta Central Filantrópica de San Carlos de Puebla*, comprising officials, churchmen and doctors.[68] In response to a request for vaccine from the southern city of Oaxaca, Balmis showed statesmanship in asking Dr García Arboleya, the Viceroy's physician, to undertake the mission. During his month in Oaxaca, he vaccinated over 500 children and oversaw the formation of a provincial vaccination board. The Bishop of Oaxaca issued a pastoral letter encouraging vaccination, distributed needles to the parish clergy so that they could take up the practice and offered indulgences to parishioners presenting themselves for treatment. Inspired by García Arboleya, the board sent a surgeon with vaccine among the Mixtec nation in the remote highlands to the west. He was successful in winning their trust and performed 16,983 vaccinations.[69]

[64] For the text, see S. F. Cook, 'Francisco Xavier Balmis and the introduction of vaccination to Latin America. Part II', *BHM*, 12 (1942), 70–101, at 95–101.
[65] *Diario de Mexico*, 1 (October–December 1805), 116.
[66] *Diario de Mexico*, 7 (May–August 1807), 393–6.
[67] Smith, 'Real Expedición', 38–40; *Gaceta de Madrid* (January–June 1805), 496–8.
[68] Smith, 'Real Expedición', 38–40.
[69] Smith, 'Real Expedición', 40–2; *Diario de Mexico*, 2 (1806), 288.

After a brief return to Mexico City, Balmis toured the northern provinces. In Celaya, he adopted a system of vaccinating children in one village to go arm-to-arm with children in another village a week's distance along the road. He divided his forces, sending Gutiérrez with two boys in the direction of Valladolid, pressing on himself to Guanajuato. In late November, Juan de Riaña, the Intendant of Guanajuato, organised a public demonstration of vaccination as he had previously done with variolation. Balmis provided training to the local physicians and, although the authorities did not set up a vaccination board, he felt confident enough in the management of the practice to advise medical men in other towns to seek vaccine and instruction there.[70] In Zacatecas, the civil and ecclesiastical authorities staged an exuberant reception, a thousand children were vaccinated, and a *junta* was established. Early in December, Balmis arrived in Durango, his furthest point north, where he was welcomed by Governor Bonavía, who had sent a report on smallpox inoculation in 1798 to the Royal Academy of Medicine in Madrid.[71] The Governor hosted a demonstration of the new prophylaxis in his house on 9 December, the birthday of Queen María Luisa. Balmis then headed back through Zacatecas, arriving at Querétaro on Christmas Eve.[72]

During his time in Mexico, Balmis was concerned about the fate of the boys who had accompanied him from Spain and the need to recruit others to carry the virus across the Pacific. Soon after his arrival in the capital, he had entrusted them to Viceroy Itirrugaray who was responsible for providing them an education until they were able to look after themselves. Temporarily placed in the *Real Hospicio de Pobres*, they were transferred to the *Escuela Patriótica*, which opened in July 1806. Several of them were subsequently given apprenticeships, but it is not known how any of them fared as adults.[73] To meet the needs of the expedition to the Philippines, the Viceroy instructed each city in the northern provinces to find three boys, either from an orphanage or from families willing to let them go. Balmis authorised Gutiérrez to offer parents up to 100 pesos. On the road back from Durango, he gathered a number of children, including six boys from Zacatecas.[74] In his last month in Mexico, Balmis continued to feel frustrated by a lack of co-operation from the government. Early in February 1805, accompanied by several members of his old team and twenty-six Mexican boys, he finally set sail from Acapulco to Manila.[75]

---

[70] Angela T. Thompson, 'To save the children: smallpox inoculation, vaccination, and public health in Guanajuato, Mexico, 1797–1840, *The Americas*, 49, no. 4 (1993), 431–55, at 445–6.

[71] Smith, 'Real Expedición', 43; Agustín Albarracín Teulón, Luis Maldonada and Susana Pinar, *Catálogo de los Fondos Manuscritos del S. XVIII de la Real Academia Nacional de Medicina* (Madrid, 1996), p. 115.

[72] Smith, 'Real Expedición', 43–7.   [73] Smith, 'Real Expedición', 33–4.

[74] Smith, 'Real Expedición', 42, 44.   [75] Smith, 'Real Expedición', 47–9. See Chapter 13.

Vaccine across the Andes

After the shipwreck, Salvany reached Cartagena on 24 May 1804 and spent two months in the city. Finding some time to convalesce, he performed nine general vaccinations in the city square, trained up some local medical men and clergy, set up a *junta de vacunación* and attempted to infect cattle with cowpox to generate a local supply of vaccine.[76] Setting out again on 24 July, with ten boys under vaccination, he arrived a week later at Mompox, where enthusiasm for the new prophylaxis was so great that he found himself exhausted from the 'great mass of arms extended to receive the good preserver of life'.[77] While Salvany continued by boat down the Magdalena River, Manuel Grajales, his assistant, took an easterly route overland, through Pamplona and Tunja, vaccinating many Indians.[78] At the village of Nares, Salvany was greeted by men from Medellín who had brought two boys to be vaccinated to provide vaccine for the western province of Antioquia.[79] By the time he reached Honda in late October he was very ill. He nonetheless performed 2,000 vaccinations and set up a vaccination board. Although his life was in danger for a time, he recovered sufficiently to resume his arduous journey. A week before Christmas 1804, he arrived at Santa Fé de Bogotá to a hero's welcome. Antonio Amar y Borbón, Viceroy of New Granada, gave him a splendid reception and the Archbishop of Santa Fé de Bogotá held a thanksgiving service with a sermon in praise of King Carlos, the philanthropic expedition, and the new prophylaxis.[80]

In few parts of the Spanish empire was the vaccine expedition so long or keenly anticipated. Smallpox had wrought havoc in the viceroyalty, with a virulent epidemic reaching its peak as recently as the spring of 1802. An account of the desperate state of affairs and appeal for assistance, sent by the former Viceroy in June 1802, was long in transit, but encouraged the new Viceroy to attempt to introduce vaccine and provided the crucial catalyst for organisation of the royal expedition.[81] On arrival in Bogotá, Salvany rapidly set to work propagating vaccine lymph and found people were well primed to partake of its blessings.[82] In the viceregal capital, too, he paused to reflect on

---

[76] Warren, *Medicine in Peru*, pp. 95–6.

[77] Renán Silva, *Las epidemias de viruela de 1782 y 1802 en el virreinato de Nueva Granada. Contribución a un análisis histórico de los procesos de apropiación de modelos culturales* (Medellín, Colombia, 2007), pp. 185–7.

[78] Andrea Catalina Gutiérrez Beltrán, 'Las epidemias de viruela en la ciudad de Tunja: 1780–1810: La junta de vacuna', Unpublished thesis, Instituto Colombiano de Antropología e Historia, Bogotá, 2007, pp. 24–5.

[79] Susana María Ramírez Martín, *La mayor hazaña médica de la colonia. La Real Expedición Filantrópico de la Vacuna en la Real Audiencia de Quito* (Quito, 1999), pp. 386–7.

[80] Warren, *Medicine in Peru*, p. 98; Ramírez Martín, *La mayor hazaña médica*, p. 388.

[81] Ramírez Martín, *La mayor hazaña médica*, pp. 194–5.   [82] Warren, *Medicine in Peru*, p. 98.

the achievements of his expedition. According to his records, he had completed 56,237 vaccinations since his arrival in Cartagena, excluding the innumerable vaccinations performed by the practitioners he had trained or to whom he had supplied vaccine.[83] He prepared rules for the conservation of vaccine in the viceroyalty with some customisation of Balmis's plan. Rather than instituting a central vaccination board, he assigned the relevant tasks to the newly constituted *Junta de Sanidad* which was responsible for public health.[84]

In early March, Salvany and his party set out on the gruelling journey across the high Andes to Quito. Salvany took the westerly route, backtracking through the province of Chocó before heading south to Popayán. Grajales traversed paths along the eastern flank of the Andes so hazardous that at times he and his party had to be carried on the backs of Indian porters. Spitting blood from a raging tubercular infection, Salvany struggled into Popayán, where the expedition's arrival was celebrated with fireworks and other festivities. News of smallpox in and around Quito forced him to take to the road again after a few days. On 16 July, he was met on the outskirts of the city, close to La Mitad del Mundo, on the Equator. The reception was again exuberant, with the boys under vaccination embraced by the local children. In the capital of the *audiencia* of Quito (now Ecuador), Salvany and his colleagues allowed themselves two months to recover, during which time they oversaw the foundation of a central vaccination board and the extension of the practice in the province.[85] Setting out in mid-September on the road to Lima, Salvany arrived in Cuenca on 12 October. If it was not, at a mere 2,500 metres, literally the high point his expedition, it proved so figuratively. A thanksgiving service set the scene for three days of celebration, including bullfights, a masked ball and a firework display. Over the following week, he presided over the vaccination of 7,000 people, making a total of over 100,000 vaccinations since leaving Bogotá. In addition to securing Indian muleteers and children to continue the mission, he found a disciple in Lorenzo Justiniano de los Desamparados, a Bethlehemite friar, who dedicated several years to the task of spreading the vaccination gospel in remote districts of the Andean cordilleras.[86]

As he descended the Andes, Salvany found the climate hot and fetid. His health worsened and his nerves were on edge. Entering the viceroyalty of Peru, he found less enthusiasm for the expedition. At Piura, he was dismayed to receive a letter from the Marquis de Avilés, Viceroy of Peru, reporting that the new practice had begun in Lima with vaccine sent from Buenos Aires.[87]

---

[83] Díaz de Yraola, *La vuelta al mundo de la expedicion de la vacuna* (Sevilla, 1948), p. 72; Ramírez Martín, *La mayor hazaña médica*, p. 389.

[84] Ramírez Martín, *La mayor hazaña médica*, p. 388.

[85] Díaz de Yraola, *Vuelta al mundo*, pp. 74–5.   [86] Díaz de Yraola, *Vuelta al mundo*, p. 75.

[87] Warren, *Medicine in Peru*, pp. 99–100.

Salvany, who had now vaccinated more people than anyone else in the world, naturally doubted that the practice in Peru was well founded. Pressing on to Trujillo, he was left stranded by his muleteers and then ran into serious trouble with the indigenous people. Initially the villagers around Chocope hailed him as the emissary of King Carlos bringing the blessed anti-pox to 'make them immaculate'. Disappointed by the simplicity of the procedure, they were soon denouncing him as the Antichrist. Salvany beat a hasty retreat to avoid injury or worse.[88] Hearing reports of smallpox elsewhere in northern Peru, he headed back along the coast to Lambayeque and then inland to Cajamarca. The ceremonies with which he was welcomed at Cajamarca included the recitation of a *loa* or poem celebrating the wonders of vaccine and some traditional Indian dances.[89] Circling back to Trujillo, he met up with colleagues who had been vaccinating in outlying districts. In the town itself, the expedition had to resort to bribery to find children to preserve the supply of vaccine. Though he attributed the lack of cooperation to the apathy of local officials, Salvany must have been concerned that the civil and medical authorities in Peru no longer regarded his mission as necessary.

Brazil and the Southern Viceroyalties

The government and medical establishment in Peru had considerable experience in the management of smallpox. From the late 1770s, there was growing recognition of the utility of variolation but also the danger of it's spreading the contagion.[90] During the epidemic of 1802, reports of the success of vaccination in Europe made the risks involved in variolation less tolerable. According to Humboldt, who visited Lima at this time, there was considerable local interest in cowpox, not least in a report of a slave on the estate of the Marquis of Valleumbroso who attributed his insusceptibility to smallpox to a disease he had caught milking cows in the Cordillera of the Andes. The arrival of some vaccine on a ship from Spain in November 1802 prompted an unsuccessful attempt to propagate it at Callao by Dr José Hipólito Unanue, Lima's leading physician.[91] In 1803, a merchant of Lima allegedly went to some trouble and expense in Cádiz to acquire vaccine, recruit twenty-four orphans and hire a practitioner to vaccinate them in succession on a voyage to Peru, but gave up on his scheme when he heard that the king planned to make 'this inestimable project a royal one'.[92]

---

[88] Díaz de Yraola, *Vuelta al mundo*, pp. 76–7; Warren, *Medicine in Peru*, p. 101.
[89] Díaz de Yraola, *Vuelta al mundo*, pp. 77–9; Warren, *Medicine in Peru*, pp. 102–3.
[90] Warren, *Medicine in Peru*, pp. 81–6.
[91] Humboldt, *Essai politique*, 1, pp. 68–9; Warren, *Medicine in Peru*, pp. 86–7.
[92] Warren, *Medicine in Peru*, p. 106.

The first of the initiatives that led to the advent of vaccination in the southern viceroyalties of Spanish America began with Dr Barboza, an enterprising physician based in Brazil. In October 1802, the Portuguese Minister of the Navy and Colonies recommended the introduction of the new prophylaxis in Brazil, but nothing was achieved until Barboza went to England in 1803 and obtained samples of vaccine. Making use of them in Lisbon, he set out for Brazil with newly propagated lymph. Finding it inert on arrival in Bahia, he proposed a scheme by which local boys were to be sent to Lisbon for vaccine and then vaccinated successively on the return voyage. With the Governor of Bahia's approval, Francisco Caldeiro Brant, a wealthy landowner, made seven slaves available for this purpose in 1804. On their return in late December, Barboza put the last of the vaccinees arm-to-arm with Brant's son and other children. In a letter to Jenner on 26 January 1805, Barboza reported that he subsequently vaccinated some 700 people in the Governor-General's palace and intended to distribute vaccine more widely.[93] Vaccination was soon established in Rio de Janeiro, the capital of Brazil, and the Governor-General appointed Barboza to oversee the practice. Antonio Machado Carvalho, a Portuguese merchant, saw the value of vaccinating the thirty-eight slaves he was taking to market in the Spanish viceroyalty of Rio de la Plata and recognised the opportunity to use them as a means of introducing vaccine. The routine notice of the arrival of his frigate *La Rosa del Rio* in Montevideo on 5 July was accompanied by the announcement of the availability of the new prophylaxis. In the following weeks, 200 people were vaccinated in and around the town.[94]

The Marquis of Sobremonte, Viceroy of Rio de la Plata, who had urged the Council of Indies to send children under vaccination directly to Buenos Aires, was delighted at the news.[95] A female slave under vaccination was brought from Montevideo to the viceregal capital and, as promised, was granted emancipation for being the means of saving many lives.[96] On 2 August 1805, the Viceroy presided over the vaccination of twenty-two children. Over the following months, Dr Argerich offered to vaccinate the poor of the city; Saturnino Segurola, the Dean of the Cathedral, preached sermons in support of vaccination; and Dr Gorman published a tract explaining the practice.[97]

---

[93] *MPJ*, 14 (June–December 1805), 512–13; Baron, *Life*, 2, p. 10; Alden and Miller, 'Out of Africa', 211–12.

[94] Jose Luis Molinari, 'Introducción de la vacuna en Buenos Aires', *Azul. Revista de ciencias y letras*, December 1930, 14–17.

[95] Molinari, 'Introducción en Buenos Aires', 14.

[96] Diego Barros Arana, *Historia jeneral de Chile*, vol. 7 (Santiago, 1886), p. 269.

[97] Molinari, 'Introducción en Buenos Aires', 17–19; Pedro L. Luque, 'Apuntes históricos sobre epidemología Americana, con especial referencia al Rio de la Plata: continuación', *Revista de la Universitad Nacional de Córdoba*, 28 (1941), 249–72, at 256–7.

Meanwhile Viceroy Sobremonte set his mind to measures to extend vaccination throughout the viceroyalty. The presence in Buenos Aires of the president-elect of Cuzco, Francisco Muñoz, proved fortuitous. He offered to cover the costs of making vaccine available in the High Andes by vaccinating his slaves successively on the journey home.[98] The Viceroy also dispatched vaccine to the captaincy-general of Chile. By September, it was in use in Santiago, where Brother Chaparro, active in inoculation since the 1760s, took up the new practice with surprising vigour.[99] The Governor of Concepción in Chile, who received vaccine from Santiago, sent a sample further south to the Governor of Valdivia.[100] Merchant ships and whalers likewise brought vaccine around Cape Horn.

In the last quarter of 1805 the medical men in Lima were expecting the delivery of vaccine from sleek frigates from the south rather than from the lumbering expedition from the north. Viceroy Sobremonte probably played a direct role in sending vaccine to Peru.[101] In September 1805, when a ship from Buenos Aires arrived at Callao with a package of vaccine matter dried between glass plates, Pedro Belomo, the medical officer at the port, knew what he needed to do. His persistence and skill elicited a genuine vaccine response on the arm of a boy named Cecilio Cortez. Dr Unanue and his colleagues were soon able to attest the inauguration of vaccination in Lima. It was the occasion of patriotic celebration in the Peruvian capital, not least as it could be presented as independent of metropolitan initiatives. The *cabildo* (town council) of Lima awarded Belomo a lucrative post and granted Cecilio Cortez an annuity of 100 pesos until he reached twenty-five.[102] In November, Viceroy Avilés announced that the medical men had made solid progress in establishing vaccination and were effectively combatting 'the ignorance and malice of those who would like to discredit it'.[103]

Entering Lima on 23 May 1806, six months later, Dr Salvany found himself in a similar situation to Dr Balmis in Mexico City. The authorities went through the motions of welcoming him, but expressed the view that his mission was no longer necessary as the *cabildo* 'had already done as much as the expedition could do'.[104] Needless to say, Salvany was not impressed by his reception and the lack of respect for the royal expedition. Though he acknowledged the work of the local physicians, he believed that it was his duty to confirm or otherwise the quality of the vaccine, the validity of the vaccinations and the adequacy of arrangements for maintaining the practice.

---

[98] Molinari, 'Introducción en Buenos Aires', 24–5.

[99] Barros Arana, *Historia de Chile*, 7, p. 271.

[100] Díaz de Yraola, *Vuelta al Mundo*, pp. 79–80.   [101] Warren, *Medicine in Peru*, p. 243, n.1.

[102] Warren, *Medicine in Peru*, pp. 78–9.   [103] Warren, *Medicine in Peru*, pp. 104–5.

[104] Díaz de Yraola, *Vuelta al Mundo*, p. 81.

He received reports of failures and observed the crass commercialisation of the practice. Some charlatans were advertising, at an inflated price, supposedly superior vaccine soaked in strips of English taffeta. At odds with the medical men and the civic authorities in Lima, Salvany appealed to Viceroy Avilés. Torn between his loyalty to the creole establishment and his obligation to assist the expedition, the Viceroy listened to Salvany's concerns and approved his scheme for a central board. The *audiencia* appointed Salvany as director and José Manuel Dávalos, a doctor active in smallpox prophylaxis, and Pedro Belomo as its medical consultants.[105] It was not until after a new Viceroy's arrival in August, however, that the *Junta* was properly established and Salvany could begin work.[106] Even then, the city council asserted its influence to secure the appointment of Dávalos and Belomo to manage the practice in the city. Increasingly in poor health and under a great deal of stress, Salvany behaved intemperately, making mistakes as well as enemies. His colleague, Grajales, caused offence by his harsh response to a mother whose child had an adverse reaction to vaccination and who had to be bribed not to agitate against the practice. It must have been galling for members of the expedition to be reminded by local officials 'to treat infants and their families with softness and love, to prevent them becoming exasperated before knowing the benefit they will receive'.[107]

During his time in Lima, Salvany at least received one honour. The University of San Marcos awarded the Catalan surgeon an honorary degree in medicine. In his discourse at the ceremony in November 1806, Professor Unanue praised the royal expedition and lauded the expertise and dedication of Salvany.[108] Outside the halls of academe, though, unseemly power games continued. In preparing for his onward mission, Salvany found that the authorities were in no hurry to assist him with the boys and equipment he needed. In turn, he delayed in responding to the board's request to leave behind a supply of the expedition's vaccine. Feeling that the medical men in Lima had made little effort to make vaccination available outside the capital, he resolved to continue his philanthropic enterprise in the provinces.[109] Setting out in January 1807, he experienced many trials, including desertions, loss of vaccine and sickness and apathy towards prophylaxis. After resting in Chincha, he resumed his southerly progress, often meeting incomprehension, fear and outright hostility. The Indians around Ica heard rumours that he was rounding up infants 'to take and populate an island,

[105] Warren, *Medicine in Peru*, p. 107.   [106] Díaz de Yraola, *Vuelta al Mundo*, pp. 83–5.
[107] Warren, *Medicine in Peru*, pp. 111–12.
[108] *Actuaciones Literarias de la Vacuna en la Real Universidad de San Marcos de Lima* (Lima, 1807), pp. 30–9.
[109] Warren, *Medicine in Peru*, p. 108.

which was so far away that they had to be all small'. Women fled with their babies to the hills and local officials and priests found it difficult to persuade them to return to have their children vaccinated. In September, however, Salvany received a hearty welcome in the city of Arequipa. Remote from and neglected by Lima, the local officials and practitioners enthusiastically supported the mission. Over two months he toured the villages of the district and vaccinated thousands of inhabitants. His visits were accompanied by shouts of 'viva', the ringing of bells and other expressions of 'the happiness that reigned among them for considering themselves freed from the destructive epidemic'.[110]

By the end of 1807, Salvany was again seriously ill. He instructed Grajales to travel by boat to Chile to inspect the progress with vaccination. After a slow start in the last months of 1805, a serious smallpox epidemic had given new impetus to the practice in the province, with Bernardo O'Higgins accepting the offer of a public-spirited merchant to take on the cost of promoting vaccination. Prior to the arrival of Grajales he oversaw some 7,600 vaccinations, but Grajales was able to assist in embedding the new prophylaxis and won the lasting regard of the Chileans.[111] In the meantime Salvany set his course inland, proposing to climb back upwards through Arequipa, traverse the high plateau of modern Bolivia and return home through Buenos Aires. His increasingly serious tubercular condition led him on arrival at Arequipa to petition the Spanish crown to be relieved of his commission and given an administrative position in La Paz by which he might support himself. In the meantime he held to his arduous course, pausing at Puno to convalesce on the shores of Lake Titicaca. In La Paz, he continued his work through 1808, sending plaintive letters to a government that no longer existed. The last letter that survives is dated March 1809. Salvany died, still in his mid-thirties, in Cochabamba in July 1810. By this stage, more than three years after his return to Spain, Balmis was back again in Mexico. After a further four years building the practice in Chile, Grajales returned to settle in Peru in 1812. The Spanish Royal and Philanthropic Vaccine Expedition had finally come to an end.

Imperial Beneficence and Creole Agency

The king of Spain's Royal and Philanthropic Vaccine Expedition played a central role in bringing vaccination to the Caribbean and Central and South America. Designed to generalise a procedure developed in England, it drew on practices and initiatives in Britain and France. It is likely, too, that the

---

[110] Warren, *Medicine in Peru*, pp. 113–14.   [111] Barros Arana, *Historia de Chile*, 7, pp. 272–7.

government took some notice of the Russian vaccine expedition, approved in spring 1802, which involved an itinerant team of medical men, the use of children to transmit vaccine, the enlistment of provincial governors to support the expedition and the establishment of committees to maintain the practice afterwards. The commonalities reflect common problems and forms of governance. Both Spanish and Russian rulers were seriously concerned about smallpox, faced similar challenges in extending vaccination over vast territories and were heavily reliant on co-opting local elites to implement their policies. Especially notable is the common concern to project images of paternalist beneficence and philanthropy. The use of the hitherto little-used epithet '*filantrópica*' to describe the Spanish expedition may have been inspired by Russian example. In April 1803, the *Gaceta de Madrid* reported the amalgamation of several Russian agencies into 'one named *Filantrópica*'.[112] It may have been known in Spain, too, that in Russia a Medical-Philanthropic Committee, established in May, assumed responsibility for the vaccination programme.[113] A further indication of Spanish awareness of Russian influence is a poem written in honour of the *Junta central de la vacuna* in Puebla, Mexico, that appears to credit Tsar Alexander, 'the Solomon of the North', with the institutional innovation.[114]

In its grand ambition, the Spanish vaccine expedition, whose aim was to carry vaccine around the world and establish vaccination through an empire on which the sun never set, was in a league of its own. In explaining his needs in June 1803, Dr Balmis stressed his zeal to bring about an expedition so glorious that it would be envied by all nations.[115] The Spanish Crown committed central funds for the salaries of Balmis and his team and the preliminary needs of the expedition and instructed the colonial governors to pay for its local expenses. From the outset, King Carlos IV was closely identified with the enterprise. In *Venezuela Consolada*, Bello hails King Carlos and asks what more precious monument can there be than to have 'his name stamped with indelible letters on the loving hearts of my children'.[116] The boys recruited to carry vaccine across the Atlantic and Pacific were given smart uniforms with the royal insignia. The insignia on the uniforms of the boys from Mexico also included the inscription 'Dedicated to María Luisa, queen of Spain and the Indies'.[117] The vaccine expedition projected an image of royal beneficence to a population, creole and indigenous, that generally saw metropolitan Spain as

[112] *Gaceta de Madrid* (1803), 305.
[113] Adele Lindenmeyr, *Poverty is not a vice. Charity, society and the state in Imperial Russia* (Princeton, NJ, 1996), pp. 104–5.
[114] *Diario de Mexico*, 7 (September–December 1807), 351–2.
[115] Perigüell and Añón, *En el nombre*, p. 108.   [116] Perigüell and Añón, *En el nombre*, p. 185.
[117] Smith, 'Real Expedición', 44.

remote, exploitative and unconcerned about their welfare. More generally, it sought to show the capacity of the imperial state to advance the cause of humanity. In the late eighteenth century, Spain sponsored several scientific expeditions, notably the Malaspina expedition of 1789–94, that laid claim to global standing as a modern state seeking to advance knowledge for the benefit of all mankind. In his eulogy of the vaccine expedition in Tenerife, the Marquis of Casa Cagigal associated it with such enterprises and pointed out that, while England and France seemed bent on war, Spain was seeking to promote humanitarian causes.[118]

The focus on the vaccine expedition, however, arguably places too much emphasis on the imperial and metropolitan initiative. In the Hispanic world, as elsewhere, there is some need to challenge and reverse assumptions of colonial backwardness and dependency.[119] Experience with smallpox and expertise in prophylaxis were as great, if not greater, in Spanish America as in metropolitan Spain. Dr Flores, the author of the first plan for the vaccine expedition, was a native of Guatemala, who had organised large-scale immunisation campaigns. If vaccination made earlier headway in British spheres of influence, it became a topic of high interest in Spanish America remarkably early. Francisco Zéa, a botanist from New Granada, who observed the early trials of vaccine in Paris in 1800, was possibly the first to suggest to the Minister of Grace and Justice that it be sent out to the New World.[120] The history of vaccination in Latin America reveals networks of information, initiative and activism in regard to the new prophylaxis prior to and independent of the royal expedition. The Economic Society of Havana offered a prize for the first person to make vaccine available.[121] The authorities in New Granada believed that it was their lobbying in 1802 that ensured the crown's commitment to the expedition. Viceroy Iturrigaray evidently felt that he and his physicians had the new prophylaxis well in hand before Balmis's arrival. The creole establishment in Peru was likewise proud of its record of self-reliance in the management of smallpox and its success in introducing vaccination independently of the Spanish initiative.

The medical men active in vaccination in Latin America were certainly not passive recipients of metropolitan expertise. Many of the prominent physicians – Romay in Cuba, Esparragosa in Guatemala and Unanue in Peru – were born and educated locally. The two who asserted creole authority over the practice in Lima, Belomo and Dávalos, reflect some of the

[118] García Nieto and Hernández, 'La vacuna en Canarias', 158.
[119] Jorge Cañizares-Esguerra, *How to write the history of the New World: histories, epistemologies, and identities in the eighteenth-century Atlantic world* (Stanford, CA, 2001).
[120] *Rapport du Comité central* (1803), pp. 47–8.   [121] Sánchez, *Romay*, pp. 84–9.

complexities of identity. Though born in Spain, Belomo was rapidly accorded the status of a creole hero. As his African ancestry prevented him enrolling at the University of San Carlos (Lima), Dávalos obtained his medical degree at Montpellier, but racial discrimination in his native land did not make him any less a patriot.[122] Creole medical men were often more conversant with the latest ideas from Europe north of the Pyrenees and from the United States than their counterparts in Spain. As early as 1804, Dr Romay was circulating information derived from De Carro in Vienna about the successful use of vaccine crusts in vaccination.[123] Furthermore, conditions in the New World gave more scope to make new observations, conduct experiments, adapt policies and practices to local circumstances and indeed devise new therapies, sometimes drawing on indigenous knowledge and local ingredients.[124] The problems inherent in obtaining and maintaining viable vaccine meant that the search for cowpox in Spanish America was more persistent than in Spain. Several reports of cowpox in Mexico were confirmed by Balmis and his colleagues.[125]

There was a broader community of interest in the new prophylaxis. In Havana, the Economic Society brought together a diverse group of men who regarded themselves as enlightened and patriotic and sought to advance the colony through the diffusion of knowledge and new ideas. In other major towns, there were similar groups who helped sustain, with some easing of censorship, a small but fragile public sphere.[126] Newspapers helped to advance the new prophylaxis. The *Gaceta de Guatemala* began including notices on cowpox, stimulating interest and allaying concerns, a year or so before its arrival in the colony.[127] The *Diario de Mexico* reported the charitable endeavours of the Viceroy and Vicereine in promoting vaccination, monthly tallies of the numbers of people vaccinated in the parish of San Miguel and details of the Viceroy's plan for the management of the practice in the capital.[128] If new ideas and political turmoil were beginning to

---

[122] José R. Jouve Martín, *The black doctors of colonial Lima: science, race, and writing in colonial and early republican Peru* (Montreal, 2014), pp. 62–3.

[123] Romay, *Vacuna en Cuba*, p. 23, n.8.

[124] Martha Few, 'Circulating smallpox knowledge: Guatemalan doctors, Mayan Indians and designing Spain's smallpox vaccination expedition, 1780–1803', *British Journal for the History of Science*, 43 (2010), 519–37, at 525–6.

[125] Smith, 'Real Expedición', 43–7.

[126] Jordana Dym, 'Conceiving Central America: a Bourbon public in the *Gazeta de Guatemala* (1797–1807)', in Gabriel Paquette (ed.), *Enlightened reform in Southern Europe and its Atlantic Colonies, c. 1750–1830* (Farnham, UK, 2009), pp. 99–118.

[127] Smith, 'Real Expedición', 50.

[128] *Diario de Mexico*, 1 (October–December 1805), 116; *Diario de Mexico*, 4 (September–December 1806), 28, 132, 152, 188, 227–8, 263, 303–4, 348, 426, 462; *Diario de Mexico*, 7 (May–August 1807), 393–6.

create fissures in the creole elite between those who feared change and those who sought to promote it, vaccination generally proved a unifying cause. In vaccination, there was always scope for subaltern agency. Fear of smallpox and opposition to quarantine measures disposed many people to vaccination, at least when contagion threatened.[129] Mothers as well as fathers informed themselves of the advantages of the new method. María Bustamente's decision to have her child vaccinated in Puerto Rico won her the prize for introducing vaccine to Cuba.[130]

The clergy were best placed to promote the practice among people who were illiterate and had little reason to trust their masters. In his plan for the expedition, Dr Flores recommended that the clergy sanctify the procedure with prayers and indulgences, require godparents to bring the children back six months after baptism for vaccination, keep a register of vaccinations and, when necessary, perform the operation themselves.[131] The Catholic Church in Latin America played an even larger role in the promotion of the new prophylaxis than in Europe. In Cuba, the Bishop of Santiago de Cuba invited Dr Romay to offer vaccination to the young people who flocked to his palace from across the island for confirmation ceremonies. By this means, he wrote in 1804, they would return home protected from a destructive illness and fortified for their spiritual progress.[132] Born in Mexico, Bishop Campillo of Puebla wrote and published a pastoral letter promoting vaccination.[133] At his consecration the week before Balmis's arrival, he presented vaccine as a blessing of God, revealed by the 'immortal Jenner', a friend of humankind, and sent as a gift from King Carlos 'as a true father' to his 'beloved vassals' for their 'health, preservation and happiness'. Addressing his clergy, he assured them that it had been found to be simple, useful and effective and by no means against divine law, exhorted them to promote and facilitate it and informed them that they might be required to practise it themselves just as, *in extremis*, they were obliged to perform Caesarean sections, albeit the latter obligation being stricter as the spiritual welfare of the unbaptised infant was at stake.[134] The curate of the parish of Acaxochitlán was sufficiently enthused to write a poem in praise of vaccination for recitation at a meeting of the vaccination committee.[135]

---

[129] Ramírez, 'Oaxaca's smallpox', 231–5.   [130] Sánchez, *Romay*, p. 237, n.147.
[131] Smith, 'Real Expedición', 13–14.   [132] Romay, *Vacuna en Cuba*, pp. 14–15.
[133] Juan Pablo Salazar Andreu and Mariana Durán Márquez, 'Manuel Ignacio González de Campillo (1803–1813): el obispo del discurso antiinsurgente', *Rivista Mexicana de Historia del Derecho*, 29 (January–June 2014), 101–19; *Exhortacion que el ilustrísimo señor Don Manuel Ignacio Gonzalez del Campillo, obispo electo de La Puebla, hace á sus diocesanos para que se presten con docilidad á la importante práctica de la vacuna* (México, 1804), p. 16.
[134] *Exhortacion*, p. 25. For context, see José G. Rigau-Pérez, 'Surgery at the service of theology: postmortem Cesarean sections in Puerto Rico and the royal cedula of 1804', *Hispanic American Historical Review*, 75 (1995), 377–404.
[135] *Diario de Mexico*, 7 (September–December 1807), 351–2.

In the viceroyalty of the Rio de la Plata, Severino Segurola was not only an advocate of vaccination, cajoling and even bribing the poor to be vaccinated, but also a mainstay of the practice until the government's establishment of a vaccine institute in 1822.[136]

Vaccination cut across racial lines. In introducing vaccination among the indigenous peoples, the clergy played a crucial role. In parishes with large Amerindian communities and on mission stations, priests and monks were often of mixed descent, familiar with the relevant languages and able to provide leadership on matters relating to the welfare of the community. In Guatemala, Dr Esparrago undertook his own vaccine missions and used priests and monks to extend the reach of his campaigns.[137] Though vaccination involved fewer risks than variolation, it presented the larger challenge of supply of vaccine. Some indigenous people resolutely refused to accept vaccination, resentful and suspicious of the requirements of the system. In his work among non-Spanish-speaking communities in South America, Salvany was greatly assisted by Brother Lorenzo who, in addition to promoting vaccination in the community languages, took up the lancet himself in the villages around Trujillo.[138] There were dangers in the church's promotion of vaccination, not least in presenting it as if it were a sacrament. Acceding to a request to include Chocope in his itinerary, Salvany may have regretted his decision when he learned that the villagers expected 'to be made immaculate'.[139]

The Spanish royal vaccine expedition made a difference. Its announcement in August 1803 prompted mobilisation across the empire. The crown's endorsement and support of vaccination cut through the hesitations and doubts that would have led members of the colonial elite to dither and bicker among themselves. The church hierarchy and lesser officials were certainly well primed to assist the new prophylaxis. While Balmis and Salvany found vaccination already in progress in Havana, Mexico City, Guatemala City and Lima, it should not be assumed that it had been established on sound foundations or that it would have been extended as widely without their stimulus. Even though vaccination had begun in Peru six months before his arrival, Salvany certainly found that there was still a great deal of work to do. The royal expedition offered a model and a body of experience to inspire, provoke and inform creole adaptations. In celebrating the advent of vaccination in Caracas and Lima, Andres Bello and José Hipólito Unanue were fulsome in their praise of King Carlos's beneficence. In his address in Lima, Unanue took

---

[136] Woodbine Parish, *Buenos Ayres and the Provinces of the Rio de la Plata*, 2nd ed. (London, 1852), p. 131.
[137] Smith, 'Real Expedición', 53.   [138] Warren, *Medicine in Peru*, p. 99.
[139] Warren, *Medicine in Peru*, p. 101.

pride, too, in the Spanish achievement in taking vaccine around the world to China.[140] Still, there can be little doubt that the introduction of vaccination in South America depended a great deal on local agency. For many activists in the cause, it was a deeply patriotic undertaking. If the royal vaccine expedition briefly strengthened the bonds of empire it certainly did not secure them. Men like Bello and Unanue, who were to play prominent roles in independent Latin America, were looking to a future based on autonomy and agency not on paternalism and dependency. Vaccination, once embedded, was an emancipatory force.

Vaccination was conducted on quite a large scale in the West Indies, Central America and South America in the first decade of the practice. It has been estimated that Balmis was responsible for some 100,000 vaccinations in New Spain.[141] Long before his death in 1810, Salvany may have given up counting, but his personal tally would have been at least double this figure. Manuel Grajales, Salvany's assistant, who remained active in Chile until 1812, claimed to have vaccinated some 400,000 people. A recent study of the Spanish royal vaccine expedition refers to 'hundreds of thousands' of people vaccinated and rightly regards the achievement as 'colossal' for the time.[142] This estimate, however, does not include the large numbers of people vaccinated in the wake of the expedition, the independent programmes in Cuba, Mexico, Peru and other European colonies, especially British Jamaica and Portuguese Brazil.[143] Overall, it is reasonable to assume a million vaccinations in the West Indies, Central America and South America between 1803 and 1812. While a million people would constitute only a small fraction of the population, it should be borne in mind that many people in the larger cities and towns would have acquired some level of resistance naturally or through variolation in recent epidemics. Furthermore, large-scale vaccination activity in gateway cities like Havana and Veracuz contributed disproportionately to the protection of the inland populations. It is likely enough that there was some loss of momentum in vaccination after the passing of the royal expedition and that there was a breakdown in the administration of the practice as the French invasion of Portugal and Spain in 1807–8 inaugurated two decades of turmoil and conflict in Latin America. Still, vaccination continued on some scale in Lima and other centres.[144] When Balmis returned briefly to Mexico in 1810, he learned from Intendant Riaño that 4,953 people in Guanajuato had been vaccinated since 1804.[145] The relocation of the Portuguese royal family to Rio de Janeiro in

---

[140] *Actuaciones Literarias de la Vacuna*, p. 11.   [141] Smith, 'Real Expedición', 49.
[142] Mark and Rigau-Pérez, 'World's first campaign', 90.
[143] Alden and Miller, 'Out of Africa', 212.   [144] Ramírez Martín, *La salud del Imperio*, p. 199.
[145] Thompson, 'To save children', 452–4.

1811 prompted the establishment of a vaccination commission that vaccinated 102,791 people over the following two decades.[146] Gautemala City showed its commitment to vaccination by commissioning a bust of Jenner to adorn the fountain in city square.[147]

[146] Alden and Miller, 'Out of Africa', 212.
[147] Henry Dunn, *Guatimala, or, the United Provinces of Central America, in 1827–8* (New York, 1828), pp. 154–5.

13   Oceanic Vaccine
The World Encircled

Few men knew the oceans so well as Amasa Delano, mariner and merchant of Duxbury, Massachusetts. He sailed around the world three times, rounding Cape Horn into the Pacific, conducting his main business in Canton (Guangzhou), before heading on westwards. Picking up provisions and trade goods in the Pacific, he was a regular visitor to the Sandwich Islands (Hawaii), where young men were eager to sail with him. In 1801, he took on one young Hawaiian but later found four stowaways. Since he knew the danger posed by smallpox to the islanders, he had all five variolated in Canton, though he found it 'very inconvenient as well as expensive' to see them through the infection. In 1805–6, he was following a similar route and had similar experiences. As he entered the Pearl River early in 1806, however, he found another American ship at anchor that had some kinepox available. The first successful vaccination had taken place in Canton, around October 1805, and over the winter of 1805–6 it had been practised on some scale. Delano's use of the term 'kinepox' raises the possibility that it had been brought directly from America, but the greater likelihood is that it simply reflected American usage. In any event, Delano did not hesitate to use it to inoculate the Hawaiians among his crew and was very satisfied with the outcome. In the narrative of his travels, he paused to advise other captains on long voyages to provide themselves with vaccine, 'which may be easily procured, and preserved in such a manner as to be carried to any part of the world'.[1]

The arrival of cowpox in Canton in 1805 marked its circumnavigation of the globe. Although there had been several unsuccessful attempts by the East India Company to deliver virus from Calcutta and Madras to its factory in Canton, the first vaccine that was successfully used on the Pearl River was brought by Dr Balmis from Mexico through the Philippines to Macao

---

[1] Amasa Delano, *A narrative of voyages and travels in the northern and southern hemispheres: comprising three voyages around the world; together with a voyage of survey and discovery in the Pacific Ocean and oriental islands* (Boston, 1817), p. 393.

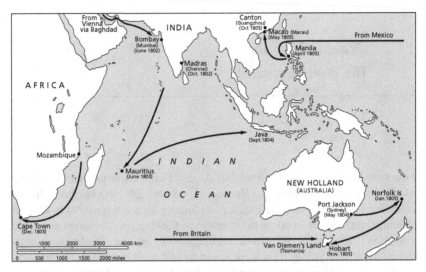

Figure 13.1 Map of the spread of vaccination in the Indian Ocean
and South China Sea

(Macau). Rather remarkably, even as Alexander Pearson, surgeon of the East
India Company, was seeking to establish the new prophylaxis in Canton, the
Russian embassy to China was waiting for permission to proceed to Beijing
and Dr Rehmann was nursing his ambition to introduce vaccine to the
Celestial Empire. More generally, 1805 was an *annus mirabilis* for global
vaccination and more specifically for oceanic cowpox. In the previous two
years, vaccine had been carried from British India into the Indian Ocean.
A French merchant brought it to Mauritius and the French governor made
special arrangements to send it to the Dutch East Indies, then under French
protection. Portuguese slavers used it along the coast of Mozambique and
brought the first viable vaccine to the Cape of Good Hope. From Rio de
Janeiro, where vaccine arrived early in 1805 on the arms of slaves vaccinated
in Lisbon, the practice spread southwards to Buenos Aires and thence to
Chile and Peru. In the meantime, a sample of cowpox had already survived
the long voyage to Sydney in 1804 and samples were subsequently sent to
Norfolk Island and, in November 1805, to the British empire's southern
outpost in Van Diemen's Land (Tasmania).[2] Its arrival in Hobart marked,
for some decades, cowpox's furthest reach from its origins on a dairy farm in
England (Figure 13.1).

---

[2] *HRA, Series III*, vol. 1 (Sydney, 1878), p. 346.

Smallpox in the Southern Latitudes

At the beginning of the eighteenth century, smallpox was still unknown in large parts of the world. Despite the increasing severity and the growing reach of the disease from the late sixteenth century onwards, the southern hemisphere remained largely untouched. Smallpox was neither as contagious nor as fast-moving as is often supposed. It had to pass from one individual to one or more people in close contact and tended to move slowly, along well-beaten paths, from settlement to settlement, needing to find a pool of non-immune individuals to sustain itself.[3] Given the long history of smallpox in Africa, it is telling that it had still not found its way overland to the more temperate lands at its southern tip. It likewise moved relatively slowly through the Indonesian Archipelago and did not reach Australia until the end of the eighteenth century. By this stage, of course, trade and colonisation were linking the world together ever more closely, especially by sea, and setting the stage for a new era in the spread of smallpox. It greatly reduced, too, its dependence on direct communication from person to person. As Dr James Lind wrote in 1761, Europeans 'carried the smallpox to almost all parts of the world, where their ships have opened a trade', pointing out that the infection 'will lie concealed for a long time in clothes, so as to be carried in them from England to the Cape of Good Hope, and even to China'.[4] It is certainly the case that smallpox arrived in southern Africa from European ships before there was any hint of the southward spread of contagion from the interior. The source of the smallpox that appeared around the British colony in 1789 cannot be established with any certainty, but the likelihood is that, as in south Africa, the contagion was brought in European ships.[5]

In Africa, smallpox had been carried over the centuries on caravan routes across the Sahara and on dhows down the east coast. It took hold in the inland kingdoms that arose on the savannah grasslands on either side of the Equator. To the north, the kingdom of Dahomey had long familiarity with smallpox, seemingly spreading from the interior.[6] To the south, smallpox was becoming a regular visitor in the Swahili kingdoms and city-states and a presence around Mombasa and Zanzibar in the 1580s.[7] There were smallpox outbreaks in

---

[3] A. B. Smith, 'Khoikhoi susceptibility to virgin soil epidemics in the eighteenth century', *South African Medical Journal*, 75 (1989), 25–6; Kelton, *Cherokee medicine*, pp. 21–4 and passim.

[4] James Lind, *Two papers on fevers and infection, which were read before the Philosophical and Medical Society, in Edinburgh* (London, 1763), pp. 110–11.

[5] Bennett, 'Smallpox and cowpox', 43–9.

[6] James H. Sweet, *Domingos Álvares, African healing and the intellectual history of the Atlantic world* (Chapel Hill, NC, 2011), pp. 20–1.

[7] Hopkins, *Greatest killer*, p. 169.

Luanda in Portuguese Angola in the 1620s, probably linked with the arrival of slaves from the interior. By this stage, Arab and European slaving and trading enterprises were increasing the disease's severity and assisting its spread. On the eastern seaboard of southern Africa, an outbreak on Kilwa Island in 1775 was attributed to inland foyers of infection.[8] Still, it does not appear that this contagion had spread much further south. The three smallpox epidemics that hit the Dutch Cape Colony and the African peoples living in and around it in 1713, 1755 and 1767 can be attributed to European trade with Asia. Since the first victims in 1713 were East India Company slaves working in the laundry in Cape Town, it is probable that the virus arrived in soiled clothes and bedding and clothes. The disease spread among the Hottentots (Khoikhoi), many of whom sought flight across the mountains and perished in Table Valley.[9] The second epidemic of 1755 followed the arrival of smallpox on Mauritius in 1754.[10] On this occasion, some 2,072 colonists, free blacks and slaves died, along with an unknown number of Khoikhoi. In 1767, the case fatality-rate in the colony itself was 32 per cent. This time, the contagion spread more widely and was probably the source of the epidemic among the Xhosa nation around 1770.[11] In 1792, there was another severe epidemic in Mauritius, again introduced on European ships. Finally, in 1805, after two millennia of smallpox in Africa, expeditioners from Cape Colony encountered smallpox that they believed was coming from the north and not, as usual, from coastal shipping.[12]

Smallpox was long known in Southeast Asia. It appeared in the archipelagos straddling the Equator in the sixteenth century. Arab, Indian and Chinese trade accounts for its early arrival in Java and Luzon, the most populous islands of the Indonesian Archipelago and the Philippines. European commercial and colonial activity added to its profile from the seventeenth century onwards. In the Philippines, Spanish sources record an epidemic that spared neither young nor old on the island of Luzon in 1574 and a serious outbreak in Manila in 1591. The opening of a road from Manila to Cagayan in northeast Luzon in 1739 was followed by smallpox among the Igorot people in 1740–1. A missionary friar observed that 'smallpox was very punctual in causing

---

[8] G. S. P. Freeman-Grenville, *The French at Kilwa Island. An episode in eighteenth-century East African History* (Oxford, 1965), pp. 120–1.

[9] Theal, *History of South Africa*, pp. 59–60; Percy Ward Laidler and Michael Gelfand, *South Africa: its medical history 1652–1898. A medical and social study* (Cape Town, 1971), p. 40.

[10] Adrien d'Epinay, *Renseignements pour servir à l'histoire de l'Île de France jusqu'à l'année 1810* (Île Maurice, 1890), pp. 140, 363–4.

[11] Jeffrey B. Peires, *The dead will arise: Nongqawuse and the great Xhosa cattle-killing movement of 1856–7* (Bloomington, IN, 1989), pp. 31–2.

[12] Henry Lichtenstein, *Travels in Southern Africa in the years 1803, 1804, 1805 and 1806*, transl. Anne Plumptre, 2 vols. (London, 1812 and 1815), 2, p. 248.

general devastation' in the island every twenty years.[13] Smallpox likewise became all too familiar in the Indonesian archipelago in the seventeenth century. A Dutch report from Batavia (Jakarta) in 1618 reported that outbreaks occurred every seven or eight years, with the most recent occasioning the death of a sixth of the population.[14] By the late eighteenth century, smallpox may have been endemic in Java and spreading more widely. Around 1780 there was an epidemic in Sumatra, in which a third of the population reportedly perished.[15] In Sulawesi and the Moluccas, there were severe outbreaks in 1763–4 and 1792.[16] Since fishermen from Makassar were making annual voyages to northwest Australia in search of *trepang* or sea slug and spending months ashore in contact with Aboriginal Australians, smallpox could have made landfall there in the late eighteenth century.[17] In April 1789, barely fifteen months after the establishment of the colony at Port Jackson (Sydney), the British authorities were alarmed to discover that smallpox was spreading among the peoples of the Eora nation living around them and that large numbers of people were suffering and dying from the disease.[18]

By the late eighteenth century, of course, Europeans had acquired greater means to manage and even contain smallpox. Smallpox inoculation was unknown in 1713, when smallpox first hit Cape Town, and in 1755, when it struck again, it was still viewed with some apprehension. In the third major outbreak in 1767, it was put into service and may have reduced mortality. It may have added to the number infected, though, and spread the epidemic more widely.[19] On the Île de France (Mauritius), the first outbreak of smallpox in 1754 prompted Governor Magon to organise the inoculation of 500 slaves over

[13] Linda A. Newson, *Conquest and pestilence in the early Spanish Philippines* (Honolulu, 2009), pp. 17–22, 239.

[14] Hopkins, *Greatest killer*, pp. 112–13; Boomgaard, 'Smallpox, vaccination, Indonesia', 591–3.

[15] Hopkins, *Greatest killer*, p. 124.

[16] Peter Boomgaard, 'Smallpox data and vaccination on Java, 1780–1860: medical data as a source for demographic history', in A. M. Luyendijk-Elshout, G. M. van Heteren, A. de Knecht-van Eekelen and M. J. D. Poulissen (eds.), *Dutch medicine in the Malay Archipelago 1816–1942* (Amsterdam, 1989), pp. 119–32, at 120; David Henley, *Fertility, food and fever: population, economy and environment in north and central Sulawesi, 1600–1930* (Leiden, 2005), p. 275.

[17] Judy Campbell, *Invisible invaders. Smallpox and other diseases in Aboriginal Australia* (Melbourne, 2002), pp. 66–82.

[18] *HRNSW*, 1, part 2 (Sydney, 1892), pp. 298–9; David Collins, *An account of the English colony of New South Wales*, 2 vols. ed. Brian H. Fletcher (Sydney, 1975), 1, pp. 53–4; Watkin Tench, *A complete account of the settlement at Port Jackson, in New South Wales, including an accurate description of the situation of the colony; of the natives; and of its natural production* (London, 1793), pp. 18–19.

[19] Laidler and Gelfand, *South Africa*, p. 57; Hopkins, *Greatest killer*, p. 180; Russel S. Viljoen, 'Medicine, medical knowledge and healing at the Cape of Good Hope: Khoikhoi, slaves and colonists', in Poonam Bala (ed.), *Medicine and colonialism: historical perspectives in India and South Africa* (London, 2014), pp. 41–60, at 46.

the following two years.[20] The advance of *variola* southwards along the Rift Valley and Swahili coast in the eighteenth century was apparently accompanied by the spread of traditional African inoculation practices. In 1775 Jean-Vincent Morice, a French slave-trader operating out of Kilwa Island, heard about smallpox and the use of inoculation in the interior. When some of the slaves he had acquired broke out with the disease, he set about inoculating the rest, congratulating himself in having saved 500 of the 700 he had bought.[21] Across the Indian Ocean, Dr Jan van der Steege made a successful trial of inoculation in Batavia, the headquarters of the Dutch East India Company, in 1779 and inoculated 200 people over the next two years.[22] Further afield, the council of the African Company at Cape Castle, Gold Coast (Ghana), resolved in 1789 to inoculate the slaves and to make the procedure available to local residents requesting it.[23] In Japan in the early 1790s, Dr Keller at the Dutch Factory in Deshima demonstrated the European mode of smallpox inoculation to Japanese medical men, two of whom wrote treatises on the practice.[24] The use of smallpox inoculation during a severe epidemic in Mauritius in 1792 reveals a real concern about its potential to spread the infection. The government's decision to permit the practice met with opposition in some hitherto unaffected districts. One plantation-owner reportedly used for preference a crude version of the Chinese practice of insufflation: he applied variolous matter to a handkerchief and held it over the patient's nose and mouth.[25] It was a risky method, guaranteeing an outcome comparable to natural smallpox. After the abatement of the epidemic, the colonists voted to destroy infective matter rather than preserve it for future prophylactic use.[26]

The First Fleet brought hundreds of soldiers and over a thousand convicts to build a settlement at Sydney Cove in 1788. Accompanied by a contingent of surgeons, it was well managed from a sanitary point of view, but some medical men brought out 'variolous matter in bottles'. Although it was not standard issue in the navy, some surgeons may have learned from experience the advantages of having smallpox matter available to begin inoculating as soon as smallpox threatened. The unusual nature of the expedition in 1788, which included so many men, women and children to establish a colony, may have made it seem prudential. Even in 1792, when he should have known

[20] *Journal de médecine, chirurgie et pharmacie*, 34 (January–June 1770), 135n.; D'Epinay, *Renseignements*, p. 363.
[21] Freeman-Grenville, *French at Kilwa*, pp. 64, 120–1.
[22] Boomgaard, "Smallpox data', pp. 121–2.
[23] *Records relating to the Gold Coast settlements from 1750 to 1874*, ed. J. J. Crooks (London, 1923), pp. 79–80.
[24] Jannetta, *Vaccinators*, p. 21.   [25] D'Epinay, *Renseignements*, p. 363.
[26] Meghan Vaughan, 'Slavery, smallpox and revolution: 1792 in Île de France (Mauritius)', *Social History of Medicine*, 13 (2000), 411–28, esp. 415–18.

better, Philip King, Lieutenant-Governor of Norfolk Island, wrote to Sir Joseph Banks to send smallpox matter to protect the children being born in the colony.[27] In regard to the epidemic around Sydney Cove, it has been claimed that any smallpox brought by the First Fleet would have lost its infective power in the almost two years between the Fleet's departure from England in May 1787 and reports of the first cases around April 1789.[28] There has been a marked preference for the theory that Makassan fishermen introduced smallpox on the coast of northwest Australia, and that it was carried by a chain of infection 4,000 miles across the continent.[29] Although this scenario cannot be entirely ruled out, consideration of the challenges of the climate and terrain in northern and central Australia, and taking into account the seasonal movements of Aboriginal Australians and the traditional pathways and meeting places between nations and clans, make it appear most improbable.[30] Conversely, there is a real possibility that smallpox particles, preserved and stored by an experienced practitioner, could have remained infective over the requisite timeframe. Since the British surgeons had access to smallpox matter in Cape Town in October 1787 and the epidemic among the Aboriginal Australians presumably took months to build, the necessary timeframe is between seventeen and twelve months. It is most unlikely that the British officers and medical men deliberately released smallpox, but it seems very probable that somehow, either through malice or misadventure, the imported smallpox was the source of the epidemic.[31] The mortality was certainly extremely high, with over half of the Cadigal clan of the Eora nation reportedly lost. Although the full horror of the catastrophe can only be imagined, its devastating impact cannot be in doubt.[32]

Planting Cowpox in Cape Colony

The Cape of Good Hope was an important hub in an increasingly networked world. Among the ships at anchor in Table Bay, news, commodities, and

---

[27] Papers of Joseph Banks, series 39, no. 4, State Library of New South Wales, Sydney.

[28] Alan Frost, *Botany Bay mirages: illusions of Australia's convict beginnings* (Melbourne, 1994), p. 202.

[29] Campbell, *Invisible invaders*, passim.

[30] Noel G. Butlin, 'Macassans and aboriginal smallpox: the "1789" and "1829" epidemics', *Historical Studies*, 21 (1984–5), 315–35; Dale Kerwin, *Aboriginal dreaming paths and trading routes. The colonisation of the Australian economic landscape* (Brighton, UK, 2010), pp. 26–34; Craig Mear, 'The origin of the smallpox outbreak in Sydney in 1789', *Journal of the Royal Australian Historical Society*, 94 (2008), 1–22, at 8–13; Christopher Warren, 'Smallpox at Sydney Cove – who, when, why?', *Journal of Australian Studies*, 38 (2014), 68–86, at 75–7.

[31] Bennett, 'Smallpox and cowpox', 48–9.

[32] Grace Karskens, *The colony. A history of early Sydney* (Crows Nest, NSW, 2009), pp. 373–6.

microbes from points east and west were exchanged. Cape Colony protected itself by rigorous quarantine. In the late eighteenth century, too, it sought to isolate itself as much as possible from European power rivalries. The establishment of the Batavian Republic in the Netherlands, closely allied with France, in 1795, however, prompted a British takeover at the Cape. In the late 1790s, the colonists were able to follow news of the cowpox discovery quite closely. Mr Woody, a surgeon *en route* to India in 1800, probably inspired some of them to petition the new governor, Sir George Young, to have samples sent from England.[33] W. S. van Ryneveld, a prominent official of Cape Colony, even wrote to the former governor, Lord Macartney, presenting 'to his humane consideration our sad situation' should smallpox break out and seeking his 'good offices that the cowpox might be introduced here, if found successful in England, as a substitute for small-pox'.[34] Early in 1801, Lady Ann Barnard observed that 'The Doctor [Jenner] will be comforted that his bottled up disease (the fine name of which I forget, but its vulgar name is cowpox) has just arrived in proper preservation', but she did not record whether it worked on the six people inoculated with it.[35] At the end of the year, when a medical man arrived with cowpox, there was a renewed buzz about vaccination.[36] After confessing that 'the idea of being inoculated from an animal makes me shudder', Lady Barnard informed her sister that 'a very few successes will render it general' and the doctor will then be 'esteemed the Guardian Angel of the Cape by preserving the lives of the *Heers* and the beauty of the *Vrouws*'.[37] The experiments again seem to have been unsuccessful.

In the Truce of Amiens in March 1802, Cape Colony was restored to Dutch rule, occasioning further delay in introducing cowpox. General Janssens, the Governor installed by the Batavian Republic in August, was aware of the potential of vaccination but, if he or a member of his party brought vaccine with them, it did not survive the voyage. Vaccination began in Cape Town not with matter brought from Britain or the Netherlands, but from an enterprising Portuguese slave-trader, who acquired it, directly or indirectly, from Goa, then under British military rule.[38] In authorising its use on *Belisario* in October

[33] Laidler and Gelfand, *South Africa*, p. 82.

[34] Helen Henrietta Robbins, *Our first ambassador to China: an account of the life of George, Earl of Macartney, with extracts from his letters, and the narrative of the experiences in China, as told by himself 1737–1806* (London, 1908), p. 450.

[35] *The letters of Lady Anne Barnard to Henry Dundas from the Cape and elsewhere, 1793–1803, together with her journal of a tour into the Interior and certain other letters*, ed. A. M. Lewin Robinson (Cape Town, 1973), p. 259.

[36] Laidler and Gelfand, *South Africa*, p. 82.

[37] Dorothea Fairbridge, *Lady Anne Barnard at the Cape of Good Hope, 1797–1802* (Oxford, 1924), pp. 249–50.

[38] Anon., 'Introducção de vaccina em Goa', *Archivo de pharmacia e sciencas accesorias da India Portugueza*, 2 (1865), 22–4, 43–5.

1803, Captain Domingo Christiadoro may have had no larger purpose than to safeguard the 342 slaves in transit to Brazil. The ship's surgeon evidently vaccinated them in batches, as there were slaves under vaccination when *Belisario* put in at Table Bay in November. Captain Christiadoro assured the health officers that there was no smallpox, only cowpox, on board and offered to make vaccine available to the colony. After Governor Janssens convened a council to consider the captain's offer, Dr Reinier de Clerk Dibbetz, director of the medical hospital, went aboard *Belisario* and confirmed the cowpox. Finding the *Belisario*'s surgeon keen to assist, Dibbetz secured approval for recently vaccinated slaves to be brought to Paarden Island to go arm-to-arm with fifteen slaves from the government's slave lodge. After demonstrating their insusceptibility to smallpox some weeks later, Dibbetz and his colleagues assured the government 'by all that is sacred, that vaccine renders the person immune'. On 12 December, Janssens issued a proclamation that affirmed the value of the new prophylaxis, encouraged all citizens to avail themselves of it and instituted a vaccine commission to maintain a supply of lymph.[39]

On New Year's Eve, the *Kaapsche Courant* reported the acceptance of vaccination by leading burgher families. Van Ryneveld led the way, having himself vaccinated and making his home available to Dr Dibbetz to vaccinate thirty-four others.[40] In January 1805, François Péron, chief naturalist on *Géographe*, part of Baudin's expedition returning from the South Seas, struck up a friendship with Dibbetz. As he had observed vaccination in Paris in 1800 and more recently on Mauritius (Île de France), he took a close interest in the practice and later published an account of its promising start in Cape Town, with the charming detail that Dibbetz presented the Portuguese surgeon with a box of surgical instrument in gratitude for his 'humane exertions'.[41] By the end of January, the vaccine commission boasted some 1,199 successful vaccinations, observing that one in three of them would otherwise have perished when smallpox next struck.[42] It was resolved to open up the practice, initially confined to Dibbetz and his team, to all accredited medical men after further training.[43] Over the first half of 1804, the practice became quite general in Cape Town and in the Platteland. Some 5,000 people were vaccinated in the first six months.[44]

[39] Edmund H. Burrows, *A history of medicine in South Africa up to the end of the nineteenth century* (Cape Town, 1958), pp. 98–99; Laidler and Gelfand, *South Africa*, p. 94.

[40] Burrows, *History of medicine*, p. 100.

[41] Edward Duyker, *François Péron. An impetuous life. Naturalist and explorer* (Melbourne, 2006), pp. 203, 208; François Péron, *Notice sur l'introduction de la vaccine au Cap de Bonne-Espérance* (Paris, 1803).

[42] Laidler and Gelfand, *South Africa*, p. 95.   [43] Burrows, *History of medicine*, p. 100.

[44] E. M. Sandler, 'Lichtenstein's vaccination tour, 1805. Introduction and extracts', *South African Medical Journal*, 48 (1974), 3–15, at 5.

Though Cape Town remained the centre of vaccination, a young physician took the initiative in the second half of 1805 to introduce the practice in the northern borderlands of the colony. A native of Hamburg and a newly minted doctor of medicine, Heinrich Lichtenstein came to the Cape in 1802 as General Janssens's physician and tutor to his son. He first gained experience in using cowpox as surgeon-major of the Hottentot infantry. Appointed in 1805 to visit settlements and missions on the frontiers of the colony and assess the condition of the San [Bushmen] and Khoikhoi in the region, he soon saw the need for vaccination. After crossing the Orange River, he and his party were warned of the presence of smallpox in settlements they were planning to visit, prompting the Khoikhoi servants, fearful of the disease, to desert.[45] The Afrikaners likewise sought to avoid contact with men coming from the settlements and kept 'windward of the missionary camp, that the infection might not be wafted to them through the air'.[46] After examining cases, Lichtenstein confirmed that it was smallpox, but was assured that it was unusually mild, with a case-fatality rate of one in twenty-five. Given the assumption that smallpox was introduced from the coast, he found it significant that the contagion was so 'very far in the interior of the country, among a people with whom the inhabitants of the coast had so little intercourse, [and who] asserted that the malady was brought to them from the north'.[47] On the journey back to Cape Town, he came across many localised outbreaks, meeting one missionary who had 'immediately [variolated] all his people, even his wife, and none of them had the disorder severely'.[48]

By this time, Lichtenstein had written to inform the government of the advance of smallpox, to recommend the use of vaccination 'to preclude, as much as possible, all danger of the disorder rising to any height in the colony', and to offer to go himself 'into the country where there was most danger of the infection being communicated, to recommend this preventative, and inoculate as many as were willing to avail themselves of it'. Prior to reaching Cape Town, he received a supply of vaccine, a commission to 'spread the vaccine inoculation as much as possible among the colonists' and letters requesting local officials to assist his work.[49] Lichtenstein proved up to the task. At the outset, he took care to vaccinate small groups to build up his stock of vaccine. He wrote to two missionaries travelling to Anderson's Institution to request that some boys be sent to him for vaccination so that they could carry the virus back to the missions.[50] In the Roggeveld, he had difficulty in persuading some conservative Boers to accept the practice but claimed some success in

[45] Lichtenstein, *Travels*, 2, p. 224.   [46] Lichtenstein, *Travels*, 2, p. 235.
[47] Lichtenstein, *Travels*, 2, p. 248.   [48] Lichtenstein, *Travels*, 2, pp. 344–5.
[49] Lichtenstein, *Travels*, 2, p. 353.   [50] Sandler, 'Lichtenstein's vaccination tour', 9.

'removing their scruples'.[51] At a settlement on the Tankwa River, they proved a tougher proposition. They were unwilling to pollute their children with animal matter and believed it wrong to tempt Providence.[52] The new prophylaxis, however, gained wide acceptance. The people in the Karoo, Lichtenstein wrote, 'brought their children, their slaves, and their Hottentots, in great numbers to undergo the operation; nay, several fathers of families themselves, with their wives, were inoculated' with cowpox.[53]

The reforming initiatives of Governor Janssens were hampered by a lack of funds, especially after the resumption of the war.[54] In January 1806, a British force invaded Cape Colony and Dr Dibbetz served as an intermediary in negotiating the surrender of the Dutch army. The British regime generally sought to strengthen Dutch initiatives to establish vaccination. Early in 1807, the vaccine commission was given a new legislative foundation, and the old secretary was kept in his post. The Earl of Caledon, the incoming Governor, issued a proclamation endorsing vaccination, requiring all householders in Cape Town to provide details of the vaccination status of members of their households and making provision for the dispatch of vaccine to all parts of the colony. He ordered the distribution of copies of Jenner's instructions and insisted on his method for the storage of vaccine, namely between two plates of glass, one with a slight cavity to contain a drop of lymph. When Caledon's proclamation led to murmuring about infringements of liberties, the government insisted that it was not intended to make the practice compulsory. The proclamation certainly produced results, with nearly 6,000 vaccinations. Even so, it remained a challenge to maintain a supply of good vaccine and make it generally available. In the country districts, there were constant complaints that the vaccine was inert.[55]

Caledon enlisted the missionaries in the enterprise. Mr Kicherer was already offering vaccination at his mission on the Sak River in the north.[56] When the Moravians from the new mission at Baviaanskloof in the eastern Cape came to Cape Town to present a congratulatory address to the new Governor in 1807, they were informed of the government's wish to encourage the practice among the Khoikhoi. They dutifully went to the town hall, where vaccination was in progress, talked to the surgeons and obtained a supply of vaccine. On leaving Cape Town, they vaccinated a Khoikhoi servant who arrived at the mission with 'several very fine pustules'. According to their report, 'our people readily

[51] Lichtenstein, *Travels*, 2, p. 354.   [52] Sandler, 'Lichtenstein's vaccination tour', 13–14.
[53] Lichtenstein, *Travels*, 2, pp. 354–5.
[54] William M. Freund, 'The Cape under the transitional governments, 1795–1814', in Richard Elphick and Hermann Giliomee (eds.), *The shaping of South African society, 1652–1840* (Middletown, CT, 1988), pp. 324–57, at 324–7.
[55] Burrows, *History of medicine*, pp. 100–1; Laidler and Gelfand, *South Africa*, pp. 112–13.
[56] Sandler, 'Lichtenstein's vaccination tour', 14–15.

consented' to the practice. Starting with a hundred people, and then five hundred more, the missionaries succeeded, according to a letter to London, 'with God's blessing ... with all'.[57] The London Missionary Society likewise instituted the practice among the Griqua, a mixed-race people who had settled north of the Orange River. William Anderson, who accepted a smallpox outbreak in his mission station in 1805 as punishment for religious turpitude, regarded the availability of vaccine to avert an 'impending calamity' in 1807 as providential.[58]

The population of Cape Town was then around 15,000 and, though growing, the population of the entire colony was only around 90,000.[59] The smallness of the population, the high number of vaccinations in 1804 and 1807 and the abolition of the slave-trade in 1806 all made it difficult for Cape Town to find sufficient non-immune subjects to maintain the supply of vaccine for the colony at large. The government began to put pressure on families to vaccinate their children in an orderly fashion and a new Vaccine Institute was established in 1811.[60] In March 1812, there was a smallpox outbreak in Cape Town, with a Portuguese slave ship the source of the infection. There were several score cases, mainly among slaves and children of the poor, but no fatalities. The crisis demonstrated the benefits of vaccination and the value of quarantine measures. It also strengthened the case for a more robust approach to promoting prophylaxis. The government instructed the ward-masters to provide a monthly list of births to the office of the fiscal, which would then determine a set quota of children from each ward to be vaccinated at the institute to maintain the supply of lymph. In addition to Cape Town, vaccine depots were maintained at George, Stellenbosch and Graaff-Reinet and the system of registering births and monitoring vaccination was extended to country towns.[61]

Cowpox in the Indian Ocean

In May 1800, Dr Jenner dispatched vaccine to India on the *Queen*, which came to grief on the coast of Brazil. It was one of many unsuccessful attempts to send viable vaccine into the Indian Ocean. Léonard Clair Laborde, chief medical officer on the Île de France (Mauritius) and veteran of the smallpox epidemic in 1792, was especially keen to make a trial of the new prophylaxis. In 1801, the newly appointed chief physician on Réunion brought some

[57] *Evangelical Magazine*, 16 (1808), 138–9.
[58] Thomas Smith, *The history and origin of the missionary societies ... in different parts of the habitable globe*, vol. 2 (London, 1825), pp. 177–8.
[59] Freund, 'The Cape under transitional governments', pp. 329–30.
[60] Laidler and Gelfand, *South Africa*, pp. 113–14.
[61] Laidler and Gelfand, *South Africa*, pp. 114–15.

vaccine to Mauritius, but it proved inert.[62] Laborde wrote directly to Dr Woodville in London, asking him 'to become the benefactor of the colony', but, as he recalled, the war 'rendered communications difficult'. The Truce of Amiens, scarcely honoured in the Indian Ocean, provided only a limited window of opportunity for the transmission of vaccine. By the end of 1802, however, Laborde would have heard of the arrival of cowpox in India. In April 1803, he received both dried vaccine and fresh lymph from a French merchant, who obtained vaccine on threads in Madras and organised the vaccination of a child prior to his departure for Mauritius.[63] Finding both sets of matter serviceable, Laborde propagated sufficient vaccine in the public hospital to distribute samples to colleagues. There was concern when some children exhibited slight fevers, sore throats and minor eruptions, but when the symptoms disappeared with the change of season, 'confidence was unanimously restored'. Laborde was keen to test the value of vaccination, but the island was largely smallpox-free. The arrival of a slave ship with smallpox aboard provided the opportunity for a robust trial. With the ship in quarantine in the Seychelles, Laborde arranged for six vaccinated children to be put on board to eat and drink using the same utensils as the smallpox patients and then to be challenged by variolation. He likewise arranged for the vaccination of forty slaves who had not hitherto fallen sick. The trials conclusively demonstrated the value of vaccination: none of the six children came to harm; none of the forty vaccinated slaves subsequently caught smallpox; and the smallpox outbreak was rapidly extinguished.[64]

During the truce, Napoleon strengthened the military and naval capacity of the Île de France. The new commander, General Decaen, strongly supported Laborde's efforts to establish the new prophylaxis. He arranged for its introduction on Réunion and sought to send it across the Indian Ocean to the Dutch East Indies, then under French military protection. After sending Jan Siborg, the Dutch Governor-General, information on the practice late in 1803, he dispatched slaves under vaccination on *Marengo*, a warship. The initiative, though unsuccessful, inspired M. Gauffré, surgeon-major of the French battalion in Java, to set out for Mauritius in May 1804 with fifteen slave children. After vaccinating the first pair in Mauritius, the infection was maintained on the return voyage to Surabaya by serial vaccination. Once vaccine became available in Java in June, the Dutch authorities organised a trial in which children were vaccinated and then tested by variolation. In September, the

---

[62] D'Epinay, *Renseignements*, p. 442.
[63] Leonard Clair Laborde, 'An account of the introduction of the vaccine disease into the Isles of France and Reunion', *Philadelphia Medical and Physical Journal*, 1, part 2 (1805), 71–5, at 72; D'Epinay, *Renseignements*, p. 457.
[64] Laborde, 'Introduction of vaccine', 71–75.

government formally authorised the practice and instructed Pieter Engelhard, commissioner for native affairs, to make children available to propagate a supply of vaccine.[65] An ambitious programme, in which vaccinated children were taken to go arm-to-arm with children in another district, was soon underway under Gauffré, who was allowed to charge for the procedure. An extant list of 165 vaccinees in Semarang in November details the vaccination of children of Dutch officials, the families of the regent of Pati and other Javanese notables and scores of slaves. There are records of children from Semarang being sent to be vaccinated in Surakarta and a surgeon travelling from Yogyakarta to Surakarta to obtain lymph.[66] By early 1805, the new prophylaxis was established in Batavia (Jakarta) and Governor-General Siberg was able to inform the British governor of Fort Marlborough (Bengkulu), in Sumatra, who had sent some cowpox, that they already had a supply of vaccine from the Île of France, which they were propagating 'with great success'. In seeking to pass on to the Governor-General of British India his gratitude 'for his humane intention' of preserving the people of Java from 'this terrible evil', he proposed that, if in future it should be necessary, he 'would send a small vessel under a flag of truce, with some people of experience in the art of vaccination, to get some fresh matter'.[67]

Between 1803 and 1810, General Decaen stoutly defended the Île de France. The destruction of the French fleet at Trafalgar in 1805 did not diminish the island's strategic importance or the capacity of French privateers to disrupt British communications and trade with the East.[68] He was no less determined to safeguard the island from smallpox. Although the import of slaves provided critical mass for the maintenance of the practice, the interest of slave-owners in vaccinating all their slaves as soon as possible threatened the supply of vaccine. Early in 1806, it proved necessary to import new vaccine. In a set of regulations to address the issue, all residents were obliged to submit lists of dependants, free and slave, with details of their age and immune status. The board of health used the information to determine the number of people to be vaccinated at set intervals and restricted the practice to the surgeon-major in each district, who was required to keep a register of vaccinations. In La Réunion, there was a little more flexibility. Whites and free blacks could be vaccinated in their homes as long as the vaccinations were reported. Slaves, on the other hand, had to be vaccinated in the hospital and returned for inspection and, presumably, to have their vesicles milked to provide vaccine. In a provision that indicates private practice on some scale,

[65] Boomgaard, 'Smallpox, vaccination, Indonesia', p. 122.
[66] Boomgaard, 'Smallpox, vaccination, Indonesia', pp. 122–4.
[67] Shoolbred, *Report 1804*, pp. 63–5.   [68] Fregosi, *Dreams of empire*.

people were forbidden to allow vaccine to be taken from their children or slaves for use by others.[69]

In 1810, the Île de France surrendered after a long siege. The British expeditionary force included a medical man, Dr Scot, who had the task of assuring the continuity of vaccination in the new British colony of Mauritius. Although not an impartial observer, Scot was unimpressed with what he found. The lack of experience of the early vaccinators was doubtless the source of some problems and recent conditions in the colony could not have been conducive to good management. Aghast at the poor state of the records, Scot doubted the validity of many of the vaccinations. Some of his criticisms reflect problems identified by the French themselves in 1806. Though plantation owners had an interest in protecting their slaves, their surgeons tended to make their own calls on when it was convenient to do so. In the towns, whites and the free blacks tended to make their own arrangements. Still, Scot credited the French medical men with a strong commitment to vaccination and found them ready to see his capacity, as an outsider, to override private interests for the public good. Mauritius was evidently one of the most fully vaccinated places in the world. According to a report in 1814, there had been 200,000 vaccinations since 1804. Since the island's population was only around 60,000, the figure cannot be right, though it may include the vaccination of sailors, soldiers and slaves in transit and revaccinations. Still, the new prophylaxis helped to keep the island free from smallpox between 1803 and 1811. The British conquest in 1810 and an influx of soldiers and civilians from India brought contagion in its wake. Though there were many smallpox cases in 1811, including people who had been vaccinated, there were few deaths and the outbreak was rapidly suppressed. The high mortality experienced in 1792 was never repeated. Under British rule, Mauritius continued as an important centre of vaccination. Prior to his departure in 1813, Dr Scot devised a plan which, if implemented, would have made vaccination virtually compulsory. The plantation system, where slaves were replaced by indentured labourers and Indian convicts, helped to maintain a high level of vaccination activity. On several occasions, Mauritius served as a source of vaccine for the British colonies in Australia.[70]

To the Ends of the Earth

The early enthusiasts for cowpox did not neglect the penal colonies of Australia. It was naturally hoped that the initiatives in respect to Cape Colony and

---

[69] *A collection of the laws of Mauritius and its dependencies. Vol. 2. 1803–1810*, ed. John Rouillard (Mauritius, 1866), pp. 400–5.
[70] J. H. L. Cumpston, *The history of small-pox in Australia, 1788–1908* (Melbourne, 1914), p. 140.

India would soon see it introduced there. One man who might have taken the opportunity to convey packets of vaccine was Philip Gidley King. He had gone to Botany Bay with the First Fleet, returned to England in 1790 and then travelled out in 1791 as Lieutenant-Governor of Norfolk Island. The birth of his first son later in the year may have prompted him to ask Banks to send variolous matter to protect children in the event of a smallpox outbreak. With his growing family, he returned to England in 1796 and presumably heard a good deal about Jenner's discovery before setting out in August 1799 to take over as Governor of New South Wales. If he had a packet of vaccine in his trunk, it did not survive the voyage. Soon after his arrival in Sydney, however, he organised an inspection of the local cattle for traces of the disease.[71] The first documented attempt to introduce cowpox to Australia occurred early in 1802. Surgeon John Savage secured vaccine in London, hoping to propagate it in a series of vaccinations on *HMS Glatton*, but was frustrated by the ship's surgeon's refusal to co-operate and the captain's unwillingness to 'take the responsibility on himself' to support the venture.[72] Aware of the failure of Savage's initiative, Governor King included in a dispatch to Lord Hobart in May 1803 a request for vaccine to be sent out as soon as possible, expressing concern about the consequences of the arrival of smallpox for 'the rising offspring of the inhabitants'. Conscious of the logistical problems, he asked that it be 'sent out in every possible way by a whaler, but not to be sent on board until the ship is on the eve of departure from England'.[73] The surgeons on *HMS Calcutta*, setting out late in April 1803, carried vaccine and one of its surgeons, William I'Anson, was trained in the procedure, but there is no record of its use.[74] For a time, there was a prospect that Australia would be supplied from British India. Asked about the feasibility of sending vaccine to Australia by the serial vaccination of children from the Orphan School in Calcutta, John Shoolbred advised Governor-General Wellesley in November 1803 that there were insufficient children for a ten-week voyage but assured him that he would continue his efforts to supply viable vaccine by sending parcels 'preserved in different ways'.[75] As William Paterson, Lieutenant-Governor of New South Wales, gratefully acknowledged in May 1804, Dr Anderson of Madras also made several attempts to send viable cowpox, 'so interesting to the welfare and happiness of this infant colony'.[76]

The arrival of *Coromandel* in Sydney on 4 May 1804, after only 154 days at sea, raised high hopes.[77] It brought a packet of vaccine addressed to Governor

---

[71] *HRA, series I*, 4, pp. 81–2.   [72] Anderson, *Correspondence*, p. 20; *MPJ*, 5 (1804), 537–8.
[73] *HRA, series I*, 4, pp. 81–2.
[74] *HRNSW*, 5, p. 406n.; *HRA, series III*, 1, p. 316; Ring, *Treatise*, 2, p. 944.
[75] IOR/F/4/169/2985, pp. 60–7, OIOC, BL.   [76] Anderson, *Correspondence*, pp. 19–20.
[77] C. Bateson, *Convict ships, 1787–1868* (Glasgow, 1959), pp. 288–9.

King, which was immediately used by Surgeon Jamison to inoculate some soldiers and children. On 12 May, the *Sydney Gazette* was upbeat in reporting the trials and the government's plan to make vaccination publicly available, and reprinted the Royal Jennerian Society's promotional leaflet outlining the advantages of vaccination over variolation.[78] By this stage, however, it was becoming evident that the vaccine had failed. Sitting down to write to Lord Hobart on 12 May, King expressed his disappointment at the latest failure and suggested that the government arrange for the vaccine to be maintained 'by inoculating the healthiest prisoners or children on the passage' and some reward to be offered to the surgeon as 'an incentive to his exertions'. Prior to sending his dispatch, however, he learned that, in addition to the official consignment, John Ring had sent a sample of vaccine 'put up in a different manner' to John Savage, who had used it to successfully vaccinate a child at Parramatta, fifteen miles upriver. He enclosed with his dispatch Chief Surgeon Jamison's letter confirming the success of the trial and affirming that the 'true vaccine pock' had now been propagated in the colony.[79] In the same post, Savage sent a letter to inform Ring of the fortunate outcome, observing that 'he had met with much jealousy' on this account.[80]

With the supply of vaccine secured, Chief-Surgeon Jamison and Surgeon Savage worked to promote and embed the practice. In a letter in the *Sydney Gazette* in June, they offered free vaccination and urged parents to obtain 'so great a blessing' for their children.[81] By August, 400 children had undergone the procedure. Once orphans and children of compliant parents were vaccinated, however, it was hard to find recruits for the procedure. In October, Jamison wrote 'General observations on the Small-pox', the first article on a medical topic published in Australia. He stressed the safety and effectiveness of the procedure. By reference to the smallpox epidemic in 1789, which he attributed to the 'French ships then lying in Botany Bay', and to the severity of smallpox in Cape Colony, he challenged the perception that 'little danger is to be apprehended from [smallpox's] effects in this climate'. Above all, he sought to make clear the real danger that the 'vaccine infection' might be lost. 'Any objection to so innocent an operation in which the very existence of our children is deeply interested', the editor of the *Gazette* added, 'must hereafter be considered as a flimsy absurdity'.[82] By the beginning of 1805, however, the tally of vaccinations had only advanced to 459.[83] Since the maintenance of the vaccine supply required more general and systematic practice, Jamison made a special effort to encourage parents in the countryside to have their children

[78] *Sydney Gazette*, 12 May 1804.   [79] *HRA, series I*, 4, pp. 647–8.
[80] Anderson, *Correspondence*, p. 15.   [81] *Sydney Gazette*, 3 June 1804.
[82] *Sydney Gazette*, 14 October 1804; Cumpston, *Small-pox*, pp. 176–7.
[83] *HRNSW*, 5, p. 429; *Sydney Gazette*, 13 January 1805.

vaccinated, identifying 'convenient places of attendance' where the procedure could be performed.[84]

By this time, Governor King had sent vaccine to Norfolk Island, 1,300 miles into the Pacific, and the new penal colony of Van Diemen's Land, 800 miles to the south.[85] The first initiatives failed. According to David Collins in Hobart, the failure 'must have been occasioned by the weakness of the virus alone', as his surgeon William I'Anson, 'had particularly attended to the practice of inoculating for the cowpox prior to his departure from England'.[86] The delivery of vaccine to the islands was finally achieved by the transport of children under vaccination. At the beginning of 1805 Lieutenant Davis used his own children to bring cowpox 'live' to Norfolk Island.[87] In November, Surgeon McMillan organised a vaccination chain aboard *Buffalo* to take vaccine from Norfolk Island to Van Diemen's Land. His reward for the enterprise was, fittingly, a grant of two cows from the public stock.[88] On 19 December, I'Anson reported that four boys and a girl had been successfully vaccinated in batches in Hobart and that other girls were undergoing the procedure. Among the vaccinees was Robert Hobart May, an Aboriginal orphan who had been found at Risdon Cove after British soldiers had fired on a band of Aboriginal Tasmanians.[89]

The history of vaccination in Australia after 1804–5 was somewhat anticlimactic. The population of New South Wales was small, a little over 10,000. Most of the settlers and convicts were smallpox survivors. Many parents were not disposed to have their children vaccinated. In January 1806, Surgeon Jamison made a last bid for their co-operation, declaring that he had 'used every persuasion and exertion' to establish 'such a laudable system' and that he trusted that 'should all the evils I have pointed out occur one day', 'the public' would agree that 'no reprehensibility can attach to me'.[90] The vaccine brought on the *Coromandel* was lost shortly afterwards. Three years later, in October 1809, Lieutenant-Governor Paterson managed to secure a new supply, perhaps from India. In reporting his successful use of this vaccine, Surgeon Redfern made recommendations that drew on the earlier experience. Assuming the support of people 'in the superior ranks of life', he stressed the need 'to impress on the minds of the poorer orders of people, whose ignorance renders them but too susceptible of the grossest and most unfounded prejudices, the usefulness, safety, and superior advantages of this new plan of inoculation'. He also observed that the supply of vaccine could be best secured 'by inoculating but a few at a time'.[91]

---

[84] *Sydney Gazette*, 8 and 15 December 1805.   [85] *HRNSW*, 5, p. 429.
[86] *HRA, series III*, 1, p. 316.   [87] *HRNSW*, 5, p. 429 n.   [88] *HRA, series III*, 1, p. 345.
[89] *HRA, series III*, 1, p. 346.   [90] *Sydney Gazette*, 19 January 1806.
[91] Cumpston, *Small-pox*, pp. 178–9.

Arms around the World

In 1805, there were moves to bring cowpox to China from all directions. After the introduction of cowpox in Bombay in June 1802, Dr Helenus Scott looked forward to its transmission through India and 'perhaps to China and the whole eastern world'.[92] From 1803, a series of initiatives led to the establishment of the practice in Prince of Wales Island (Penang) and Fort Marlborough (Bengkulu), 2,000 miles to the east, which, it was hoped, would make it possible to deliver viable vaccine to the East India Company factory in Canton. Some British medical men, who professed to believe that infanticide was common in China, sardonically expressed doubts as to whether the Chinese empire would welcome the novel procedure which, if adopted, might necessitate more brutal forms of family limitation.[93] In Penang, though, it was observed that, whereas the Malays 'display too much apathy' in regard to vaccination, the Chinese 'gladly avail themselves of its blessings'.[94] In April 1805, the chief surgeon at Fort Marlborough wrote excitedly to his colleague in Calcutta that he was sending a vaccine scab and, he hoped, a 'living subject' under vaccination on a ship about to depart for China.[95] Although there were several initiatives to deliver vaccine to Canton, none appear to have met with any success. Alexander Pearson, the Company surgeon, who was well-informed about the new prophylaxis, was doubtless frustrated by the failures.

Across the Pacific, Dr Balmis already had his sights set on China. Setting sail from Acapulco in February 1805, he still had in his company several members of his original team, including Antonio Gutiérrez, Francisco Pastor, Pedro Ortega and Isabel Zendara y Gómez, who had looked after the boys from La Coruña. The twenty-six boys recruited in Mexico, almost all aged between five and six, were mainly of Spanish descent, but included two Mestizos and one Indian. The *Magellanes*, the season's only Manila galleon, made a relatively swift nine-week crossing, entering Manila Bay on 15 April, Easter Sunday. Though the arrival of the Manila Galleon always caused excitement, there was no formal welcome for the royal vaccine expedition. Rafael Aguilar, Governor-General of the Philippines, gave priority to attending to the dispatches from Spain that arrived with the *Magellanes*. Prompted by Balmis, he instructed the city council to arrange accommodation, but was otherwise disinclined to fall in with Balmis's timetable, claiming that it was unwise to proceed immediately with a public demonstration of vaccination as,

[92] Keir, *Introduction*, pp. 19–20.   [93] Shoolbred, *Report 1804*, p. 29n.
[94] James Low, *A dissertation on the soil and agriculture of the British settlement of Penang, or Prince of Wales Island, in the Straits of Malacca* (Singapore, 1836), p. 318.
[95] Shoolbred, *Report 1804*, pp. 58–60.

if it did not go well, it could permanently damage the practice's reputation. A week after Easter, he invited Balmis to the palace to vaccinate his five children. Over the following fortnight, he observed the progress of the infection, read about vaccination and satisfied himself as to the success of the procedure. On 16 May, he received Balmis's plan for a *Junta central de la vacuna* and rules for managing vaccination. On 27 May, six weeks after the arrival of the *Magellanes*, Aguilar announced his formal sanction for the practice, reporting that over 6,000 adults and children had already been vaccinated. He appointed Dr Bernardo Rivera, a Manila-based physician, to organise vaccination in and around the capital and advertised the availability of training for other healers. Archbishop Zulaibar instructed the clergy 'to fully commit themselves' to the task of promoting and establishing vaccination in the islands.[96]

Eager to finish up his work in Manila and press on westwards, Balmis instructed Gutiérrez and the rest of the team to escort the Mexican boys back home. As the *Magallanes* required a total refit, however, their departure was postponed until spring 1806.[97] In the meantime, the Governor-General put the skills of the stranded medical men to good use. Appointed temporary head of the programme, Guitérrez vaccinated large numbers of children in the clinic at the City Hall, while Dr Rivera undertook vaccination tours in the provinces of Bulacan and Pampanga in late 1805 and in three southern provinces early in 1806. By the end of 1805, the tally of vaccinations in the Philippines reached 20,000. For their part, Pastor and Ortega were dispatched with guides and ten Filipino boys to Misamis in Mindanao, the furthest reach of Spanish rule, and then to the Visayan Islands, where Ortega perished. The departure of *Magellanes* was postponed twice more, once to avoid a predatory British frigate, giving Guitérrez the opportunity to participate in the inauguration of the central vaccine board in December 1806. Guitérrez, Pastor, the matron and the Mexican boys did not arrive back in Mexico until August 1807. An account of vaccination in the Philippines published in Mexico on their return reported that the suppression of smallpox on one island prompted rebel chiefs to lay down their arms and make peace with the Spanish government.[98]

In early September, Dr Balmis set out with Filipino boys under vaccination and arrived a fortnight later in the Portuguese colony of Macao. Vaccine from the stock that he had brought across the Pacific had preceded him. Pedro Huet, a Portuguese merchant, had brought a recently vaccinated boy from Manila in May and the practice had been rapidly established in Macao. Alexander Pearson, surgeon of the East India Company in Canton, then temporarily

---

[96] Thomas B. Colvin, 'Arms around the world. The introduction of smallpox vaccine into the Philippines and Macao in 1805', *Revista de Cultura*, 18 (2006), 71–88, at 75–9.
[97] Colvin, 'Arms around the world', 81.   [98] Colvin, 'Arms around the world', 82–5.

located in Macao, played a leading role. He found a Chinese boy to go arm-to-arm with the Filipino lad and conducted a series of vaccinations to show the utility of the practice. While his Portuguese colleagues confined their business to members of their own community, Pearson worked almost entirely with the Chinese. He wrote a brief account of the history and practice of vaccination for translation into Chinese by George Staunton, a writer for the East India Company and orientalist scholar. According to Pearson, Staunton found it difficult to 'adapt Chinese idioms and phraseology to the observations meant to be conveyed', but did a good job, 'judging from a literal re-translation and the conversation of the Chinese respecting it'. Between May and November, Pearson completed more than 600 vaccinations in Macao and among Chinese boat people. The presence in Macao of two French missionaries planning to travel to Beijing offered the chance to send vaccine into the heart of China. Pearson instructed one of them, Jean-François Richenet, in vaccination and supplied him with ivory points dipped in vaccine. The missionaries, who set off in July, however, were denied admission to the imperial capital and shipped back to Macao.[99]

The honour of introducing cowpox to China is contested. Vaccination in Macao and Canton began with Balmis's vaccine. Its introduction in Macao, however, was primarily the work of the Portuguese merchant and medical men in Macao, notably Alexander Pearson. Although his commission from the Spanish crown gave him no formal authority in Macao, Balmis was welcomed by the Portuguese authorities and helped to set the practice on firm foundations. The Bishop of Macao and the Chief Judge Miguel Arriaga lent their support, setting an example to hundreds of others by accepting vaccination from Balmis.[100] In October, Balmis took a boy under vaccination to Canton and was probably the first to vaccinate there successfully. While acknowledging that the Spanish physician was the source of the vaccine used in China, however, Pearson stressed the longer history of British activity in sending vaccine to Canton and his own role in vaccinating hundreds of Chinese in Macao, preparing a treatise on vaccination for publication in Chinese and teaching the procedure to Chinese assistants.[101] A letter written in Macao in 28 June 1805, three months before Balmis's arrival, documents all this activity.[102] In addition, Pearson insisted, probably correctly, that Balmis achieved little in Canton. During his eight-week stay, he only vaccinated twenty-two people.[103] Balmis, of course, knew that Pearson was already vaccinating among the Chinese and that Pearson was only waiting for the Company's return to Canton to establish vaccination there. The likelihood is that Balmis,

[99] Smallpox Committee, MS. 4091/22a/151, RCP.   [100] Smith, 'Real Expedición', 59.
[101] A. Pearson to Editor, 8 March 1808: *MPJ*, 20 (June–December 1808), 488–90.
[102] Baron, *Life*, 2, pp. 82–4.   [103] MS. 4091/22a/151, RCP.

who had been thwarted of the honour of being the first to introduce vaccine in Puerto Rico, Cuba and Mexico, seized the opportunity to pre-empt him.

With his experience of China, Pearson was prepared to be patient. Once back in Canton in November 1805, he helped Balmis to find the patients necessary to continue the supply of vaccine. On his advice, the East India Company established a public clinic for vaccination in December. A smallpox epidemic encouraged many Chinese to seek the new prophylaxis. By the end of the year, Pearson and his assistants had vaccinated more than 1,500 people.[104] Back in Macao, Balmis may have felt that the epidemic gave Pearson a lucky break. For his part, Pearson was under no illusions. He took the view that vaccination would make no solid progress among the Chinese people unless it was adopted by their own practitioners. He noted with satisfaction that some Chinese healers, observing the success and appeal of the practice, were beginning to take it up. He nonetheless expected that, once the epidemic was over, the popular demand for vaccination would give way to inertia. Despite his best efforts over the following years, he lost his supply of vaccine several times and had to obtain new samples from Manila and Macao. One striking indication of the success of his work, however, is that he sometimes replenished his stock with vaccine from Chinese operators who had built up practices in the countryside.

Early in 1806, Balmis set out on the *Bom Jesus de Alem*, bound for Lisbon, on the final stage in his circumnavigation of the globe. The ship's only call was at St Helena in the south Atlantic. Relishing the irony that the island was a British colony and that the Governor of St Helena stated that vaccination was unnecessary, Balmis enjoyed a last opportunity to reprise his role as the agent of the new prophylaxis.[105] Governor Patton was 'a philosopher and man of letters' as well as a soldier and responsible for several innovations on the island, including a system of telegraphic communication.[106] Balmis may have misunderstood Patton's point. It had been long observed that, although St Helena was visited by ships with smallpox cases on board, the islanders never caught the disease, but when they went to live in Britain or India they proved highly susceptible. Medical opinion was that the island's salubrious climate resisted contagion.[107] Patton may also have been teasing Balmis. On his departure, he handed him a packet of vaccine sent by Dr Jenner that had never been opened.[108]

Arriving in Lisbon in August 1806, Dr Balmis hired a coach to Madrid and, shortly afterwards, knelt before King Carlos to present a report on his mission.

[104] Smith, 'Real Expedición', 59.   [105] Smith, 'Real Expedición', 60–1.

[106] *New Monthly Magazine and Universal Register*, 14 (July–December 1820), 242.

[107] *GM*, 25 (1755), 502; Holwell, *Account of inoculating*, pp. 4–5.

[108] Smith, 'Real Expedición', 61.

In the past three years, a great deal had changed. Even as he set out across the Atlantic, Spain was being drawn by France into the war against Britain. As he moved from colony to colony, he heard about the escalation of conflict and observed the preparations being made for defence against British attack. In Macao, he would have learned for the first time of the destruction of the Spanish fleet at Trafalgar. At St Helena, he received intelligence of the British reconquest of Cape Colony and the plan for the army to cross the Atlantic to invade the Rio de la Plata.[109] Back home, Balmis found little joy in a regime that was bankrupt and demoralised. In spring 1808, Napoleon forced the abdication of King Carlos and then dethroned his son Ferdinand VIII. In the civil war that ensued, Balmis's house outside Madrid was sacked. During this time, Balmis remained deeply committed to the work of the vaccine expedition. He was anxious to receive reports from Dr Salvany, who remained in Chile and Upper Peru until his death in 1810. Remarkably, in the circumstances of the time, Balmis secured some funds to visit Mexico in 1810–11. Apart from the summary report published in the *Gaceta de Madrid* in 1806, however, he left no account of the great expedition and his own papers may have been lost when his house was sacked. By the time of his death in 1819, the empire he had served was falling apart.

Worldwide but Skin Deep

The arrival of vaccine in Canton (Guangzhou) in 1805 completed its encirclement of the globe. The global success of the new prophylaxis since its public endorsement by physicians and surgeons in London in 1800 is quite astonishing. In a mere five years, medical men and lay supporters of the practice met the challenge of using and storing vaccine, organising its propagation and distribution and delivering it to all corners of the world. Although measures like sealing lymph between glass plates offered fair prospects of success, there were no certainties and often enough only sheer persistence won the day. The first successful delivery of viable vaccine to Sydney in 1804 was attributable to good fortune as well as good management. Its survival on the voyage of *Coromandel* was a record of sorts and the delivery of viable vaccine in the Antipodes is a rare example of its direct transmission from metropolitan centre to colonial periphery. Almost all the other vaccine used in the Indian Ocean and Pacific had been propagated in India and Mexico and passed from arm-to-arm by children and slaves. As remarkable as the rapidity of vaccine's spread in the southern latitudes, then, is its multi-directionality. The old world of trade centred on the Indian Ocean, expanded and amplified by European commerce

---

[109] Smith, 'Real Expedición', 61.

and colonialism, formed the matrix for a complex web of exchange and connection that served, in the late eighteenth century, to spread smallpox southwards and, in the early nineteenth century, to circulate cowpox. Although not all the children used to carry cowpox were slaves, the institution of slavery played a significant role in establishing vaccination south of the Equator.

Needless to say, there were definite limits to the early globalisation of the new prophylaxis. Apart from in European enclaves, vaccination remained unknown in much of the vast continent of Africa. If children and slaves carried cowpox around the Indian Ocean and across the Pacific from Acapulco to Manila and if vaccination became a relatively familiar practice in Table Bay and at the mouth of the Pearl River, the new practice often failed to spread far beyond its initial arrival points. Still, in Mauritius, Java and the Philippines, colonial governors and plantation-owners established the practice in gateway cities and had some success in extending it in the countryside. The embedding of vaccination in major population centres provided an important foundation for the practice. Furthermore, given that the spread of smallpox in the southern latitudes was often by sea, the establishment of the new prophylaxis in port cities was of great benefit. In sparsely populated regions, like the British colonies in Australia, the supply of vaccine was hard to maintain. The commitment to the practice by the authorities, however, ensured that the import of vaccine was a priority. The relatively compact population of Mauritius, with its large numbers of slaves and indentured servants, on the other hand, made it more feasible to maintain a robust system of vaccination. Interestingly, the European colonies around the Indian Ocean and South China Sea supported each other in maintaining the supply of vaccine and extending vaccination. The Roaring Forties made for fast voyages in an easterly direction, with South America serving as a source of vaccine for Cape Town in 1811, and Cape Colony and Mauritius replenishing the vaccine stock in New South Wales and Van Diemen's Land in 1818.[110]

In and around Canton in 1805–6, the arrival of vaccination was a matter for some reflection. For Qiu Xi, a merchant who was vaccinated and trained in the procedure by Alexander Pearson, it was the beginning of a long career vaccinating thousands of his fellow countrymen in Guandong.[111] Even before Dr Balmis's arrival, Pearson reported that the Chinese were 'now sensible of the importance of the discovery', and that he had 'no doubt of its being shortly practised throughout the Chinese empire'.[112] He rapidly became aware, however, that the establishment of the practice in China would be a long struggle and depend entirely on the Chinese themselves taking up the practice. In the event, he would remain in Canton, encouraging and reporting on the progress

---

[110] Laidler and Gelfand, *South Africa*, pp. 113–14; Bennett 'Smallpox and cowpox', 59.
[111] Chang, 'Aspects of smallpox', 161.   [112] Baron, *Life*, 2, p. 83.

of vaccination in China for three decades.[113] One visitor to the Pearl River who acknowledged his work was Admiral Krusenstern, commander of a Russian convoy that had sailed from St Petersburg around Cape Horn and through the Pacific. His recent experience in ordering the variolation of his men, after one of them caught smallpox in Japan, and discovering that all the others were secure, either from prior infection or variolation, sharpened his interest in the new prophylaxis.[114] He evidently spent some time with Pearson. He took the view that the English surgeon had been 'almost robbed' by the Spanish physician 'of the honour of having introduced the cowpox among the Chinese', an honour which belonged 'exclusively' to him. Describing Pearson's practice of vaccinating each day and training Chinese assistants, he expressed his belief that Pearson had 'already been the means of rescuing thousands, and the lives of millions may in future be saved by him'. He doubted that the Chinese would ever show gratitude for 'this humane undertaking'. On the contrary, he mused, if Pearson 'should have the misfortune, by any accident, to lose one of his Chinese patients' he would 'be severely punished'.[115] For his part, Amasa Delano, another visitor to the Pearl River in 1806, had nothing to report on the progress of vaccination in China. In its way, his reticence on the matter is as revealing as Krusenstern's exuberance. For Delano, kinepox brought benefits so obvious that its widespread adoption could be taken for granted. For him, it was a modern amenity that had become globally available.[116]

The transmission of cowpox through the southern latitudes and vaccine's circumnavigation of the globe were attended with little fanfare in a world at war. The escalation and extension of the Napoleonic Wars from 1805 broke lines of communication and consumed most attention. The delivery of cowpox to Sydney in 1804, vaccine's longest journey, should have been newsworthy. John Ring noted it in his account of the progress of cowpox but offered no detail and little comment. The introduction of vaccination in Canton in late 1805 went unreported for some time. It is not known when Jenner read Pearson's letter from Macao in June 1805 and he seems not to have seen Pearson's report on the practice in 1806. John Barrow at the Admiralty had a copy of Pearson's Chinese treatise on vaccination. He lent it to Jenner for his perusal but asked for its return as it was the only copy in England. Ironically, Britain's victory at Trafalgar in 1805 led French privateers to regroup in Mauritius, making Britain's maritime links with the East very vulnerable. In 1809, the East India Company lost fourteen of its large ships to enemy attack

---

[113] *Chinese Depository*, 2 (1833–4), 35–41; *Sixth Report of the Hankow Medical Mission Hospital* (Shanghai, 1870), p. 20.

[114] A. J. von Krusenstern, *Voyage round the world in the years 1803, 1804, 1805, and 1806*, transl. R. B. Hoppner, 2 vols. (London, 1813), 2, pp. 101–3.

[115] Krusenstern, *Voyage round the world*, 2, pp. 316–18.

[116] Delano, *Narrative of voyages*, p. 393.

or storms.[117] It was not until after the British capture of the French colony in 1810 that lines of communication were re-established. The wider crisis enveloping Spain likewise meant that Balmis's story was never fully told. His brief report in the *Gazeta de Madrid*, however, was known in England and translated into English by the end of 1806. Though short in detail, it was pressed into the service of the cause of vaccination in Britain. 'What a delightful narrative is here!', Jenner wrote to a friend in December 1806, 'What lover of vaccination can feel himself at war with his Catholic Majesty after its perusal!'[118]

[117] Stephen Taylor, *Storm and conquest. The battle for the Indian Ocean, 1809* (London, 2007).
[118] Baron, *Life*, 2, pp. 355–6.

14 The World Arm-to-Arm

Jenner and the Vaccination Revolution

After an extremely cold winter in England, spring came early in 1814. The invasion of France by the Allied armies brought the end of war into sight and there were soon rumours that Napoleon had been overthrown. Celebrations began in early summer with the signing of the Treaty of Paris and culminated in June with the arrival in London of Tsar Alexander of Russia, the king of Prussia and other Allied leaders. Though concerned to restore the old world, Europe's statesmen acknowledged the massive changes in circumstances and aspirations since 1789 and were beginning to entertain visions of a new world order. At odds on some issues, they were united in regarding vaccination as one of the most beneficial innovations. In vaccination circles, there was some hope that peace would release energies for the struggle against one of mankind's greatest scourges and provide a suitable occasion to honour the man whose discovery had saved so many lives. To this end, Jenner was called on by his friends to come to London to take part in the celebrations. In a letter to Jenner in late 1813, James Moore, Director of the National Vaccine Establishment [NVE], wrote expansively about 'the amelioration of the world [being] at hand'. 'Till now, our views of what the twenty years' commotion in Europe was to bring forth, were dim and obscure', Jenner replied, 'but the "still small voice" has ordered the mists and clouds to be dispersed, and through a clear and serene atmosphere we see a beautiful order of things gradually rising, as it were, out of chaos'. He then informed Moore, who was writing a history of smallpox and vaccination, that he intended to come to London to attend to numerous matters and then hear his account of 'the rise, progress, and downfal [sic] of a monster still more horrible than Bonaparte'.[1] Shortly before his sixty-fifth birthday, he set out for London for the last time.

In the previous five years, Jenner had retired to Berkeley and professed a desire to withdraw from public life. Even if he had wanted to withdraw entirely from the fray, there was little real prospect of his being left at leisure. At his home, The Chantry, he allocated time to vaccinate charitably and he continued

---

[1] Baron, *Life*, 2, pp. 391–4.

to receive correspondence that drew him back into the business. As he told an old friend in 1810, far from giving him peace of mind and leisure to sit down and smoke a cigar under the hawthorn tree, the government's new vaccination establishment proved, initially at least, a 'source of embarrassment & vexation'.[2] Two years later, he complained about the incessant calls on his time as a country doctor and 'the multifarious toils of Vaccination', not least 'a correspondence that knows no limits'.[3] He appears to have been less close to some of his earlier comrades, some of whom like 'poor John Ring' may have felt burnt out by their labours in the vaccination cause.[4] Still, Jenner was attracting a new generation of acolytes who looked to him for leadership. A recent graduate from Edinburgh, John Baron met Jenner in London in 1808, became one of his closest friends and, in time, his somewhat hagiographical biographer.[5] More immediately useful was James Moore at the NVE. The son of a Scots physician and brother of General John Moore, he held Jenner in high regard, kept him informed and appreciated his counsel. In addition to accolades from overseas, there was some belated recognition in England, including a doctorate from the University of Oxford in 1813 and appointment as Physician Extraordinary to the Prince Regent, requiring his presentation at a *levée* at Carlton House in May 1814.[6] His other business in the capital was more appealing. He would enjoy the illuminations with his younger son, discuss vaccination with Moore and meet up with old friends, some for the last time. Above all, he would be introduced to the 'European potentates' who, he hoped, might be inclined to make some larger commitment to the advance of vaccination.

A great deal hung in the balance in 1814–15, especially in the Hundred Days between Napoleon's return from Elba and his defeat at Waterloo. Disengagement, demobilisation and the winding back of expenditure brought not a peace dividend but a suite of new problems and stresses. The vaccination cause was only one frazzled thread in a complex tapestry. In retrospect, the coming of peace marks the end of the heroic phase in the history of vaccination. There was still some expansionary momentum, important initiatives to strengthen and embed the practice and above all some strengthening of the resolve to defeat smallpox. As Samuel Coleridge, who saw Jenner's achievement as emblematic of the highest human endeavour, wrote, 'what need we deem unattainable, if all the time, the effort, and the skill, which we waste in making ourselves miserable through vice, and vicious through misery, were embodied and marshalled to a systematic War against the Evils

---

[2] MS. 5240/18, WLL.   [3] *Letters of Jenner*, ed. Miller, pp. 75, 78.   [4] MS0016/2/7, RCS.
[5] Baron, *Life*, 2, pp. 136–41.
[6] *Letters of Jenner*, ed. Miller, p. 83; MS. 5240/50, WLL; *Bury and Norwich Post*, 18 May 1814; MS 5240/52, WLL.

of Nature?'[7] As the guns were stilled, the clouds of war dispersed, and communications restored, it was at least possible for the friends of vaccination to gain a more comprehensive picture of its remarkable global progress. The coming of peace in 1814–15 certainly provides a suitable vantage point from which to review the progress of vaccination worldwide, to observe the developments in generalising the practice and embedding it in systems of public health, and to explore the scale and significance of the vaccination revolution.

Global Receptions and Responses

From the outset, there was a keen sense of cowpox as a boon for mankind. Given hardening conceptions of race from the late eighteenth century, the firm assumption of a common humanity to which smallpox posed a common threat is noteworthy. It was recognised, of course, that climate, diet and sanitation introduced variability in the occurrence and severity of the disease and that peoples less familiar with the disease were likely to suffer more severely than peoples who encountered the disease more frequently, but such differences were understood in environmental and biological terms that were universally applicable. Since cowpox was unknown in most parts of the world, it could not be assumed that it would behave in an identical fashion everywhere, but the points at issue related more to the capacity of the vaccine virus to survive in different climatic conditions rather than to the susceptibility of other races to vaccine infection. Race, in terms of skin colour and physiology, was remarked by vaccinators, but almost entirely in relation to the practical matters of making a firmer incision in coarser skin and identifying a vaccine response on darker skin. In the practice of vaccination, there was little apparent concern among Europeans about transferring lymph across racial lines. The crucial issue was the health of the donor child. In 1803, when a high-ranking British official offered his children to be the first to be vaccinated in Calcutta he was using cowpox that had been first propagated on a black-skinned child in Bombay and had passed most recently through the bodies of a Tamil child, a Malay child and a boy from Botany Bay.[8]

The universal dread of smallpox made for commonality of interest in avoidance, prevention and control, but there were cultural differences in response to the disease. In hunter-gatherer and pastoral communities, the strategy that often made most sense was avoidance and flight. Some peoples well acquainted with smallpox, on the other hand, viewed it with a degree of

---

[7] Tim Fulford and Debbie Lee, 'The Jenneration of disease: vaccination, romanticism and revolution', *Studies in Romanticism*, 39 (2000), 139–63, at 157.

[8] Shoolbred, *Report 1802–3*, p. 4.

fatalism, integrating it into their lives and attempting to manage it through religious and magical observances. Fatalistic attitudes were most common among the poorer and more powerless segments of most societies. Elite physicians deplored the fatalism of the urban poor in Britain, the peasants in the Russian empire and the masses in China in remarkably similar terms, even alleging that they welcomed smallpox as a form of family limitation. Naturally enough, there was cultural variation in responses to smallpox prophylaxis. Given that all the forms entailed some element of risk, cost and inconvenience, even educated people had reason to be cautious in adopting them. Some religious traditions, notably Christianity and Islam, saw smallpox in providential terms and found the idea of deliberately infecting a child with a disease, not least an animal disease, rash and impious. While variolation involved higher risks and costs that made sense only if there was a real and immediate threat of smallpox, vaccination was relatively risk free, inexpensive and, since it did not make people ill or infective, relatively convenient. On the other hand, it was hard for people to be certain of its safety and effectiveness, especially over the long term. Prior experience with smallpox inoculation was naturally an important variable in the reception of cowpox. Overall, experience with the older form of prophylaxis made it easier to accept the surgical procedure and appreciate the advantages of cowpox. Awareness of the high level of protection provided by variolation, however, led some people, not least in England, to prefer the old method. In India and China, too, traditional forms of prophylaxis made it both easier and harder for people to accept vaccination. In many parts of the world, of course, it was recognised that smallpox inoculation had the capacity to spread the disease and consequently the practice was either banned or confined, in practice, to elite families. The promise of cowpox was that it both eliminated the risk to the individual and presented no danger to the wider community.

Given its dependence on the availability of vaccine, the speed with which the new prophylaxis spread around the world is astonishing. Divided by war, Europe was united by a common culture of learning, including an emphasis on empirical knowledge, a readiness to apply it to human affairs and a belief in progress. In the late eighteenth century, medical practitioners and the lay intelligentsia found the practice of variolation a matter of interest and debate. The cowpox discovery was widely reported and Jenner's writings were rapidly translated into the major European languages. The clinical trials at St Pancras in 1799 and the public endorsement of cowpox by leading physicians and surgeons in London in 1800 guaranteed it a favourable hearing in many parts of the world. Britain's medical men were soon distributing samples of cowpox and information on its use through wider networks of medical, scientific and literary correspondence and exchange. Once the medical men in Paris took up vaccination, there emerged a robust consensus on the continent about the value of new prophylaxis and a range of initiatives to support and extend the practice. Beyond Europe, the spread of vaccination followed the lines of European trade and empire, carried through networks of power and knowledge and common sets of ideas and values. Medical networks played an important role: the pioneers of vaccination in British India were mainly Scots, long-standing colleagues in the service of the East India Company. Within a few years, there arose a number of centres of vaccination activity, like Vienna, Madras and Philadelphia, that served as subsidiary hubs for the distribution of vaccine and the advancement of the practice. There was also a complex, multi-directional web of exchange not reliant on simple diffusion from Europe. The professional elites in Cuba, Mexico and Peru did not wait for Spain but procured vaccine and advice from elsewhere, including the United States. Naturally enough, the new prophylaxis spread less rapidly beyond the zones of European influence, but there are hints, most notably in India and China, that non-European practitioners took up vaccination in their own communities and beyond the ken of the European chroniclers of the practice.

The first medical men outside England to use cowpox wrestled with the difficulties of identifying a genuine cowpox response, generating a supply of vaccine, devising techniques for storing and distributing it and developing protocols for the organisation and oversight of the new practice. With reports from Britain to inform them, the physicians of Hanover, Vienna, Geneva, Paris and Milan, however, were soon making their own contributions to the under-standing and management of the practice. In seeking to establish vaccination, there were demonstrations of its simplicity and safety and formal trials to prove its effectiveness by the 'counter-proof' method of challenging patients who had been vaccinated by inoculating them with smallpox. Naturally enough, medical men and interested laymen living some distance from England played the leading part in evaluating and refining the various methods of storing and transporting vaccine lymph. In Vienna, De Carro provided feedback to London and publicised the latest ideas and, in Virginia, President Jefferson applied his mind to the problem. It was James Bryce, a Scot, who first begged to differ from Jenner's view that cowpox was not serviceable in crust form.[9] Experi-mentation with this mode of storage, a useful back-up in remote regions, soon followed in France, Spain, India and North America. In the meantime, searches for indigenous cowpox and attempts to propagate cowpox on healthy cows continued in countries around the world. Reports of success in these endeav-ours are hard to assess and there is little evidence of such strains being used over time. The exception is Luigi Sacco, who found cowpox among cattle in the fairs of Lugano, tested it carefully and used it fairly extensively.

---

[9] James Bryce, *Practical observations on the inoculation of cowpox* (Edinburgh, 1802), pp. 128–36.

His experimental work on animal viruses is the best early example of the science and practice of vaccination being constructed on a transnational stage. He had some success in using horse-grease, presumably horse-pox, as a form of prophylaxis and sent samples to De Carro and Jenner.[10]

The vaccination cause was often carried on a wave of enthusiasm. For physicians, it was an opportunity to show themselves up to date with beneficial innovations. In putting the procedure to the test, pronouncing on its merits and engaging with its philosophical and social implications, the university-educated medical elite in Europe showed itself erudite and up-to-date, scientific, socially concerned and humane. Several made their name from their commitment to the new prophylaxis. In addition to vaccinating on some scale and his scientific experimentation, Dr Sacco made broad-ranging contributions to the promotion, organisation and cultural identity of the practice, including collaborating in the production of elegant wax models to illustrate the vaccine pustule.[11] Some of the surgeons who wielded the lancet likewise found it a procedure that gave them a sense of social mission. The new prophylaxis certainly fitted the agenda of social medicine so politically relevant in the wake of the French Revolution and was well suited to the ethos and skill set of the *officiers de santé*. Around the world, there were many individuals in the lower echelons of the medical profession who found a vocation in the new practice. José de Salvany vaccinated hundreds of thousands of people in South America before his death in 1810, but Sawmy Naik, another military surgeon active in the presidency of Madras over several decades, probably had the honour of vaccinating more people than anyone else in the world. Notable, too, is the humanitarian enthusiasm for the new prophylaxis of people from outside the medical profession. Aristocrats and merchants, women and men, lent their names and raised subscriptions to establish and extend the new prophylaxis, though perhaps accepting some return in gratitude and deference for their humane endeavours. Far from opposing the practice, the clergy of the Catholic and the major Protestant churches, whether on their own account or on direction from government, presented the practice as a gift of God and associated it with Christian rites of passage. Many monarchs saw in the promotion of vaccination not only a means of increasing population and productivity but also a means of showing themselves to be loving fathers of their people. The Buttats vaccination expedition in Russia and the Balmis expedition in the Spanish empire were presented as philanthropic enterprises. In making vaccine available to the world, of course, there were less creditable interests at play, including the protection of plantation economies, the creation

---

[10] Sacco, *Osservazioni*, pp. 60–158; Baxby, *Jenner's vaccine*, pp. 132–3, 176.
[11] Fabio Zampieri, Alberto Zanatta and Maurizio Rippa Bonati, 'Iconography and wax models in Italian early smallpox vaccination', *Medicine Studies*, 2 (2011), 213–27.

of new forms of control and dependency and the projection of images of western scientific supremacy.

While the global spread of vaccine was an multinational effort, Britain remained at the heart of the enterprise. The new practice began with cowpox from England and its reputation owed much to its provenance. Even after vaccine had been propagated elsewhere, practitioners in other countries and climes often sought to get the edge on their colleagues by seeking vaccine and the latest words of advice from Jenner. In Britain, there were certainly moves to present a public image of Jenner as a kind country doctor who had made known to the world the blessings of cowpox. It was in continental Europe, however, that the cult of 'immortal' Jenner took root and flourished. The friends of vaccination in France were fulsome in their praise of Jenner's genius and paid handsome tribute to England's medical men for holding to the principle that the sciences are never at war. Festivals were established in Germany to commemorate Jenner's discovery and there was a proposal in Spain to call the new procedure 'yennerización' in his honour.[12] Foreign acclaim helped to shore up the standing of Jenner and the vaccination cause in Britain. In the debate on a second premium to Jenner in 1807, Lord Petty reminded his parliamentary colleagues that 'we are now acting in the view of other nations'.[13] Given his role in the abolition of the slave trade, William Wilberforce spoke with some authority when he stated as evidence of Jenner's international esteem that no one 'is so much inquired after by foreigners when they arrive in this country [and] has so extensive a correspondence from all quarters and corners of the globe'.[14] Accounts of the success of vaccination in foreign parts served to show the benefits of supporting the practice more wholeheartedly in Britain. In parliament in 1807, William Smith read out a translation of Balmis's report of the Spanish vaccine expedition and then a letter from Marseille, reporting that vaccination had freed the city from smallpox and that its citizens could not believe that in Britain, 'the original seat of the discovery', smallpox was 'not exterminated'.[15] From Ceylon, Dr Christie wrote to report how vaccination had kept the island clear of smallpox for eighteen months in 1808–9.[16] In retirement in Cheltenham, he expressed great surprise that 'some degree of scepticism and incredulity still existed about the efficacy of the practice'.[17]

The end of the war was an opportune moment to celebrate the global success of vaccination. The arrival in London in 1814 of the Allied leaders, all interested in meeting Jenner, appeared a glorious opportunity to advance the

---

[12] *Gaceta de Madrid*, 23 November 1801; Murray, *Debates*, pp. 71–2; Blasco Martínez, 'Higiene y sanidad', 343.
[13] Murray, *Debates*, pp. 71–2.   [14] Murray, *Debates*, p. 97.   [15] Murray, *Debates*, p. 125.
[16] *Edinburgh Medical and Surgical Journal*, 7 (1811), 234–5; Baron, *Life*, 2, pp. 364–8.
[17] Christie, *Ravages in Ceylon*, pp. i–ii.

cause. Tsar Alexander of Russia had taken measures to establish the practice across his vast empire. Frederick William III, king of Prussia, the first sovereign to have his own children vaccinated, had founded a state-of-the-art vaccine institute in Berlin that held annual festivals on Jenner's birthday. Count Orlov, a Russian diplomat, and Dr Hamel, a Russian physician, met Jenner in Cheltenham and urged him to come to London to meet the Tsar and his sister, the Grand Duchess of Oldenburg. There was reportedly some design by Jenner's friends to address a memorial on his behalf to the sovereigns in London, but Orlov advised Jenner that he should 'memorialise' them himself 'on the score of his claims as an universal benefactor'. According to Dr Baron, Jenner 'shrank from such a project'.[18] Jenner's idea for a memorial was presumably no mere petition for honour and reward but involved a call for some collective endorsement of vaccination and commitment to action. In a letter on 14 June, he explained that he had in mind a plan for some 'some great man', perhaps Henry Petty, now Marquis of Lansdowne, to present a copy of the memorial and 'explain its purport' to each ambassador of a foreign court.[19] By this time, Jenner was himself in London, waiting for an audience with the sovereigns who had arrived in London on 6 June. When he finally met Tsar Alexander on 19 June, he heard fine words on the success of vaccination in Russia, but embarrassed himself by denying that he had received 'the gratitude of the world' for his discovery.[20] To add to the awkwardness, when Orlov later called on Jenner to ask him if a Russian order would be acceptable, he replied by observing that such an honour could only go to someone who had the means to support it.[21] Jenner was likewise presented to King Frederick William and met Marshal Blücher and other foreign notables, but as there is no record of the conversations it is not known if anything of substance was discussed.[22] Back in Berkeley, some months later, however, Jenner still had in mind a memorial, now to be presented at the Congress of Vienna. In September, he wrote to a colleague that 'nothing is yet fully determined on respecting my affairs with the monarchs, but tho' I shall outdare Bonaparte himself they must be attack'd, & in their entrench'd camp at Vienna'. His hope was to get the ear of Lord Castlereagh, the leader of the British delegation, 'and find that ear harmonis'd to vaccination'.[23] If Castlereagh was approached to present a proposal in the cause of vaccination, he seems not to have taken it up. Dr De Carro, who in his memoir recalled assisting Castlereagh in Vienna in translating a memorial on the slave trade, makes no mention of it.[24]

---

[18] Baron, *Life*, 2, p. 209.
[19] Jenner to Rev. Joyce, 14 June 1814: Associated photocopies of letters, Royal Society of Medicine, London.
[20] *Letters of Jenner*, ed. Miller, p. 86.   [21] Fosbroke, *Berkeley manuscripts*, pp. 236–9.
[22] Fosbroke, *Berkeley manuscripts*, pp. 239–40; *Letters of Jenner*, ed. Miller, p. 86.
[23] MS 5240/53, WLL.   [24] *Annals of Philosophy*, 10 (July 1817), 4–5.

Salus Populi: **Public Health and Compulsory Vaccination**

In the late eighteenth century, it was assumed that heads of families were responsible for the health of themselves and their households. Still, European states were beginning to anticipate a role in the promotion of public health, especially in relation to contagious diseases. In addition to imposing quarantine, government agencies concerned themselves with the isolation of smallpox cases and sometimes the provision of nurses. The use of smallpox inoculation as a containment measure complicated matters, as inoculated smallpox could pose as great a risk to other people as natural smallpox. Many towns in Britain and elsewhere took steps to inhibit the practice when smallpox was not an immediate threat. Once the contagion took hold, the risks involved in inoculation became more acceptable and the practice was permitted and even actively promoted. The Republic of Geneva, a city-state, was the first government to make provision for inoculation in 1754. The adoption of the practice by European princes in the late 1760s likewise involved promotion of the practice, especially in the armed services and in hospitals under royal patronage. Rulers were very reluctant to override the rights and responsibilities of individuals to decide for themselves and for their children. In ordering the inoculation of children in state institutions, of course, rulers were acting in *loco parentis*. Still, in issuing an edict for the inoculation of children in royal orphanages in 1798, Carlos IV of Spain showed more resolution than most rulers.

Initially, cowpox seemed set to prosper in England without state support. The new inoculation appeared to be a simple procedure and less costly and inconvenient than the old method. It was assumed, then, that the extension of vaccination could be left to the marketplace and self-help. Popular hesitancy about inoculating an animal disease and problems in obtaining genuine vaccine and ascertaining a true vaccine response, however, made it more necessary for medical men to be involved in managing the business. The early vaccine institutes and clinics in England were not government-funded and supported themselves by fees and charitable subscription. Outside of Britain, where cowpox was not readily available and the new prophylaxis appeared more alien, there was more need for state support to introduce vaccine and establish the practice. In the British empire, governors and medical men in their service played a much more active role than was necessary or appropriate for state functionaries in Britain. Ferdinand, king of the Two Sicilies, was the first of many princes to lend their authority to the introduction of vaccination. The French state, increasingly under Napoleon's direction, proved a formidable ally of the new prophylaxis, albeit more in the promotion and organisation of the practice than in the provision of funding. In Russia, Tsar Alexander rapidly built on his mother's sponsorship of vaccination to extend the practice throughout the empire. Even more remarkable, King Carlos IV of Spain sponsored a vaccine expedition that established the practice around the world.

If Jenner and his colleagues did not initially see the need for public support, early controversies over cowpox made high level endorsement highly desirable, especially if it strengthened their authority over the practice. Members of the royal family and the aristocracy had already privately acknowledged Jenner's pre-eminence in the field. The parliamentary premium awarded Jenner in 1802, which at least reimbursed him for some of his labours in the vaccination cause, set the scene for the formation of the Royal Jennerian Society in 1803, a private charity under royal patronage, which gave the appearance of state support, though its only cost to the public purse was its exemption from postal charges. In the meantime, old prejudices against cowpox and reports of vaccination mishaps and failures were mobilised by anti-vaccinists in a scare campaign that led many Londoners in 1805 to abandon vaccination and seek variolation. Foreign observers were shocked by the savagery and mendacity of the tracts that attacked vaccination. In Germany, the intemperate denunciations of *Brutalimpfung* disappeared as the leading medical men forged a consensus on the practice. In France, the medical men who had doubts about the safety and the effectiveness of vaccination soon found that they could not get their observations and warnings published in the newspapers. From 1809, nothing could be published on vaccination without the approval of the *comité central de vaccine*.[25] The friends of vaccination in Britain had no wish to inhibit freedom of expression but continued to look to Parliament to reaffirm, as it did in 1807, its endorsement of the new practice. In reflecting on the greater salience of anti-vaccine sentiment in England than elsewhere in Europe, James Moore saw English liberty as 'permitting empiricism, and many species of impostures, to flourish'. As he ruefully observed, more arbitrary regimes were better able to punish knaves.[26]

The strong tradition of smallpox inoculation in England added to the problems. The continuation of the old practice caused a great deal of confusion. Offering their patients a choice between the old and the new, some practitioners variolated and vaccinated interchangeably. As early as 1799, Jenner viewed smallpox inoculation as 'a private blessing, but a general curse'.[27] Once cowpox inoculation was shown to be safe and effective, the old practice, with the danger of cross-infection, began to appear less acceptable. The friends of vaccination in England were aware that the British rulers in Bengal had moved early on to suppress variolation in Calcutta by police

---

[25] Fressoz, *L'apocalypse joyeuse*, pp. 100–1.   [26] Moore, *History of vaccination*, p. 115.
[27] MS0016/6 [Transcript from Royal College of Physicians, Edinburgh], RCS; Baron, *Life*, 2, pp. 153–4.

measures.[28] Still, Jenner did not feel it was wise or feasible to ban it, though he probably would not have argued the point with the Duke of Bedford who, in a letter to him, argued that freedom to variolate 'surely cannot be consistent with the principles of a wise government, or even of a free one'.[29] In 1807, Sir Edmund Carrington, a former Chief Justice of Ceylon, likewise took a firmer line than Jenner, publishing a tract in which he presented English precedents for legislative intervention for the *salus populi* that might 'startle the prejudices of a jealous liberty, though it would convey no terror to a reforming mind'.[30] Increasingly, though, Jenner and his allies were looking to inhibit the practice of inoculation. In May 1808, a parliamentary bill 'to prevent the spreading of the infection of the smallpox' by restricting inoculation to houses outside towns, requiring the notification of neighbours and imposing the strict isolation of patients lapsed for lack of support.[31] Later in the year, Charles Murray, secretary of the Royal Jennerian Society, distinguishing between an adult's right to be variolated and a parent's right to variolate a child, came to the view that variolation 'ought to be put down by law'. 'Every infant born', he argued, 'is the child of the state: and, however, extensive parental power and influence may be, it is a known rule of our law, to restrain that power, and prevent its being exercised to the injury or destruction of our offspring'. Given the safety and effectiveness of vaccination, he could not see 'on what principle of reason or right, it can now be argued, that we are entitled to compel our infants to undergo a disease, from which they must at all events, suffer greatly; and which may destroy them'.[32]

Across continental Europe, royal and republican regimes moved more purposefully to support vaccination. Early vaccination in Germany, Austria and Italy depended on private initiative, but the practice soon engaged the attention of rulers and professional bodies. The king of Naples made institutional provision for vaccination at the outset, and the Cisalpine Republic appointed Dr Luigi Sacco as director of vaccinations and published his instructional leaflet on the practice in 1801.[33] After a late start, the French state rapidly pushed ahead of other countries in its strong public endorsement of vaccination. Though the French government provided little funding, it laid down a nationwide infrastructure for the practice in 1804, with *comités de*

---

[28] Shoolbred, *Report 1802–3*, pp. 66–9.   [29] Baron, *Life*, 2, p. 61.

[30] [Sir Codrington Edmund Carrington], *A letter to the right honourable Spencer Percival ... on the expediency and propriety of regulating by parliamentary authority the practice of variolous inoculation, with a view to the extermination of the small-pox* (London, 1807).

[31] Deborah Brunton, *The politics of vaccination. Practice and policy in England, Wales, Ireland, and Scotland, 1800–1874* (Rochester, NY, 2008), p. 16.

[32] Charles Murray, *An answer to Mr Highmore's objections to the Bill before Parliament to prevent the spreading of the infection of the small-pox* (London, 1808), pp. 52–3.

[33] Luigi Sacco, *Istruzione sui vantaggi, e sul metodo d'innestare il vajuolo vaccino pubblicata per ordine del comitato governativo della Repubblica Cisalpina* (Milan, 1801).

vaccine in the *départements* reporting to a *Comité central de vaccine* in Paris. In Prussia, Denmark and Sweden, kings and ministers worked with medical colleges to assess the new prophylaxis, set up specialised institutes to propagate vaccine and oversee the practice and used local government agencies to make the procedure generally available. The Emperor of Russia and the king of Spain both integrated vaccination into older forms of imperial and royal philanthropy and supported much larger enterprises for the spread of the practice in their empires. Several rulers went beyond simply encouraging vaccination by legislating measures to contain smallpox, suppress variolation and make vaccination obligatory. In August 1805, the new Principality of Hesse, a Napoleonic creation, was the first major state to make vaccination compulsory. A month later, the king of Bavaria approved legislation for the control of smallpox that included a requirement that all infants should be vaccinated. By 1807, vaccination was generally available and the vaccination of infants was mandatory.[34] Legislation in Denmark in 1810–11, while not making vaccination strictly compulsory, made it almost impossible to avoid.[35] In most parts of continental Europe, smallpox inoculation was suppressed and only practised on any scale in remote areas during epidemics. Although authoritarian rulers like Napoleon and the king of Prussia were reluctant to make vaccination compulsory, believing that people should be free to act on their conscience and recognising that compulsion would provoke resistance, the citizens of Napoleonic France and the subjects of the 'Iron Kingdom' knew what was expected of them and that opportunities would be denied their children if they were not vaccinated.

In Britain, Jenner and his allies continued to give priority to winning over public opinion, encouraging friends to use the press and other means to promote the practice. Early in 1808, there was a coordinated campaign to publicise the measures taken in continental Europe to suppress smallpox and generalise vaccination, with newspapers across the British Isles packaging brief notices of the king of Sweden's prizes for leading vaccinators, the ban on variolation and compulsory vaccination in Piombino-Lucca, and the king of Bavaria's ordinances for the vaccination of all infants.[36] The Royal Jennerian Society nonetheless held to the line that the promotion of vaccination 'should be confined to measures or recommendation only' and looked for no more than the sort of institutional support and incentives for the practice offered by many European states, 'in consequence of which they have there almost annihilated the Small-Pox'.[37] The government's decision in 1809 to fund a National

---

[34] Giel, *Schutzpocken-Impfung in Bayern*, pp. 96–105.   [35] Bonderup, *En kovending*, pp. 95–6.
[36] *Morning Chronicle*, 4 January 1808; *Royal Cornwall Gazette*, 9 January 1808; *Caledonian Mercury*, 11 January 1808.
[37] Murray, *Debates*, pp. xix–xx.

Vaccine Establishment (NVE), which opened in 1810, raised new possibilities. Although he chose not to associate himself formally with the new institution, Jenner responded to the diplomatic overtures of James Moore, the Director, and was soon offering advice. In 1812, for example, he sent Moore a copy of Luigi Sacco's latest book on vaccination in Italy, passed on reports of the practice in Berlin and Cuba and asked him to observe how 'our clever neighbours the French have organised their vaccine Institutions'.[38] In 1812–13, epidemic smallpox in London and Norwich, associated with 'the rash and inconsiderate manner in which inoculation has been conducted', led the vaccination lobby again to press for the restriction of variolation.[39] Observing the spike in mortality in London, Jenner attributed 'the horrid slaughter in the metropolis' to the backstreets inoculators.[40] The epidemic in Norwich, fuelled by hasty recourse to the old prophylaxis, prompted Dr Edward Rigby to call for severe penalties on anyone 'directly or indirectly concerned in variolous inoculation'.[41] In January 1813, Jenner informed a friend that penal measures instituted in the Cape Colony were being considered for implementation in Britain.[42] Later he helped to draft a bill to regulate the practice by requiring practitioners to notify the local authorities of their activity and warn the public by placing red flags around their houses.[43] Introducing the bill into the House of Lords in June, Lord Boringdon argued that, though in principle everyone 'had a right to do what he pleased with his own person and property', there were precedents, as with the quarantine, for limiting such rights when their exercise was hazardous to others.[44] After opposition from the law lords, the bill was withdrawn. Lord Ellenborough, the Lord Chief Justice, who infuriated Jenner with the observation that vaccination provided only temporary security, argued that the bill was ill-conceived and unnecessary because there was a remedy available in the common law of nuisance for the reckless spread of disease.[45]

Acting on the Chief Justice's advice, the NVE began to look for a test case in which the practice of smallpox inoculation had been directly responsible for the spread of the disease. In summer 1814, Charles Murray received a report of a smallpox outbreak in Paddington that was blamed on Mrs Sophia Vantandillo who, after having her baby inoculated at an apothecary's shop, carried it around with her on the streets, including among the crowds gathered

---

[38] Baron, *Life*, 2, pp. 376–9.   [39] *Christian Observer*, 1814, p. 535.
[40] Jenner Letter 12, 10a/142, College of Physicians, Philadelphia.
[41] Edward Rigby, 'Report of the Norwich pauper vaccination', *Edinburgh Medical and Surgical Journal*, 10 (1813), 120–6, at 124.
[42] MS. 5240/49, WLL.
[43] Fisher, *Jenner*, pp. 244–6; Brunton, *Politics of vaccination*, pp. 16–17.
[44] *New Annual Register for 1813* (1814), 190–1.
[45] Jenner Letter 13, 10a/142, College of Physicians, Philadelphia.

to watch the exiled king of France pass by on his return to France. Her neighbours attributed the spread of smallpox, including nine fatal cases, to her refusal to keep her child indoors. Several parents also bore witness to the negligence of the apothecary, Gilbert Burnett, and alleged that two children inoculated by him had died. In September, the Grand Jury of Middlesex formally indicted Mrs Vantandillo for unlawfully and injuriously exposing her child in public and the apothecary for causing inoculated children 'to be exposed improperly in the public streets and highways, to the imminent danger of communicating the infection'.[46] Despite an affidavit from Mrs Vantandillo and her husband that four of their six children had been vaccinated with adverse outcomes, she was found guilty and sentenced to six months' imprisonment. Even though Burnett issued printed instructions to parents not to take their children outside during the infective stage, he was likewise found guilty and given a three-month sentence. *Rex versus Vantandillo* was a victory of sorts for vaccination and the judgement was widely reported in newspapers. The imprisonment of a mother of six and a struggling apothecary may have served to make mothers seeking inoculation or individuals providing the service exercise greater caution. It did not make variolation illegal and did not bring the practice to an end. It was still the general view that parents were free to make their own decisions with respect to their children's health and that prohibiting variolation would implicitly make vaccination compulsory. Few would have agreed with Murray's proposition that 'every infant born is a child of the state'.[47]

There were measures elsewhere in the English-speaking world around this time to provide support for vaccination. In a rare intervention in health matters, the United States Congress passed an act for 'the encouragement of vaccination' in 1812 that made provision for a vaccine agency to provide, at fixed rates, vaccine matter to anyone, anywhere in the country, who requested it.[48] A smallpox outbreak in the British province of Lower Canada in 1813 and its return in 1815 led to the mandatory vaccination of soldiers and their families, and the Vaccine Act of 1815 which provided £1,000 for a vaccine institute and the payment of practitioners for each procedure, conditional on their attendance on the patient to confirm a successful outcome. Conducted between 1815 and 1816, the programme led to hundreds of vaccinations. The programme was refined in 1817 and was run again in 1821.[49] In the meantime, there had been a similar attempt in the British Parliament to make general provision for vaccination. A bill was introduced in June 1815 to make vaccination freely available to the poor. The scheme was to be administered locally

---

[46] *MPJ*, 34 (July–December 1815), 84.   [47] Murray, *An answer*, pp. 52–3.
[48] Bell, 'Smith and vaccination', 500–16.
[49] Tunis, 'Public vaccination in lower Canada', pp. 264–78.

by the overseers of the poor who would make contracts, as some of them already did, with local surgeons. A national board, however, would oversee the scheme, make vaccine available, approve the practitioners and receive reports. Though it was well received in the House of Commons, the bill was rejected in the Lords on the grounds of cost, government interference and the scope that the board's scrutiny of practitioners offered for jobbery.[50] The defeat of the bill for the vaccination of the poor in Britain brought an end to the initiatives of the age of Jenner. There were no further moves on behalf of vaccination for twenty-five years.

'Take a survey of Europe', Jenner wrote in 1815, 'and you will find that while we [have been] fighting our battles with antivaccinists, they have been fighting with the smallpox & have vanquish'd the monster'.[51] On the continent, too, the coming of peace set the scene for a reinvigoration of the practice. In France, the foundations laid in the Napoleonic era proved quite robust and vaccination was rapidly re-established. In northern Europe, the systems established prior to 1812 largely continued in force. After the Swedish parliament indicated its support for compulsory vaccination, the king approved a law in 1816 that required the vaccination of children by the age of two years.[52] In southern Europe, there was some loss of provision, especially in Spain, where war and civil commotion revealed the practice's shallow roots. If some Italians had resisted vaccination as a French innovation, Italian commitment to vaccination remained surprisingly strong, with three times the number of people vaccinated in Otranto in 1817 than any previous year.[53] Overall, Liberal Europe proved less robust in championing vaccination than the enlightened absolutisms of the Napoleonic era. Britain, then, was not alone in its failure to make progress in enlisting state power in support of vaccination in the 1820s and 1830s. There were new initiatives in some German states. In Hanover, compulsory vaccination was introduced in the 1820s. In Prussia, where there was some experimentation with compulsion in 1810 and in the late 1820s, the door was firmly closed on compulsion in 1829.[54] In Britain, a smallpox epidemic that caused 40,000 deaths in 1837 finally provided the impetus for action. Though controversial and limited in the practice, legislation passed in 1840 finally provided for universal vaccination and prohibited variolation.[55]

[50] Brunton, *Politics of vaccination*, p. 18.   [51] Fisher, *Jenner*, p. 245.

[52] Sköld, *Two faces*, pp. 444–7.

[53] Bercé, *Chaudron et lancette*, pp. 89–91; Lorenzo Carlino, 'Cenni sull'opera di Antonio Miglietta e Cosimo de Giorgi in terra d'Otranto', in Antonio Tagarelli, Anna Piro and Walter Pasini (eds.), *Il vaiolo e la vaccinazione in Italia*, vol. 2 (Villa Verucchio, 2004), pp. 551–9, at 552–3.

[54] Baldwin, *Contagion and state*, p. 262.   [55] Brunton, *Politics of vaccination*, pp. 20–38.

The Vaccination Revolution

By 1801, medical men discerned a revolution in the making. Acknowledging the advances in philosophy and science in the eighteenth century, they observed that one of the greatest, Jenner's cowpox discovery, had come right at the century's turn. His thesis that cowpox provided a security against smallpox found support in clinical trials in London in 1799 and similar trials around the world in the first years of the nineteenth century. Inoculating cowpox, however, proved far less straightforward than first anticipated. The rarity of the relevant cattle disease presented major challenges to the establishment and extension of new prophylaxis. Overcoming the challenges of propagating, preserving and distributing good vaccine was the collective achievement of scores of pioneers, some in contact with Jenner, most others dependent on observing or reading about the practice. In the first decade of the nineteenth century, a vast number of people were engaged in a conversation about cowpox, sharing their experiences of the new prophylaxis, conducting their own trials and experiments and addressing the technical, organisational and political issues that it raised. This global conversation proved sufficiently productive for vaccination to rapidly become a well-recognised, largely effective and widely available prophylactic measure. Parents in many parts of the world discovered that they could protect their children from a terrible disease with no danger and at minimal cost or inconvenience. As the large-scale use of vaccination was seen to have the capacity to suppress smallpox and banish it from whole districts, it became possible to envision a wider extirpation of the scourge. Jenner initially hesitated to give public utterance to the idea of eradicating smallpox but, after reviewing the success of vaccination in 1801, he declared that 'it now becomes too manifest to admit of controversy, that the annihilation of the small pox, the most dreadful scourge of the human species, must be the final result of the practice'.[56] He would have been disappointed had he known that the achievement would be delayed until 1977, when the last natural case of smallpox was detected in Somalia.[57]

The number of vaccinations grew dramatically. In Britain, hundreds in 1799 became thousands in 1800, and in spring 1801 Jenner claimed that a 'hundred thousand persons, upon the smallest computation, have been inoculated [with vaccine] in these realms'.[58] By 1803, vaccination was well-established in western Europe, was becoming available in many parts of

---

[56] Jenner, *Origin*, p. 8.

[57] Williams, *Angel of death*, pp. 353–4; D. A. Henderson, 'The global eradication of smallpox: historical perspectives and future prospects', in Sanjoy Bhattacharya and Sharon Messenger (eds.), *The global eradication of smallpox* (Hyderabad, 2010), pp. 7–35.

[58] Jenner, *Origin*, p. 7.

North America and was being put into service in Sweden, Russia and India. Early in 1803, Dr Sacco reported 50,000 vaccinations in Italy.[59] Even in India, where cultural sensitivities about the practice were acute, thousands of people were vaccinated in the presidency of Madras during 1803. From 1804, vaccination was conducted on a massive scale in Spanish America and in 1804–5 the practice was introduced in ports and colonial outposts from Cape Town and Mauritius to Sydney, Jakarta, Manila and Canton. The spread of cowpox around the world, largely by successive vaccinations, was astonishingly rapid. The initial momentum, of course, could not be sustained, not least because in the early years many adolescents were vaccinated along with children. The early surge in vaccination was generally followed by a slackening of activity, picking up some years later when smallpox reappeared. In encouraging routine vaccination, the promoters of the practice were not simply concerned with protecting children but also the propagation and maintenance of the local supply of vaccine. Even in England, recourse to the cow was rarely an option. From the outset, the global practice largely depended on the procedure itself, with vaccinations conducted literally arm-to-arm. If the procedure was neglected by parents until there was a smallpox outbreak, there would be little good vaccine available to meet the spike in demand. In some quarters, the dependence of the practice on humanised vaccine raised concerns that the vaccine in circulation, many generations from cow, was losing its prophylactic power. Jenner, who was not himself very successful in cultivating a stock of good vaccine, was inclined to attribute deficiencies in the quality of vaccine to lack of care in propagation. Dr Christie supported this line, reporting that the vaccine he was using in Ceylon in 1810 was performing exactly as it did in 1803, even though it had passed through 399 generations.[60] Still, the perception of a decline in the quality of vaccine became more general. Jenner himself experimented with cowpox and horsepox as it became available and there were a range of initiatives to reinvigorate the stock of vaccine by recourse to the farm.

As the first decade of the practice came to an end, the more pressing problem was the increasing number of reported cases of smallpox after vaccination. Rumours of other adverse outcomes led to an upsurge in anti-vaccinist sentiment in England, especially in London. In Europe, too, the return of epidemic smallpox, in which some people who had been vaccinated caught the disease, put trust in the procedure to the test. Jenner held that true vaccination provided lifetime security and pointed out that, in the first years of the practice, many people had been exposed to smallpox shortly before they were vaccinated and that inexperienced doctors had often used vaccine of dubious quality and

[59] Baron, *Life*, 1, pp. 250–1.   [60] Christie, *Ravages in Ceylon*, p. 98.

neglected to confirm the success of the operation. Reflecting on his early practice, he himself confessed to a friend that 'when I consider how many I merely punctured without any further inspection of their arms, I almost tremble for the result'.[61] Jenner based his belief in the permanent protection provided by cowpox on an assumed equivalence with smallpox and on his evidence of people who had been casually infected with cowpox resisting smallpox decades later. Even as the number of cases of smallpox after vaccination continued to rise, the supporters of vaccination pointed to cases of smallpox after variolation and argued that the vaccination failures represented only a small fraction of the rapidly rising tally of vaccinations. After receiving testimonials from across Britain in 1807, the Royal College of Physicians declared that the practice provided a near-perfect level of security, although, since the data related to relatively recent vaccinations, any claim in relation to permanent protection was manifestly premature. Jenner and his allies continued to hold the line against recommending routine revaccination, believing that it would undermine confidence in the procedure. Most cases of smallpox after vaccination, in any case, were not especially severe. For this reason, they proved difficult to diagnose, with confusion and debate as to the identity of what was sometimes termed 'varioloid' or 'modified smallpox'. By 1821, the National Vaccine Establishment pulled back from claiming that vaccination provided absolute and permanent security, but pointed out that in the small minority of cases in which it disappointed expectations, it nonetheless exercised a significant 'controlling power' over smallpox.[62] After large numbers of apparent vaccination failures in epidemics in 1818 and the early 1830s, vaccinators in continental Europe began to build the case for periodic revaccination. German physicians took the lead in recommending revaccination, though as late as 1838 a slight majority of French medical men doubted its necessity.[63]

The vaccination revolution did not involve major conceptual breakthroughs. The success of the practice, the expansion in activity, the mass of experimental data and the broad address to anomalies and problems all helped to prepare the ground for the later microbial revolution. Jenner played a crucial role in familiarising the use of the term 'virus' to refer to a disease agent. Though the term itself is Latin for poison, he appears to have used virus in a more neutral and perhaps abstract sense. While he described smallpox as a poison and for a short time presented cowpox as an 'antidote', he almost always referred to cowpox as a virus.[64] Jenner, of course, lacked the technical means to observe microbes. There is indeed no firm evidence that he regarded viruses

---

[61] MS. 5240/22, WLL.   [62] *MPJ*, 48 (July–December 1822), 191.
[63] Bercé, *Chaudron et lancette*, pp. 259–63.
[64] Baron, *Life*, 1, p. 266; Jenner, *Continuation*, p. 42.

as entities that were potentially observable. It is probable, though, that, like
Cotton Mather in the 1720s, he imagined them figuratively as living things.[65]
He certainly took viruses seriously, assigning them agency, noting their
specific properties, and describing the responses that they elicited. He observed
that when a person was simultaneously inoculated with smallpox and cowpox
the latter delayed or even halted the smallpox infection. He found that herpetic
skin conditions often disrupted the process of vaccination.[66] Unfortunately, he
lacked the technical means to make a firm determination of the identity of
cowpox. Aware that the cow was not the original source of the infection, his
theory that it was derived from the horse, though insightful, was poorly
formulated and met with great scepticism. Drawing attention to the similarities
as well as the differences between smallpox and cowpox, he evidently
supposed that, like the wolf and the dog, they shared a common ancestry.[67]
Dr Coxe of Philadelphia followed up on Jenner's supposition but argued that,
given 'the length of time' necessary for the variation between them, it was
more plausible to regard them as distinct diseases.[68] In practice, medical men
seeking to confirm a case of cowpox remained dependent on observing the
progress of the vesicle at the inoculation site and comparing it with Jenner's
description and depiction of them. Dr Luigi Sacco, who discovered cowpox in
Italy, also proved able to build on Jenner's work by inoculating horsepox and
putting it into service on some scale.[69] Jenner also resumed his experimentation with horsepox, sending samples to the NVE in 1813 and 1817.[70] Over
the following decades, the issue of the identity of cowpox became even more
confused, with even Dr Baron, Jenner's biographer, taking the line that it was a
modified smallpox. The practice of retro-vaccination, in which calves were
inoculated to serve as reservoirs of cowpox lymph, added considerably to the
strains in circulation in the late nineteenth century. Advances in microscopy
brought some clarification in the 1930s when it was established that *vaccinia*
was not only different from *variola* but also from extant forms of cowpox. In
the late 1970s, Derrick Baxby raised the possibility that horsepox was the
source of *vaccinia* and Jenner's cowpox.[71] Genomic sequencing of horsepox
virus isolated in Mongolia, and the discovery of ancestral horsepox genes in
vaccinia, have recently provided compelling support for this hypothesis.[72] It
needs to be noted, of course, that neither the cow nor the horse appear to have
been the natural reservoir of this virus and the likelihood is that the host

[65] Mather, *Angel of Bethesda*, pp. 47, 94.
[66] Jenner, 'On effects of cutaneous eruptions', 97–102.
[67] Jenner, *Inquiry*, p. 2n; Hunter, 'Observations', 262–4.
[68] Coxe, *Practical observations*, p. 75.
[69] Sacco, *Osservazioni*; Sacco, *Trattato*, pp. 131–43; Baron, *Life*, 1, pp. 250–1.
[70] Baxby, *Jenner's vaccine*, pp. 176–7.   [71] Baxby, *Jenner's vaccine*, pp. 171–8.
[72] Damaso, 'Revisiting Jenner's mysteries', e56–8.

species of early *vaccinia* was a small mammal.[73] Given his interest in hedge-hogs and the popular belief that they sucked on the teats of cows, Jenner would have been delighted by the idea.[74]

The age of Jenner had no comprehension of the workings of the immune system. How smallpox made a victim insusceptible to subsequent infection was a problem of long standing. The assumption that smallpox was innate and the humoral paradigm in which it was embedded provided an explanation of sorts. It interpreted the sharp fever and violent ebullition in smallpox as evacuating the variolous poison in the body leaving no 'fuel' for a return of the disease. In explaining vaccination, Jenner would have probably been inclined to fall back on the position that cowpox inoculation worked in a similar fashion to smallpox inoculation, acting as a stimulus to bring out the poison. For many people, of course, the mildness of cowpox made them doubt that the procedure had truly made them secure. For medical men, who no longer believed that smallpox was innate, there was the need to replace the old theory with another explanation of how smallpox and cowpox infection made a person, in the formulation of the time, insusceptible to smallpox. While he often used metaphors of defence and resistance, describing vaccine as 'the guardian fluid' in 1806,[75] Jenner did not use the term 'immunity' in the modern sense. Drawn from law and political theory and connoting exemption from outside interference, it came only slowly into medical use in the nine-teenth century, beginning the obsession of the biosciences with boundary maintenance.[76] Still, he would have understood the modern term well enough. The expansion of its semantic range from the exemption of place to the body's resistance to disease took place during his own lifetime. In 1806, for example, Jenner described Cheltenham, where vaccination was well practised, as having 'immunity' from smallpox.[77] Shortly before Jenner's death in 1823, Dr Gregory, physician at St Pancras, used the term, presumably not for the first time, to refer to people insusceptible to smallpox.[78] Jenner regarded vaccin-ation as effecting 'specific change in the constitution necessary to render the contagion of the small pox inert'.[79] His observation of the hypersensitivity to variolation of a woman previously infected by cowpox is more obviously pertinent to modern understandings of cellular immunology. 'It seems', he wrote, 'as if a change, which endures through life, has been produced

---

[73] Baxby, *Jenner's vaccine*, p. 168; Fenner, Witteck and Dumbell, *Orthopoxviruses*, ch. 6.

[74] He described 'how the hedgehog has recourse to the cow's belly, when lying down, for warmth': Fosbroke, *Picturesque account*, p. 285.

[75] Thornton, *Vaccinæ vindicia*, p. 277.

[76] Ed Cohen, *A body worth defending. Immunity, biopolitics, and the apotheosis of the modern body* (Durham, NC, 2009), p. 64.

[77] Willan, *Vaccine inoculation*, appendix, p. ii.

[78] *Medico-Chirurgical Review*, 4 (1824), pp. 807–8.   [79] Baron, *Life*, 1, p. 294.

[by smallpox or cowpox] in the action, or disposition to action, in the vessels of the skin'.[80] The lack of awareness of another key finding of modern immunology had especially unfortunate consequences for the early reputation of vaccination. Jenner and his contemporaries should have realised that the insusceptibility to smallpox of people who had been exposed to cowpox decades earlier was not good evidence that cowpox infection provided life-long protection. After all, most of them would have been subsequently exposed to smallpox and in some cases variolated. James Phipps, the subject of the first experiment in May 1796, was variolated twice in the following months, and twenty times more over the next two decades.[81] Still, they can be forgiven for not appreciating that immunity to smallpox required periodic stimulus by exposure to the disease itself. Rather perversely, the retreat of smallpox in the first decade of vaccination not only made many people complacent about having their children immunised but also reduced the length of time that vaccinated children remained immune. Although people who caught smallpox after vaccination generally had mild symptoms, sub-clinical cases, undiagnosed and not isolated, posed a significant threat to public health.[82]

In Britain, the grand vision for vaccination faded rapidly. The hope that, once its advantages were recognised by doctors and patients, there would be sufficient interest to ensure the permanence of the practice proved a little forlorn. In some places, there was steady demand, and medical and philanthropic activism provided the support for its continuance. Vaccination failures and plebeian mistrust of patrician and professional condescension, however, often checked the practice's progress. The ups-and-downs in the numbers of vaccinations, however, tell a simpler story. Many parents sought vaccination for their children only when smallpox appeared to be an immediate threat. Even in Gloucestershire, the nursery of the practice and proposed as the showcase for its success, it was by no means routinely practised.[83] When smallpox broke out in the village of Ablington in December 1814, it took nine days for a surgeon to obtain vaccine from Northleach and begin vaccinating the many people at risk.[84] In the city of Norwich, where the poor had been offered free vaccination in 1805 and paid half-a-crown to be vaccinated in 1816, apathy and prejudices against the practice persisted. In 1819, when smallpox again broke out in the city and recourse to variolation added to the contagion, the medical men organised a general vaccination, each one assuming responsibility for a specific parish and vaccinating hundreds of people in their homes. Dr Cross collected data on the epidemic that showed the value of

---

[80] Jenner, *Inquiry*, p. 13n; Fenner, Wittek and Dumbell, *Orthopoxviruses*, p. 25.
[81] Saunders, *Cheltenham years*, pp. 390–1.   [82] Glynn and Glynn, *Rise and fall*, p. 59.
[83] Baron, *Life*, 2, pp. 371–3; Saunders, *Cheltenham years*, pp. 354–62.
[84] D269/B/F95, Gloucestershire Record Office, Gloucester.

vaccination for the quarter of the population who had embraced it.[85] The responses he received to a questionnaire he sent to surgeons in other towns and villages in Norfolk illustrate the challenges still facing the new prophylaxis. Almost all his ninety-three correspondents practised or recommended vaccination, but there was widespread demand for variolation. Forty of the surgeons refused to variolate on principle, but thirty-eight of them variolated some people, generally on their insistence. In Thetford, a well-organised town, the mayor managed to keep smallpox at bay by securing lists of people liable to infection and threatening them with 'public exposure' if they did not seek vaccination.[86]

In parts of continental Europe, vaccination had an immediate impact. Some cities and states proved able to banish smallpox for periods of time. In the largest Dutch cities, smallpox declined rapidly as a cause of mortality in the decade after the beginnings of vaccination, and it was wholly banished from Milan for some twenty years.[87] In the 1810s, several German states and the Scandinavian kingdoms achieved rates of compliance that seemed set to control the disease entirely. In the kingdom of Bavaria, Dr G. F. Krauss reported over 160,000 vaccinations in the Anspach and Rezat circles by 1818 and, with no smallpox deaths since 1809, claimed that smallpox had been eradicated in the region.[88] When smallpox threatened Denmark in 1808, Copenhagen was well protected. Nine out of ten of the population of around 100,000 had immunity to smallpox either from prior infection or through vaccination and the rapid vaccination of nearly 3,000 children gave the city an enviable level of herd immunity. In the event, there were only 200 cases in the city, but the case fatality rate of over one in five indicates how devastating the outbreak might otherwise have been.[89] High smallpox mortality elsewhere in Denmark prompted a further raft of measures that came close to making vaccination mandatory. In parts of Germany, vaccination rates not only remained high, but there was also early recognition of the need to make provision for revaccination.[90] Leadership in the science as well as the management of vaccination was becoming more widely diffused. The French and the Italians led the way in discovering new sources of cowpox, propagating it on calves and stabilising it with glycerine.[91]

[85] John Cross, *A history of the variolous epidemic which occurred in Norwich in the year 1819* (London, 1820), pp. 1–8, 13–14, 28–39.

[86] Cross, *History of variolous epidemic*, pp. 264–71.

[87] Willibrord Rutten, 'The demographic history of smallpox in the Netherlands, 18th–19th centuries', in Theo Engelen, John R. Shepherd and Yang Wen-shan (eds.), *Death at the opposite ends of the Eurasian subcontinent. Mortality trends in Taiwan and the Netherlands 1850–1945* (Amsterdam, 2011), pp. 183–197, at 193–4; Bercé, *Chaudron et lancette*, p. 256.

[88] Krauß, *Schuzpockenimpfung*, pp. 547–52.   [89] Bonderup, *En kovending*, pp. 44–5, 89–97.

[90] Baldwin, *Contagion and state*, pp. 316–19.   [91] Bercé, *Chaudron et lancette*, pp. 276–86.

Vaccination played a significant role in population growth in Europe in the early nineteenth century.[92] Scholars have found it hard to establish its precise contribution to the demographic shift in Europe, a key feature of which was the decline in infant mortality rates, which began before large-scale smallpox prophylaxis. It is perhaps more relevant to see the contribution of vaccination in Europe from 1800 as helping to sustain the decline in mortality at a time of demographic expansion and urbanisation and in the face of increasing resource pressures and epidemiological challenges. In terms of the numbers of people variolated or vaccinated, of course, it is unlikely that they were ever more than a modest proportion of the number of live births, though presumably a somewhat larger proportion of the children who survived their first years. The statistics from some other parts of Europe appear more impressive. In France in 1811–15, the ratio of vaccinations to live births was subject to some variation: over 90 per cent in some *départements*, over 50 per cent in more than half, and less than 20 per cent in some others.[93] In Sweden, the ratio rose from around 40 per cent to around 80 per cent in the decade after 1815.[94] In the kingdom of the Two Sicilies, the number of vaccinations between 1808 and 1819, over a third of a million, represented only 15 per cent of the number of live births.[95] It needs to be borne in mind, however, that most adults in the first decade of vaccination would have already been exposed to smallpox, casual or inoculated. If one adds the proportions of babies who did not survive infancy or were infected casually by smallpox, the proportion of people who had immunity would have been quite high in some places. It needs to be recognised, too, that 'partial coverage might have had a more than proportionate effect on reducing the impact of the disease, as the presence of some vaccinated persons would inhibit its spread to the non-vaccinated'.[96] Furthermore, there is a qualitative dimension to partial coverage, as is evident in the French statistics, with low take-up being most associated with remote districts. In other word, the people most at risk of catching smallpox and in turn communicating it – especially young people living close to population centres – were more likely to be vaccinated than their country cousins. In the early nineteenth century, it was certainly assumed that the adoption of the new prophylaxis was having demographic consequences. Thomas Malthus famously predicted that the decrease in smallpox deaths would be counter-balanced by mortality from other crowd diseases and Robert Watt, a physician in Glasgow, presented data to show that measles was

---

[92] Mercer, 'Smallpox and epidemiological-demographic change', 287–307.
[93] Darmon, *La longue traque*, p. 208.   [94] Sköld, *Two faces*, p. 473.
[95] Gianni Iacovelli, 'Antonio Miglietta, *il vero apostolo della vaccinia*, e il vaiolo a Napoli tra 700 e 800, in Antonio Tagarelli, Anna Piro and Walter Pasini (eds.), *Il vaiolo e la vaccinazione in Italia*, vol. 2 (Villa Verucchio, 2004), pp. 561–80, at 568.
[96] Michael Drake, *Population and society in Norway, 1735–1865* (Cambridge, 1969), p. 53n.

taking the place of smallpox as the major child killer.[97] Most contemporaries, however, saw the lives saved from smallpox as real gains. In 1806 Emmanuel Duvillard drew up life tables for the French government, demonstrating the loss to smallpox in each cohort and calculating that, if infants were vaccinated at birth, 12.5 per cent more of them would survive to age sixteen, with the likelihood of becoming productive citizens and parents.[98] It needs to be noted, too, that vaccination significantly reduced the costs to local economies and family budgets associated with quarantines and general morbidity.

In the early years of the nineteenth century, a solid constituency was established for vaccination around the world. Although there was coercion in some contexts, it was largely a matter of parental or personal choice. For the first time, there was the means to provide, at little cost and risk, protection against a disease that, a generation earlier, afflicted most of the population and caused around 10 per cent of deaths. For parents and children, and especially for young people seeking to make their way in life, it was an emancipatory force that freed them from a major cause of disfigurement, disability and death and from a corresponding fear and anxiety for themselves and their loved ones. This quiet revolution may have been especially significant for women. Mothers often appear to have been centrally involved in decisions relating to smallpox prophylaxis. Aristocratic women promoted the practice and in several countries midwives were involved in vaccination.[99] It made so large a difference to people that they ceased to remember what it was like to live with the fear of smallpox. T. B. Macaulay, who in his history of England described smallpox in the late seventeenth century as 'chief among the ministers of death ... leaving on those whose lives it spared the hideous traces of its power [and] turning the babe into a changeling at which the mother shuddered', was a member of the first generation of children who were vaccinated.[100] Edward Ballard, though two decades younger than Macaulay, still recalled seeing many people badly scarred from smallpox. The benefits of vaccination, he wrote in the late 1860s, 'are patent enough to everybody who is old enough to recollect what he was in the habit of seeing in society and in the streets some 30 or 40 years back. I allude to the number of persons whose faces were scarred and seamed by a previous attack of smallpox. How rarely is this

[97] Robert Watt, *Treatise on the history, nature and treatment of Chincough ... with inquiry into the relative mortality of the principal diseases of children in Glasgow* (Glasgow, 1813), pp. 333–84.

[98] E. E. Duvillard, *Analyse et tableaux de l'influence de la petite vérole sur la mortalité à chaque âge, et de celle qu'un préservatif tel que la vaccine peut avoir sur la population et la longévité* (Paris, 1806), p. 149.

[99] Bennett, 'Jenner's ladies', 497–513; Tisci, 'Le levatrici', 37–41.

[100] Thomas Babington Macaulay, *The history of England from the accession of James II*, vol. 4 (Cambridge, 1855), p. 530; Knutsford, *Life of Zachary Macaulay*, p 247.

observed now!'[101] The common concern was that people were becoming complacent about prophylaxis. The appearance of smallpox, of course, usually prompted mothers to rush to have their children immunised. While this approach worked well enough for some people, the problem for the wider community was that the supply of good vaccine was rarely sufficient for a sudden spike in demand. Major smallpox outbreaks in England in the late 1830s demonstrated the limitations of voluntarism, prompting legislative support for the practice in 1840 and compulsory vaccination in 1853.

In the meantime, vaccination was continuing its global expansion. In some European colonies, not least in British India and Mauritius, it was used on a considerable scale. It could be presented as a benefit conferred by Europe on colonial subjects to set alongside the record of imperial predation.[102] The idea had special resonance in the Americas where smallpox followed the arrival of European conquest and colonisation. In his *Tale of Paraguay*, Robert Southey presents vaccination as balm to the Christian and specifically the British conscience.[103] There are indications that the practice served to reduce smallpox mortality in parts of the Philippines and Indonesia in the first half of the nineteenth century.[104] Beyond imperial frontiers, its progress was slow. European penetration of the interior of Africa opened new lines of transmission for smallpox long before vaccine could be made available. In several non-European countries, however, modernising rulers and their advisers took an interest in vaccination. In 1819, Muhammad Ali, ruler of Egypt, ordered the introduction of vaccination in Egypt and recruited French doctors to establish a nationwide programme in the late 1820s using midwives trained in the procedure.[105] Soon after his accession in 1820, Minh Mang, Emperor of Vietnam expressed a desire 'to establish [vaccination] in his country and save all the misfortunes that smallpox raised up each year'. After a French doctor in his service returned with vaccine from Macao in 1821, the practice began on a modest scale.[106] Given its success in keeping foreign influences at bay, Japan presents remarkable testimony to the utility of vaccination. In 1812, a Japanese scholar obtained a Russian pamphlet on vaccination and, after hearing positive

---

[101] Edward Ballard, *On vaccination: its value and alleged dangers. A prize essay* (London, 1867), p. 74.

[102] Ainslie, 'Observations', 72.

[103] Tim Fulford, *The late poetry of the Lake Poets. Romanticism revised* (Cambridge, 2013), pp. 98–9.

[104] Ken De Bevoise, *Agents of apocalypse: epidemic disease in the colonial Philippines* (Princeton, NJ, 1995), p. 99. Boomgaard, 'Smallpox, vaccination, Indonesia', 603–4, 610.

[105] LaVerne Kuhnke, *Lives at risk: public health in nineteenth-century Egypt* (Berkeley, CA, 1990), pp. 113–21.

[106] Léopold Cadière, 'Documents relative à l'époque de Gia-long', *Bulletin de l'Ecole française d'Extrême-Orient*, 12 (1912), 1–82, at 64–5; C. Michele Thompson, *Vietnamese traditional medicine: a social history* (Singapore, 2015), pp. 31–2, 38–44.

reports of the practice, embarked on translation. By the mid-1820s, Japanese medical men who were receiving instruction in Dutch medicine in Nagasaki recognised the potential value of cowpox. After obtaining permission for a trial of vaccination in the 1840s, they obtained viable vaccine in 1849 and succeeded in propagating it. Using the arm-to-arm method and the movement of children, the practice spread rapidly. The success of the new prophylaxis assisted the broader assimilation of western medicine in Japan.[107]

Vaccination introduced new principles and new possibilities. Unlike variolation, it could be made safely available to all. It signalled a major advance in preventive medicine and expanded conceptions of social medicine and public health. It has been presented as a first step in the medicalisation of society.[108] Like baptism, it came to mark the entry of most children into medical records and government statistics. It has been argued that the new prophylaxis differed from the old in terms of risk management. Unlike variolation, a matter of probabilities, with all its ethical and emotional concerns, vaccination was a seemingly simple technique, mandated by science and policy, with no moral implications. Though the pressure from medical men and governments should not be overstated, vaccination opened a new chapter in the alliance of science and the state and represented the pointy end of the expanding control over individuals and their bodies.[109] Conceptually, too, vaccination strained old paradigms, presented challenging questions of theory and practice and raised new hopes and ambitions. Jenner went a long way in addressing practical issues and offering speculative insights. The cowpox discovery and the rapid expansion of the practice created 'a fast-moving research front'.[110] From the obscurity and confusion, there emerged a body of data, knowledge and insight that marked the beginnings of the discipline of virology. It was not until the 1880s, however, that there was a major breakthrough in understanding the role of microbes as infective agents and in adding to the number of diseases that could be controlled by inoculation.[111] Louis Pasteur, who inoculated attenuated anthrax to protect cattle, honoured Jenner by extending the term 'vaccination' to refer to all forms of prophylactic inoculation. It was not until the 1930s, a century after Jenner's death, that the invention of the electron microscope made it possible for the first time to see the viruses whose identities and impact on the human constitution Jenner described and sought to understand. For Frank Fenner, Jennerian vaccination also laid the foundations of the modern science of immunology.[112] It was not until the late

---

[107] Jannetta, *Vaccinators*, esp. chs. 3–6.   [108] Huerkamp, 'Vaccination in Germany', 617–35.
[109] Fressoz, *L'apocalypse joyeuse*, ch. 2.
[110] Collins, *Sociology of philosophies*, pp. 352–3; Bennett, 'Note-taking', 431.
[111] Michael Worboys, *Spreading germs: disease theories and medical practice in Britain, 1865–1900* (Cambridge, 2000).
[112] Fenner, Witteck and Dumbell, *Orthopoxviruses*, p. 25.

twentieth century, however, that advances began to be made in understanding the workings of the immune system.

The End of an Age

Sixty-five years old and world-weary, Jenner left London for the last time in July 1814. In Berkeley, his beloved wife, whose health was often a concern, was seriously ill. Her death in autumn 1815 left him distraught.[113] His only surviving son Robert was at Oxford and his daughter, who had looked after her mother, married and moved away. The intimate family life that meant so much to him came to an end. Jenner passed most of his practice to his nephew Henry who still lived with him at The Chantry, and he had a close circle of friends in the neighbourhood, including Dr John Baron at Gloucester. He threw himself into the life of the community as a justice of the peace, Freemason and founder of the local branch of the Bible Society.[114] He enjoyed the pleasures of country life, including natural history excursions with old friends. He increasingly had a sense of himself as the last of his generation. Dr Caleb Parry, an old school-friend and dedicatee of the *Inquiry*, died in 1822.[115] He struggled through the winter of 1822–3. On returning home from delivering firewood to a poor neighbour, he had a stroke. He managed to drag himself into his library, but was not found until the next morning. He died in the early hours of 26 January 1823.

Almost to the end, Jenner was bound to the mast of vaccination. After his return to Gloucestershire, he was kept informed of the progress of the practice and his advice was actively sought. On his visits to Cheltenham, he was button-holed on the topic of vaccination and he continued to be burdened by correspondence. Still, he must have been gratified by expressions of esteem from admirers around the world. In autumn 1814, Dr S. T. von Sömmering wrote from Munich presenting an award from the Royal Academy of Sciences of Bavaria and adding his hope that 'the blessings of so many millions whose lives you saved, or whose deformities you prevented, contribute to exhilarate the days of their benefactor'.[116] A letter in broken English from medical men in Brünn, presenting the Moravian town as a seat of war from the time of the Huns until the French invasion, informed him that they held an annual festival on his birthday to celebrate the cowpox discovery and that on his sixty-fifth birthday the youth of the town raised a permanent monument to him, 'with the most cordial sentiments of gratitude', even as the 'great English nation' brought liberty to Europe.[117] On leave from the East Indies, Sir Thomas

---

[113] Fosbroke, *Picturesque account*, p. 290.   [114] Saunders, *Cheltenham years*, p. 337.
[115] Fisher, *Jenner*, pp. 236–7, 289.   [116] Baron, *Life*, 2, pp. 215–17.
[117] Fisher, *Jenner*, p. 243; Baron, *Life*, 2, pp. 213–14.

Stamford Raffles made a special effort to meet Jenner to report on his work in establishing a system of vaccination in Java, temporarily under British rule, in which a key feature was a corps of native vaccinators known as Jennerian sawahs.[118] Jenner enjoyed the company of Americans, several of whom he befriended in Cheltenham. He was distressed to learn from William Dilwyn, an American visitor, that a smallpox outbreak in Philadelphia had been the occasion of some loss of faith in the practice, prompting him to write a short pamphlet, published in Philadelphia in 1818, addressing some of the concerns that had arisen and affirming that his 'confidence in the efficacy of the vaccine ... is not in the least diminished'.[119] As late as February 1821, he addressed an open letter to the medical profession seeking responses to his observations on vaccinating children with herpetic conditions, and, in July, replied at length to one of his respondents.[120]

After his death, Jenner's family and friends made the arrangements for his funeral and commemoration. He was buried alongside his wife in Berkeley, but a committee was formed to organise a memorial in Gloucester cathedral and an appeal was launched for a statue. The newspapers that reported his death did so in a rather perfunctory fashion and there is no evidence of a groundswell of support for commemoration. In London, the appeal was presented as a 'provincial monument to Dr Jenner', and it is probable that his friends and admirers outside Gloucestershire may have been expecting moves for a national memorial.[121] For a time, it appeared that there would be insufficient money for a statue in Gloucester. The Royal College of Physicians subscribed £50 and Freemasons attending a service in his honour contributed £90.[122] In the end, £640 was raised, sufficient to tempt Robert Sievier, a rising talent, to take on the commission. There was some issue, too, as to how Jenner's life and achievement would be commemorated in print. The Rev. Thomas Fosbroke, an old friend, had anticipated writing his biography. He appended a brief account of Jenner's life to his history of Berkeley and John Fosbroke included some biographical notes in his appendix to his father's history of Cheltenham.[123] It was Dr John Baron, Jenner's disciple, who took on the task of working through the jumble of Jenner's papers to craft a reverential biography, including a selection of letters, published in two volumes in 1827 and 1838.[124]

Jenner was a new sort of hero, a humanitarian counterpart to the men of war and an inspiration to subsequent generations of health workers. For a time, his

---

[118] Saunders, *Cheltenham years*, pp. 366–7.   [119] Jenner, *Letter to Dilwyn*.
[120] *MPJ*, 45 (January–June 1821), 277; *MPJ*, 48 (July–December 1822), 190–5.
[121] *MPJ*, 48 (January–June 1823), 359
[122] *Bath Chronicle and Weekly Gazette*, 28 August 1823.
[123] Fosbroke, *Berkeley manuscripts*, pp. 219–42; Fosbroke, *Picturesque account*, pp. 272–300.
[124] Baron, *Life*, 1, pp. ix–xxiv.

name and his *persona* – not entirely contrived – as a kindly country doctor were usefully linked to the powerful idea of a simple remedy, a gift of Providence, for one of mankind's greatest scourges. The early anecdotes that supported this image were put into circulation by Dr Lettsom who solicited them from Jenner's circle.[125] No one deserves to be the centre of a cult and Jenner, tongue-tied and awkward with strangers, probably never quite lived up to the expectations that people had of him. Few of the admirers who met him after the cowpox discovery left reminiscences of him. The French physician Dr Valentin visited him in 1803, but Dr de Carro, who was eager for Valentin's report of the visit, had to be satisfied with generalities about his kindliness.[126] On hearing of Jenner's death, the Rev. F. E. Witts, who had known him for over twenty years, described him in his diary as 'a man of distinguished talents, an original thinker, sometimes rather eccentric, but always kind hearted'. He also presented a striking image of him as a 'broad, thickset, clumsy' man, whose countenance was 'coarse, though very intelligent, when lighted up by the talent within'.[127] On seeing Sievier's statue of Jenner sometime later, he reported that he found it elegant but not a good resemblance: Jenner's appearance, he wrote, 'was a very unsuitable study for a sculptor'.[128]

Jenner was indeed a genius. If his claims to discovery can be overstated, they remain compelling. He was not the fount of all wisdom on vaccination, but in his observation and theorising about cowpox he remained the master of his field. He worked tirelessly for the cause and gained little materially from making vaccination his life's work. He was prickly and arrogant and by no means blameless for the problems that emerged, not least the ructions that divided the vaccination movement, but he evidently felt duty-bound to uphold the validity and the integrity of a demonstrably valuable practice. As the Rev. Witts observed, Jenner 'lived to see the test of experience applied to his great discovery, and though, perhaps, the high expectations originally entertained … may have been disappointed, yet the wonderful controlling power of vaccination over [smallpox] has been most clearly ascertained', adding that his 'fame was, perhaps, more extensively established in all quarters of the globe, than in his native country'.[129] It certainly seemed that way in the following decades. Moves to honour Jenner as a national hero were slow. The centenary of Jenner's birth in 1849 may have prompted Calder Marshall to set to work on a statue. Subsequent developments sadly reprise themes of Jenner's public career. Some members of the committee formed to raise funds for a

---

[125] MS. 1277, New York Academy of Medicine.
[126] Louis Valentin, *Notice historique sur le Docteur Jenner, auteur de la découverte de la vaccine: suivie de notes explicatives*, 2nd ed. (Anvers, 1824), pp. 35–40.
[127] *The diary of a Cotswold parson. Reverend F. E. Witts 1783–1854*, ed. D. Verey (Stroud, UK, 2008), p. 53.
[128] *Diary of Cotswold parson*, pp. 31–2, 53.   [129] *Diary of Cotswold parson*, pp. 31–2.

monument resigned when they learned that the appeal was to pay for Marshall's statue not a new work. In 1857, the committee found it necessary to enlist physicians in Europe and America in the fund-raising. In writing to colleagues, the octogenarian Dr De Carro anticipated their surprise 'that Albion's rich children should seek beyond their three kingdoms and their vast colonies contributions to such an insignificant sum as £4,000', but urged Jenner's 'immense claims to universal gratitude'.[130] The Americans proved most responsive, contributing twice as much as Britain, and the Russians, with whom Britain had recently been at war, also gave generously.[131] Finally, in 1858, Marshall's statue was erected in the southwest corner of Trafalgar Square.[132] In death as in life, Jenner was not allowed to enjoy his laurels undisturbed. In controversial circumstances, the statue was moved in 1862 to the relative obscurity of Kensington Gardens.[133]

---

[130] 'The late Chevalier Jean de Carro, M.D.', *BMJ*, 1, no. 24 (13 June 1857), 504–5.

[131] *BMJ*, 1, no. 18 (2 May 1857), 383.   [132] *BMJ*, 1, no. 73 (22 May 1858), 421–2.

[133] John Empson, 'Little honoured in his own country: statues in recognition of Edward Jenner MD, FRS', *Journal of the Royal Society of Medicine*, 89 (1996), 514–18.

Select Bibliography

This list includes the repositories of unpublished sources and a selection of the published primary and secondary sources cited in the footnotes.

Primary Sources

Unpublished

Letters, reports and records relating to vaccination from libraries and archives in Australia, France, Ireland, Italy, the United Kingdom and the United States, including New South Wales State Library, Sydney; Archives nationales, Paris; Royal College of Physicians of Ireland, Dublin; Archivio de stato, Siena; British Library (including Oriental and India Office Collections), Royal College of Physicians, Royal College of Surgeons, Royal Society of Medicine, The National Archives, and Wellcome Library, London; Countway Library of Medicine, Massachusetts Historical Society, Boston; New York Academy of Medicine, New York; American Philosophical Society, Philadelphia College of Physicians, Philadelphia.

Published

Anderson, James, *Correspondence for the extermination of small-pox* (Madras, 1804).

Baron, John, *The life of Edward Jenner*, 2 vols. (London, 1827 and 1838).

Batt, William, *Giustificazione dell'innesto della vaccina di Jenner, specialmente nella Centrale nella Liguria* (Genova, 1801).

Bryce, James, *Practical observations on the inoculation of cowpox* (Edinburgh, 1802).

Calcagni, Franceso, *A letter on the inoculation of the vaccina practised in Sicily*, transl. Edward Cutbush (Philadelphia, 1807).

Carneiro, Heleodoro, *Reflections and observations on the practice of vaccine inoculation, and its melancholy consequences; with a true account of the late events which happened in Portugal and Brazil to the persons vaccinated* (London, 1809).

Carro, Jean de, *Observations et expériences sur la vaccination* (Vienna, 1801).

Carro Jean de, *Histoire de la vaccination en Turquie, en Grèce, et aux Indes Orientales* (Vienna, 1804).

Christie, Thomas, *An account of the ravages committed in Ceylon by small-pox previous to the introduction of vaccination; with a statement of the circumstances*

381

attending the introduction, progress and success of vaccine inoculation in that island (Cheltenham, 1811).

Colon, François, *Histoire de l'introduction et des progrès de la vaccine* (Paris, 1801).

Coxe, John Redman, *Practical observations on vaccination: or inoculation for the cow-pock; embellished with a coloured engraving, representing a comparative view of the various stages of the vaccine and small-pox* (Philadelphia, 1802).

Dunning, Richard, *Some observations on vaccination or the inoculated cow-pox* (London, 1800).

Epps, John, *The Life of John Walker, M.D.* (London, 1831).

Fancher [Fansher], Sylvanus, 'Progress of vaccination in America', *Massachusetts Historical Society Collections*, Series 2, Vol. 4 (1816).

Faust, Bernhard Christoph, *An den Herrn Dr. Eduard Jenner, über einige Versuche zur weiteren Untersuchung der Wirkungen und zum Beweise der Unschädlichkeit der Kuhpocken-Materie* (Hannover, 1802).

Giel, Franz Seraph, *Die Schutzpocken-Impfung in Bayern, vom Anbeginn ihrer Entstehung und gesetzlichen Einführung bis auf gegenwärtige Zeit, dann mit besonderer Beobachtung derselben in auswärtigen Staaten* (Munchen, 1830).

Hernández, Pedro, *Origen y descubrimiento de la vaccina* (Madrid, 1801).

Husson, Henri Marie, *Recherches historiques et médicales sur la vaccine*, 3rd ed. (Paris, 1803).

Jenner, Edward, *An inquiry into the causes and effects of the variolæ vaccinæ, or cow pox, a disease discovered in the western counties of England, and known by the name of the cow pox* (London, 1798).

Jenner, Edward, *Further observations on the variolæ vaccinæ, or cow pox* (London, 1799).

Jenner, Edward, *A continuation of facts and observations relative to the variolæ vaccinæ, or cow pox* (London, 1800).

Jenner, Edward, *On the origin of vaccine inoculation* (London, 1801).

Jenner, G. C., ed. *Evidence at large, as laid before the committee of the House of Commons, respecting Dr Jenner's discovery of vaccine inoculation* (London, 1805).

Krauß, Georg Friedrich, *Die Schutzpockenimpfung in ihrer endlichen Entscheidung als Angelegenheit des Staats, der Familien und des Einzelnen* (Nürnberg, 1820).

Keir, George, *Account of the introduction of the cowpox into India* (Bombay, 1803).

Lettsom, John Coakley, *Observations on the cow-pock* (London, 1801).

Miller, Geneviève, ed. *Letters of Edward Jenner, and other documents concerning the early history of vaccination* (Baltimore, 1983).

Murray, Charles, *An answer to Mr Highmore's objections to the Bill before Parliament to prevent the spreading of the infection of the small-pox* (London, 1808).

Murray, Charles, *Debates in Parliament respecting the Jennerian discovery, including the late debate on the further grant of twenty thousand pounds to Dr Jenner* (London, 1808).

Olagüe de Ros, Guillermo and Mikel Astrain Gallart, 'Una carta inédita de Ignacio María Ruiz de Luzuriaga (1763–1822) sobre la diffusion de la vacuna en España (1801)', *Dynamis. Acta Hispanica ad Medicinæ Scientiarumque Historiam Illuminandam*, 14 (1994), 305–37.

Pearson, George, *An inquiry concerning the history of the cowpox, principally with a view to supersede and extinguish the smallpox* (London, 1798).

Pearson, George, *An examination of the Report of the Committee of the House of Commons on the Claims of Remuneration for the Vaccine Pock Inoculation* (London, 1802).

Rapport du comité central de vaccine, établi à Paris par la société des souscripteurs pour l'examen de cette découverte (Paris, 1803).

Ring, John, *A treatise on the cow-pox; containing the history of vaccine inoculation*, 2 vols. (London, 1801 and 1803).

Romay, Tomás, *Memoria sobra la introduccion y progreso de la vacuna en la isla de Cuba* (Havana, 1805).

Rowley, William, *Cow-pox inoculation, no security against small-pox infection* (London, 1805).

Sacco, Luigi, *Osservazioni pratice sull'uso del vajuolo vaccino come preservativo del vajuolo humano* (Milan, 1801).

Sacco, Luigi, *Trattato di vaccinazione con osservazioni sul giavardo e vajuolo pecorino* (Milan, 1809).

Shoolbred, John, *Report on the progress of vaccine inoculation in Bengal from the period of its introduction in November, 1802, to the end of the year 1803* (Calcutta, 1804).

Shoolbred, John, *Report on the state and progress of vaccine inoculation in Bengal during the year 1804* (Calcutta, 1805).

Sigerist, Henry E., ed. *Letters of Jean de Carro to Alexandre Marcet, 1794–1817* (Baltimore, 1950).

[Smith, Juan], *Progresos de la vacina in Tarragona ó instrucciones y reflexiones sobre la inoculacion de la vacina dirigidas á los padres de familia y á los sugetos que sin ser facultativos se quieran dedicar al fomento y propagacion de este admirable descubrimiento, en beneficio de la humanidad* (Tarragona, 1801).

Thornton, Robert John, *Facts decisive in favour of the cow-pock, including an account of the village of Lowther* (London, 1802).

Thornton, Robert John, *Vaccinæ vindicia: or, defence of vaccination . . .* (London, 1806).

Walker, John, *Fragments of letters and other papers written in different parts of Europe, at sea, and on the Asiatic and African coasts or shores of the Mediterranean* (London, 1802).

Waterhouse, Benjamin, *A prospect of exterminating the small-pox. Part II. Being a continuation of a narrative of facts concerning the progress of the new inoculation in America* (Cambridge, MA, 1802).

Contemporary Periodicals

Contemporary journals and newspapers, notably medical journals that were founded at the end of the eighteenth century, e.g. *Annals of Medicine* (Edinburgh), *Archiv der Aerzte und Seelsorger wider die Pockennoth* (1796–9), *Hufelands Journal der practischen Heilkunde* (Jena), *Medical and Physical Journal* (London), *Medical Repository* (New York) and *Journal général de médecine, de chirurgie et de pharmacie* (Paris).

Secondary Sources

Published

Archila, Ricardo, 'The Balmis expedition in Venezuela. Part II: Founding of the Central Vaccination Board, 1804', in J. Z. Bowers and Elizabeth F. Purcell (eds.), *Aspects of the history of medicine in Latin America* (New York, 1979), pp. 142–77.

Balaguer Perigüell, Emilio and Rosa Ballester Añón, *En el nombre de los niños: la Real Expedición Filantrópica de la Vacuna (1803–1806)* (Madrid, 2003).

Baldwin, Peter, *Contagion and the state, 1830–1930* (Cambridge, 1999).

Baxby, Derrick, *Jenner's smallpox vaccine. The riddle of vaccinia virus and its origin* (London, 1981).

Bennett, Michael, 'Passage through India: global vaccination and British India, 1800–05', *Journal of Imperial and Commonwealth History*, 35 (2007), 201–20.

Bennett, Michael, 'Jenner's ladies: women and vaccination against smallpox in early nineteenth-century Britain', *History*, 93 (2008), 497–513.

Bennett, Michael, 'Smallpox and cowpox under the Southern Cross: the smallpox epidemic of 1789 and the advent of vaccination in colonial Australia', *BHM*, 83 (2009), 37–62.

Bennett, Michael, 'Note-taking and data-sharing: Edward Jenner and the global vaccination network', *Intellectual History Review*, 20 (2010), 415–32.

Bercé, Yves-Marie, *Le chaudron et la lancette. Croyances populaires et médecine preventive (1798–1830)* (Paris, 1984).

Bhattacharya, Sanjoy, Mark Harrison, and Michael Worboys, *Fractured states: smallpox, public health and vaccination policy in British India 1800–1947* (London, 2005).

Biraben, Jean-Noël, 'La diffusion de vaccination en France au xixᵉ siècle', *Annales de Bretagne et des pays de l'Ouest*, 86 (1979), 265–76.

Boddice, Rob, *Edward Jenner* (Stroud, 2015).

Bonderup, Gerda, *En kovending: koppevaccinationen og dens udfordring til det danske samfund omkring 1800* (Aarhus, 2001).

Boomgaard, Peter, 'Smallpox, vaccination, and the *Pax Neerlandica*, Indonesia, 1530–1930', *Bijdragen tot de Taal- en Volkenkunde*, 159 (2003), 590–617.

Brimnes, N., 'Variolation, vaccination and popular resistance in early colonial south India', *MH*, 48 (2004), 199–228.

Brunton, Deborah, *The politics of vaccination. Practice and policy in England, Wales, Ireland, and Scotland, 1800–1874* (Rochester, NY, 2008).

Carpanetto, Dino, 'Buniva e il governo della sanità nel Piemonte Napoleonica', in Giuseppe Slaviero (ed.), *Michele Buniva introduttore della vaccinazione in Piemonte. Scienza e sanità tra rivoluzione e restaurazione* (Torino, 2002).

Cash, Philip, *Dr. Benjamin Waterhouse. A life in medicine and public service (1754–1846)* (Sagamore Beach, MA, 2006).

Colvin, Thomas B., 'Arms around the world. The introduction of smallpox vaccine into the Philippines and Macao in 1805', *Revista de Cultura*, 18 (2006), 71–88.

Da Silva, Carlos, *A Vaca Imortalizada a Vacina Antivariólica e as Vacinas de Wright no Brasil* (Rio de Janeiro, 1972).

Díaz de Yraola, Gonzalo, *La vuelta al mundo de la Expedición de la Vacuna (1803–1810). Facsimil de la edición de 1948 y versión inglesa traducida y editada por Catherine Mark* (Madrid, 2004).

Fenner, Frank, Riccardo Wittek, and Keith R. Dumbell, *The orthopoxviruses* (San Diego, CA, 1989).

Ferrario, Giuseppe, *Vita ed opere del grande vaccinatore Italiano Dottore Luigi Sacco e sunto storico dello innesto del vajuolo umano del vaccino e della rivaccinazione* (Milan, 1858).

Few, Martha, *For all of humanity. Mesoamerican and colonial medicine in Enlightenment Guatemala* (Tucson, AZ, 2015).

Fisher, Richard B., *Edward Jenner 1749–1823* (London, 1991).

Fressoz, Jean-Baptiste *L'apocalypse joyeuse. Une histoire du risque technologique* (Paris, 2012).

Fulford, Tim and Debbie Lee, 'The Jenneration of disease: vaccination, romanticism and revolution', *Studies in Romanticism*, 39 (2000), 139–63.

Gins, H. A., *Krankheit wider den Tod. Schicksal der Pockenschutzimpfung* (Stuttgart, 1963).

Glynn, Ian and Jennifer Glynn, *The rise and fall of smallpox* (London, 2004).

Green, Rebecca Fields, '"Simple, easy, and intelligible": Republican political ideology and the implementation of vaccination in the Early Republic', *Early American Studies: An Interdisciplinary Journal*, 12 (2014), 301–37.

Gubert, V. O., *Ospa i ospoprivivanie* [*Smallpox and inoculation*] (St Petersburg, 1896).

Hackett, Paul, 'Averting disaster: the Hudson's Bay Company and smallpox in Western Canada during the late eighteenth and early nineteenth centuries', *BHM*, 78 (2004), 575–609.

Heydon, Susan, 'Death of the King: the introduction of vaccination into Nepal in 1816', *MH*, 63 (2019), 24–43.

Hopkins, Donald R., *The greatest killer. Smallpox in history* (Chicago, 2002).

Huerkamp, Claudia, 'The history of smallpox vaccination in Germany: a first step in the medicalization of the general public', *Journal of Contemporary History*, 20 (1985), 617–35.

Jannetta, Ann, *The vaccinators. Smallpox, medical knowledge, and the 'opening' of Japan* (Stanford, CA, 2007).

Lee, Debbie and Tim Fulford, 'The beast within: the imperial legacy of vaccination in history and literature', *Literature and History* 9 (2000), 1–23.

Mark, Catherine and José G. Rigau-Pérez, 'The world's first immunization campaign: the Spanish smallpox vaccine expedition, 1803–1813', *BHM*, 83 (2009), 63–94.

Mercer, Alex J., 'Smallpox and epidemiological-demographic change in Europe: the role of vaccination', *Population Studies*, 39 (1985), 287–307.

Munch, Ragnhild (ed.), *Pocken zwischen Alltag, Medizin und Politik. Begleitbuch zur Ausstellung* (Berlin, 1994).

Pammer, M.,'Vom Bleichzettel zum Impfzeugnis. Beamte, Ärzte, Priester und die Einführung der Vaccination', *Österreich in Geschichte und Literatur*, 39 (1995), 11–29.

Ramírez Martín, Susana María, *La mayor hazaña médica de la colonia. La Real Expedición Filantrópico de la Vacuna en la Real Audiencia de Quito* (Quito, 1999).

Ramírez Martín, Susana María, *La salud del Imperio. La Real Expedición Filantrópico de la Vacuna* (Madrid, 2001).

Razzell, Peter, *Edward Jenner's cowpox vaccine: the history of a medical myth* (Firle, 1977).

Rigau-Pérez, José G., 'The introduction of smallpox vaccine in Puerto Rico in 1803 and the adoption of immunization as a government function in Puerto Rico', *Hispanic American Historical Review*, 69 (1989), 393–423.

Rusnock, Andrea, 'Catching cowpox: the early spread of smallpox vaccination, 1798–1810', *BHM*, 83 (2009).

Rutten, Willibrord, *Pokkenepidemieën en pokkenbestrijding in Nederland in de 18e en 19e eeuw* (t' Goy-Houten, Netherlands, 1997).

Seth, Catriona, *Les rois aussi en mouraient. Les Lumières en lutte contre la petite vérole* (Paris, 2008).

Sköld, Peter, *The two faces of smallpox. A disease and its prevention in eighteenth- and nineteenth-century Sweden* (Umeå, 1996).

Smith, J. R., *The speckled monster. Smallpox in England, 1670–1970, with particular reference to Essex* (Chelmsford, 1987).

Smith, Michael M., 'The "Real Expedición Marítima de la Vacuna" in New Spain and Guatemala', *Transactions of the American Philosophical Society*, new series 64 (1974), part 1, 1–74.

Thompson, Angela T., 'To save the children: smallpox inoculation, vaccination, and public health in Guanajuato, Mexico, 1797–1840', *The Americas*, 49, no. 4 (1993), 431–55.

Tisci, Caterina, 'Le levatrici e la diffusione della vaccinazione antivaiolosa nel Regno di Napoli', *Revista Internacional de Culturas & Literaturas*, 3 (2005), 37–41.

Warren, Adam, *Medicine and politics in colonial Peru. Population growth and the Bourbon reforms* (Pittsburgh, 2010).

Williams, Gareth, *Angel of death. The story of smallpox* (Basingstoke, 2010).

Wolff, Eberhard, *Einschneidende Maßnahmen. Pockenschutzimpfung und traditionale Gesellshaft im Württemberg des frühen 19. Jahrhunderts* (Stuttgart, 1998).

Unpublished

Unpublished theses from universities and institutes in Australia, Great Britain, Colombia, Spain and the United States, by Luis Blasco Martínez, Deborah C. Brunton, Chia-Feng Chang (Jiafeng Zhang), Dianne Ecklund Farrell, Jacqueline Gratton, Andrea Catalina Gutiérrez Beltrán, Laura Martínez González, Adrián López Denis, Jennifer Penschow and Núria Pérez Pérez.

Index

Printed in the United States
By Bookmasters